Amyotrophic Lateral Sclerosis

A Guide for Patients and Families

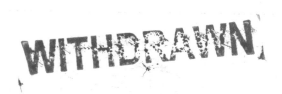

Amyotrophic Lateral Sclerosis

A Guide for Patients and Families

Second Edition

Hiroshi Mitsumoto, MD

and

Theodore L. Munsat, MD

EDITORS

New York

Demos Medical Publishing, Inc., 386 Park Avenue South, New York, New York 10016

Library of Congress Cataloging-in-Publication Data is available from the publisher on request and on our web site: www.demosmedpub.com

ISBN: 1-888799-28-5

Printed in Canada

Preface

The first edition of this book, published in 1992, was intended for health care professionals. However, patients and their families were frequent readers of the book because no comprehensive book on ALS management was available for them. For that reason the current edition has been extensively revised and rewritten to address the concerns of everyone living with the disease in an accessible, straightforward way.

Since publication of the last edition, our understanding and treatment of ALS have changed dramatically. The many puzzles of this disease are being steadily solved. One cause of familial ALS has been identified, and the mechanisms of motor neuron cell death are much better understood. The FDA has approved riluzole, the first drug available for the treatment of ALS. Additional drugs are being tested and others are on the horizon. Several consensus conferences have resulted in improved patient care and management. In addition, the World Federation of Neurology, Committee of Motor Neuron Disease, has introduced revised international diagnostic criteria and clinical trial guidelines for ALS. The American Academy of Neurology, Quality Assurance Subcommittee, ALS Practice Parameter Task Force recently published recommendations for the care and treatment of patients with ALS. The recommendations were developed using an evidence-based approach, an approach that uses detailed and uniform analysis of the medical literature. ALS Clinical Assessment Research and Education (ALS C.A.R.E.) is an ambitious North American ALS database project established to identify the current status of patient care and management, including the medical, psychosocial, and financial issues of both patients and caregivers. Finally, non-profit voluntary organizations such as the ALS Association and Muscular Dystrophy Association have become instrumental in supporting research and have increased their efforts to improve public awareness of this disease.

In the past, medical management has been the sole domain of health care professionals. Recently, however, patients and families have taken a much more active role in disseminating medical and related information. Although the Internet provides information in an unprecedented manner, much of this information is fragmented and of uncertain validity. We feel strongly that a carefully and critically edited book written by experts in the field is the best information resource for patients and their families. This is the main thrust in our revision of the first edition. Theodore L. Munsat, MD, joined Hiroshi Mitsumoto, MD, in the editing, and several new authors have contributed chapters. We also have updated all chapters to reflect new information and expanded the chapters dealing with quality of life for both patients with ALS and their caregivers. We trust readers will find those chapters discussing unique topics such as mourning and bereavement informative and useful.

v

Acknowledgments

We would like to acknowledge Terese Wheeler, who was a great help in compiling the manuscripts, figures, and diskettes in a timely manner. We are particularly appreciative of the excellent chapters written by all our contributors. Diana M. Schneider, Ph.D., President of Demos Medical Publishing, Inc., reviewed the entire manuscript to ensure that the language was suitable for patients. We also thank Joan Wolk, Managing Editor, for her editorial and production work. Finally, we are always grateful to all our patients and their families for their courage and trust in sharing and discussing the many medical and psychosocial issues with us. We have learned much about the disease from them.

Contents

Living with the Reality of ALS

Managing Advanced Disease and End-of-Life Issues

Where You Can Turn to For Help

Foreword

Amyotrophic lateral sclerosis commands public attention these days. *Tuesdays with Morrie,* a book about the last year of a patient with ALS, is in its fourth year at the top of best-seller lists. It is difficult to account for the general interest except that ALS is a clear reminder of human mortality. And ALS is one of few diseases where drug therapy has not altered the inexorable progression of symptoms, at least not in any way visible to the patient or family.

Amyotrophic lateral sclerosis cannot be cured, but it can be treated. Research efforts have expanded in the past decade and progress in the basic science of ALS has been phenomenal. An effective treatment must be coming soon.

What to do in the meantime? There has been a profusion of books about ALS for physicians and scientists, but there has not yet been one specifically designed for patients. This handbook fills a major void.

Patients and families now usually know about "Lou Gehrig's disease." At least they have heard of it, and they know the prognosis is ominous. At the start, however, they know nothing about coping because they do not know what, specifically, to expect. And physicians are not all equally skilled in transmitting the information, partly because there is no single correct way to do it. Physicians differ in personality and so do patients; each encounter involves different people. Few patients seem to want a detailed overview of the future, but some do.

Therein lies a paradox. The principle of patient autonomy requires freedom of choice for the person. But true freedom of choice requires detailed information about what lies ahead. Maintaining hope is a major goal and is not aided by too much information given too soon. How much to tell and when to tell are challenges for the health care workers.

Regardless of their views about long-range events, almost all patients and families want to know what to do at the moment. Almost all patients and families want to participate in therapeutic trials. Patients are sometimes given contradictory advice about rehabilitation exercises. Patients need guidance about the only FDA-approved drug for the treatment of ALS, riluzole (Rilutek), as well as new experimental preparations and drugs like gabapentin (Neurontin)) that have been approved for some other disease and are being used for patients with ALS. They also need help to deal with the maze of alternative remedies: antioxidants, creatine, anabolic steroids, vitamins, and dietary supplements. They need help emotionally; many physicians believe erroneously that any patient with ALS must be depressed and therefore needs antidepressant medication. Patients need help in learning about the use of therapeutic drugs to control symptoms of salivation, difficulty sleeping, aches and pains, trouble voiding, and sexual activity. Options for

ix

relieving difficulty swallowing range from dietary adjustment to a simple operation. Speech therapy or computerized voice synthesizers can ameliorate difficulty
speaking. Wheelchairs and other devices require choices. Patients need direction
in choosing the site of their care—single physician or multidisciplinary clinical
center. Patients desire help in dealing with end-of-life issues and, confronted with
major options, they differ in their ultimate choices about mechanical ventilation.
Patients and their families want to know about financial issues for their personal
situation. Many want to learn how they can support biomedical research, by
raising money or by giving permission for postmortem examination.

That is quite a list of serious considerations, but in this book experienced contributors provide the essential information. Readers will recognize that the writers
are not all neurologists or even physicians in other specialties. Some are nurses, or
clergy or have some other background that helps all of us—patients, families,
caregivers—meet the challenges of ALS.

Drs. Mitsumoto and Munsat are to be congratulated and thanked for a handbook that has been sorely needed and is therefore especially welcome.

Lewis P. Rowland, MD

Contributors

Lisa Adams, MA, CCC-SLP, LD, Communication Independence for the Neurologically Impaired (CINI), New York, New York

Fred A. Anderson, PhD, The Center for Outcomes Research, University of Massachusetts Medical Center, Worcester, Massachusetts

Patricia L. Andres, MS, PT, Research Physical Therapist, Reading, Massachusetts; Formerly of Neuromuscular Research Unit, New England Medical Center, Boston, Massachusetts

Carmen Blakely-Adams, RD, LD, Cleveland Clinic Foundation, Cleveland, Ohio

Gian Domenico Borasio, MD, Department of Neurology and Interdisciplinary Palliative Care Unit, University of Munich, Klinikum Grosshadern, Munich, Germany

Mark M. Bromberg, MD, PhD, University of Utah, Department of Neurology, Salt Lake City, Utah

Eileen M. Carr-Davis, RD, LD, MBA, Cleveland Clinic Foundation, Cleveland, Ohio

Patricia Casey, MS, OTR/L, Department of Neurology, University of Chicago, Chicago, Illinois

David A. Chad, MD, University of Massachusetts Medical Center, Department of Neurology, Worcester, Massachusetts

Marlene Ciechoski, MS, RN, Wilmington, Delaware

Ann Kuckelman Cobb, RN, PhD, University of Kansas School of Nursing, Kansas City, Kansas

Valerie A. Cwik, MD, The University of Arizona, University Medical Center, Department of Neurology, Tucson, Arizona

Vanina Dal Bello-Haas, BScPT, MEd, Cleveland Clinic Foundation, Cleveland, Ohio

Maura L. Del Bene, MS, RN, NP-P, Columbia University, Neurological Institute, New York, New York

Karen J. Fernengel, RN, PhD, University of Kansas School of Nursing, Kansas City, Kansas

Dallas A. Forshew, RN, BSN, University of Utah, Salt Lake City, Utah

Deborah Gelinas, MD, California Pacific Medical Center, Department of Neurology, San Francisco, California

Michael C. Graves, MD, University of California at Los Angeles, Department of Neurology, Los Angeles, California

Rhoda R. Jacobs, RN, BSN, Cleveland Clinic Foundation, Cleveland, Ohio

Marta Kazandjian, MA, CCC-SLP, New York Hospital Medical Center Queens, Department of Speech Pathology, Flushing, New York

Lisa Krivickas, MD, Spaulding Rehabilitation Hospital, Harvard Medical School, Department of Physical Medicine and Rehabilitation, Boston, Massachusetts

Gary LaFontaine, MSc, University of New Mexico School of Medicine, Department of Neurology, Albuquerque, New Mexico

Mary Lyons, RN, MN, Vice President, Patient Services, The Amyotrophic Lateral Sclerosis Association, Calabasas Hills, California

Raul Mandler, MD, University of New Mexico School of Medicine, Department of Neurology, Albuquerque, New Mexico

Evelyn R. McDonald, MS, The New Road Map Foundation, Seattle, Washington

Martha Meister, RN, BSN, University of New Mexico School of Medicine, Department of Neurology, Albuquerque, New Mexico

Robert G. Miller, MD, California Pacific Medical Center, Department of Neurology, San Francisco, California

Hiroshi Mitsumoto, MD, DSc, Columbia University, Neurological Institute, New York, New York

Theodore Munsat, MD, Tufts University School of Medicine, New England Medical Center, Neuromuscular Research Unit, Boston, Massachusetts

N. Michael Murphy, MD, St. Peter's Hospice, Albany, New York

JoAnn B. Reckling, RN, MA, PhD, University of Kansas School of Nursing, Kansas City, Kansas

Catherine Balsdon Richer, OTR/L, Cleveland Clinic Foundation, Cleveland, Ohio

Robert Schilz, DO, PhD, Cleveland Clinic Foundation, Department of Pulmonary Medicine, Cleveland, Ohio

Linda Boynton De Sepulveda, RN, DNSc, University of California at Los Angeles, Department of Neurology, Los Angeles, California

John Sharp, LSW, The Cleveland Clinic Foundation, Web Administrator, Information Technology Division, Cleveland, Ohio

Linda T. Skerry, AS, PTA, Research Coordinator, Reading, Massachusetts; Formerly of Neuromuscular Research Unit, New England Medical Center, Boston, Massachusetts

Susan J. Stagno, MD, Cleveland Clinic Foundation, Cleveland, Ohio

Mark J. Stillman, MD, Cleveland Clinic Foundation, Cleveland, Ohio

Robert Sufit, MD, Northwestern University School of Medicine, Department of Neurology, Chicago, Illinois

Barbara Thompson, OTR/L, CSW, ALS Regional Center, St. Peter's Hospital, Albany, New York

Brenda J. Thornell, AS, PTA, Research Coordinator, Reading, Massachusetts; Formerly of Neuromuscular Research Unit, New England Medical Center, Boston, Massachusetts

Joan Werner, MA, University of New Mexico School of Medicine, Department of Neurology, Albuquerque, New Mexico

Mary Wooley, LSW, Cleveland Clinic Foundation, Cleveland, Ohio

1

What Is Amyotrophic Lateral Sclerosis?

Valerie A. Cwik, M.D.

Historical Perspective

*"Fans, for the past two weeks you have been reading about the bad
break I got. Yet today I consider myself the luckiest man on the face of
the earth . . . I may have had a tough break, but I have an awful lot to
live for." (1)*

With those words, Lou Gehrig announced his retirement from the New York Yankees on July 4, 1939, at the age of 36, ending one of the most remarkable careers
in the game of baseball. During his 17 years with the Yankees, Gehrig played in
2,164 regular season games, hitting 493 home runs. His consecutive game record
of 2,130, which earned him the nickname "Iron Horse," stood until 1995, when it
was broken by Baltimore Orioles shortstop Cal Ripken, Jr. Most Americans had
probably never heard of amyotrophic lateral sclerosis (ALS) before Lou Gehrig.
Yet disorders of motor neurons, including ALS, were starting to be recognized
nearly a century before Gehrig developed his first symptoms.

Case reports describing the clinical motor neuron syndromes of progressive
muscular atrophy, primary lateral sclerosis, progressive bulbar palsy, and "classic" ALS began to appear in the French and British medical literature in the 1830s,
authored by such renowned physicians as Sir Charles Bell, Francois Aran, and
Amand Duchenne (2–4). One of the earliest cases of ALS was reported in considerable detail in 1853 by Cruveilhier (5). The patient, Prosper Lecomte, was an
unfortunate 30-year-old circus proprietor whose problems began in September

1

1848 with weakness of the right hand. By the following July he had weakness of both legs; walking became tiresome and he tripped over small objects. This was followed two months later by weakness of the left hand and slurred speech. He had to give up working by the end of 1849. Over the next three years his symptoms progressed steadily, so that by February 1853 he was bedridden and not able to speak or swallow. On February 12, 1853, M. Lecomte died at the age of 35, 4.5 years after the onset of his first symptom. In that early paper Cruveilhier clearly described many features of classic ALS, including progressive wasting, weakness and spasticity of the limbs, speech and swallowing difficulty, and death within five years of symptom onset.

In 1874 a French physician, Jean Martin Charcot, who was regarded as the founder of modern neurology and perhaps the most successful teacher of clinical medicine, established the clinical and pathologic characteristics of ALS (6). Charcot stressed the importance of meticulous observation to his students. To that end, Charcot is reported to have employed a housemaid with ALS and therefore was able to systematically observe the clinical manifestations of her disease (7). She was later admitted to the Salpêtrière infirmary so that Charcot could obtain an autopsy and define the pathologic features of the disease. His descriptions of ALS remain amazingly accurate to this day, and as a result ALS is referred to as Charcot's disease in some parts of the world (8). In the United Kingdom it is known as motor neurone disease. Americans are familiar with the terms *Lou Gehrig's disease* and *ALS* and know that it is a devastating, rapidly fatal disorder. However, most people are not aware of what a diagnosis of ALS truly means until an individual or family member is affected.

Where are we today with ALS and how did we get there from those early descriptions of the nineteenth century? This chapter provides an introduction to ALS with an emphasis on the historical aspects that have brought us to our current state of understanding about this disease, including epidemiology, research, cause(s), and treatment. Classification of the disease and some thoughts about future directions are presented in the latter part of the chapter. Many of the topics introduced here are covered in considerably more detail in subsequent chapters.

Epidemiology

With few exceptions, ALS has had a uniform distribution worldwide over the past 40 to 50 years, despite differences in climate, geography, race, cultures, and diet. ALS strikes approximately 1 to 2 in every 100,000 adults annually worldwide, and it has long been apparent that men are at somewhat higher risk for developing the disease than are women, although this gender difference disappears at older ages. The prevalence of the disease—the number of persons who will have the disease at any given time—is estimated to be 1 to 7 per 100,000 population.

For the first half of the twentieth century exceptional clusters of ALS, 50 to 100 times higher than worldwide rates, were reported in residents of three islands in the western Pacific. These included the Japanese villagers of the Kii peninsula of

Honshu Island, Japan; the Chamorro people on the islands of Guam and Rota of the Marianas chain of Micronesia; and the Auyu and Jakai people of West New Guinea, Indonesia (9–11). For the past 40 years, new cases of ALS have declined steadily in these regions to rates closer to those in the rest of the world. Although the cause(s) of these clusters is not known, environmental factors, such as exposure to neurotoxins in the diet and mineral imbalances in drinking water, have been postulated (12,13).

There have been reports of smaller ALS concentrations. ALS occurring in both (unrelated) partners of a married couple (conjugal ALS) has been reported in the United States and Italy (14–16). Conjugal ALS also affected two couples in southern France (17). One person developed the disease in 1977; the other three became symptomatic in 1990 and 1991. The question of genetic susceptibility or an environmental etiologic factor was raised because all four individuals were from the same geographic region (Languedoc-Roussillon). In the case of nonidentical twin brothers developing ALS within two years of one another, an intrauterine "toxic" or infectious exposure was postulated as a causative factor (18).

Small geographic clusters of ALS have also been reported. Between 1975 and 1983 six residents of Two Rivers, Wisconsin, were diagnosed with ALS. Physical trauma, consumption of fish from Lake Michigan, and a family history of cancer occurred more frequently in these patients than in non-ALS subjects from the same community (19). Additional small clusters include three patients, all Ashkenazi Jews, in a single apartment building in Montreal who developed ALS within an 18-month period, and three unrelated men living within a block of one another in Burlington, North Carolina (20,21). In the North Carolina cluster, all three men had speech and swallowing difficulty at the onset of their disease, and two of the men were diagnosed within a two-month period. Kilnes and Hochberg reported four patients in rural South Dakota, three of whom lived within a three-kilometer radius for all of their lives, who developed ALS within a 10-year period. High selenium content in the regional soil was noted (22).

Although these and other small clusters continue to raise the specter of a toxic cause of ALS, to date no definite cause and effect relationship between any environmental toxin or transmissable and/or infectious agent and the development of ALS has been firmly established.

A few countries, including Mexico, Poland, and Italy, actually report lower than average rates of ALS (23–26). The reason for the apparent lower risk is not known. However, if areas of low risk do indeed exist, explanations for those should be sought.

Research

The number of yearly publications in professional journals loosely reflects the amount of active research about a given disease. In searching *Cumulated Index Medicus, Current List of Medical Literature,* and MEDLINE by the key words *amyotrophic lateral sclerosis,* one finds almost 4,700 papers for the years

1920–1998; more than half have been published in the past 15 years alone (Figure 1-1). For the year 1920, there were no publications about ALS listed in *Index Medicus*. From 1921 through the mid-1960s, the number of yearly publications about ALS was generally fewer than 25; this number essentially tripled for the years 1966–1981. By 1993–1998, there were more than 200 annual publications about ALS. These numbers reflect only the papers published in referenced journals. They do not include oral and poster presentations at scientific and professional meetings, and neither do they include other publications, such as books about ALS.

A review of the literature from 1920 through the 1940s reveals that most publications about ALS were single case reports or small series of patients, descriptions of the pathologic findings in the various ALS clinical syndromes, or reports about putative causative factors. There also were sporadic reports about treatments, particularly vitamin therapies. The 1950s and 1960s saw increasing interest in the epidemiology of ALS, particularly with regard to ALS on Guam and in the western Pacific. Since 1970 there has been a substantial increase in the number of papers about the possible etiologies and pathogeneses of ALS, and about therapeutic trials. Over this same period, the focus of research shifted from strictly clinical observations and patient-based research to include the development of animal models for ALS and investigation of the molecular and genetic bases for motor neuron diseases.

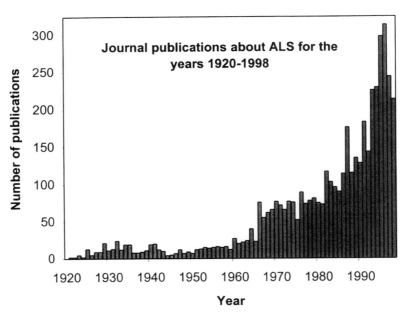

Figure 1-3. The number of publications about ALS in scientific and medical journals has increased substantially over the past 30 years.

Etiology and Pathogenesis of ALS

Despite all that we have learned about ALS over the past 150 years, some of the questions that were raised by our neurologic forefathers about the cause of ALS have only recently been resolved, and others remain unanswered.

Charcot in 1875 may have been the first to question the relationship between remote poliomyelitis infection and the subsequent development of ALS (27). Although there is little evidence to implicate the poliovirus or any other virus as a cause of ALS, this question remains open at this time (28–30).

Interest in heavy metal intoxication as a cause of ALS has been high for nearly a century. Wilson in 1907 is credited as being the first to raise the question of whether lead poisoning causes ALS (31). Further support for a heavy metal hypothesis came from the finding of increased levels of aluminum and manganese and diminished levels of calcium and magnesium in the soil and drinking water of the regions of the western Pacific, where the incidence of ALS was particularly high (13). Additionally, Currier and Haerer in 1968 and Roelofs-Iverson and colleagues in 1984 reported increased lead and heavy metal exposure in people with ALS compared with controls (32,33). We now know that lead and mercury intoxication may cause reversible ALS-like syndromes (34,35). Although the relationship between toxic environmental factors and the development of ALS remains somewhat unsettled in the year 2001, it is likely that heavy metals play only a marginal role, if any, in the development of this disease.

In 1944 Wechsler, Sapirstein, and Stein summarized the prevailing theories of the time for the cause of ALS (36). Based on their personal observations of 81 patients, they concluded that ALS was not a single disease entity but a syndrome of varying causes. The putative causes included:

1. Dietary deficiency and gastrointestinal dysfunction.

2. Inflammatory disorders, including syphilis, remote poliomyelitis, or a severe upper respiratory tract infection at onset.

3. Vascular disorders such as generalized atherosclerosis and coronary artery disease (at the time, the authors did not recognize the coincidence of a rare disease, ALS, with very common vascular diseases).

4. Toxic exposures, including gasoline, lead, heavy metals, and spinal anesthesia.

The deficiency syndrome hypothesis persisted for more than another decade, championed by Dr. Ask-Upmark in Sweden based on his personal observations of several patients who developed ALS after undergoing gastric resection (37). He theorized that the common nutritional problems that followed surgical resection of the stomach led to a "certain malnutrition" and the subsequent development of ALS. He also acknowledged, however, that some cases of ALS may be due to system atrophy or abiotrophy (premature aging) (38).

ALS is now considered a neurodegenerative disease, but the underlying cause (or causes) that initiates the degenerative process remains unknown. Over the past several decades, a multitude of putative causes have been suggested, investigated, and often refuted or discarded (Table 1-1). However, significant insights into the pathogenetic mechanisms of sporadic and familial ALS have developed over the past decade. These include:

1. Identification of a mutation in the superoxide dismutase gene on chromosome 21 in approximately 15 percent to 20 percent of people with familial ALS in 1993 (39,40). This suggests that ALS in some people arises from a disturbance in free radical homeostasis.

Table 1-1: Putative Causes and Etiologic Factors for Amyotrophic Lateral Sclerosis

Altered immunity	**Heavy metals and trace minerals**
Antibodies to calcium channels	Aluminum
Antineuronal antibodies	Copper
Antisprouting antibodies	Lead
	Manganese
Disordered neuronal metabolism	Mercury
or function	Selenium
Abnormal neurotransmitter function	
Abnormal thyrotropin releasing hormone	**Nutritional disorders**
Altered axonal transport	Dietary deficiencies
Defects in neuronal membrane structure	Gastrointestinal dysfunction
or function	Vitamin deficiencies
Defects in the urea cycle	
Disordered calcium, phosphate,	**Physical injury**
and bone metabolism	Pneumatic tools
Hyperparathyroidism	Prior surgery
Loss of cholinergic receptors	Prior trauma
Loss/dysfunction of androgen receptors	Radiation
Excitotoxicity	**Toxic agents or exposures**
Alterations in serum and spinal fluid	Animal carcasses and hides
amino acids	Endogenous "toxins"
Glutamate transporter protein deficiency	Gasoline
Seed of *Cycas circinalis*	Household pets
	Spinal anesthesia
Genetic disorders and abnormalities	
Defect in superoxide dismutase gene	**Other**
DNA and RNA abnormalities	Abiotrophy (premature aging)
Genetic markers/HLA antigen	Malignancy
Hexosaminidase deficiency	Neurotrophic factor deficiencies
	Paraproteinemia
Infectious or inflammatory disorders	Vascular disorders
Severe upper respiratory infection	
Syphilis	
Viruses, especially poliovirus	

2. The discovery, in 1995, of deficiency of a specific glutamate transporter protein, EAAT2, in the motor cortex and spinal cord in ALS, supporting the excitoxicity theory of neurodegeneration (41).

3. Identification of antibodies to calcium channels in ALS patients, in support of a role for autoimmune mechanisms (42).

Treatment of ALS

The comprehensive treatment of ALS is the main theme of this book. As of 2000 there was no treatment that effectively stopped or slowed the progression of ALS. This should not be interpreted to mean that there is no treatment for ALS. In fact, there is a tremendous amount that can be done to maintain independence and quality of life for people with the disease. The multitude of therapies available—drug and nondrug, medical and nonmedical—are reviewed in substantial detail in subsequent chapters, and only a few background comments are made here.

Drug Therapies

The failure to find an effective drug therapy for ALS has not been for lack of trying. To date, more than 60 different medications (and a few nondrug therapies) have been anecdotally reported or tested in therapeutic trials and found to be ineffective in halting or significantly slowing the course of this disorder (Table 1-2). Over the past several decades the treatments tested have spanned the gamut from antiviral agents and antibiotics to chemotherapies, from immunomodulating agents to neurotrophic factors.

Probably the most ubiquitous treatment for ALS over the past century has been vitamin E (tocopherol). Anecdotal reports of the use of this vitamin appear in the literature as early as the 1920s, and daily injections of vitamin E were given to Lou Gehrig for treatment of his disease (43). At that time the rationale for using vitamin E was not for its antioxidant properties, but in part because ALS was thought to be the result of a deficiency state. In 1940 Wechsler reported remarkable beneficial responses to vitamin E therapy in 14 of 20 patients (44). Unfortunately, several subsequent series failed to obtain any good results with vitamins E or B6 (45–47). Despite such discouraging results, many neurologists continue to recommend vitamins, particularly those with antioxidant properties, for the treatment of ALS. Although it is no longer believed that ALS is caused by a nutritional deficiency, the rationale for such therapy is based on the discoveries that (1) a mutation in the gene for copper/zinc superoxide dismutase, an endogenous antioxidant, is one cause of familial ALS; and (2) vitamin E appears to delay the onset and slow progression of clinical symptomatology in a mouse model of familial ALS (40,48).

Following years of negative results from multiple clinical trials testing a wide variety of therapies, a significant breakthrough for the treatment of ALS occurred in 1995, when riluzole was shown to have a modest effect on prolonging survival

Table 1-2: Therapies Tried for ALS

Antiglutamate/antiexcitotoxic agents
Branched-chain amino acids
Dextromethorphan
Gabapentin (currently in clinical trials)
Glycine
Lamotrigine
L-threonine
Naloxone
Riluzole

Immune system modulators
Azathioprine
Cyclosporine A
Cyclophosphamide
Hydrocortisone (oral and intrathecal)
Interferon (subcutaneous and intrathecal)
Intravenous immune globulin
Levamisole
Plasma exchange
Prednisolone
Whole-body lymphoid irradiation

**Agents that may act on
   neuronal metabolism**
Growth hormone
Lecithin
Testosterone
Thyrotropin-releasing hormone
   (intravenous, intrathecal,
   intramuscular, oral)

Antioxidants
Beta-carotene
Centrophenoxine
Coenzyme Q
Cytochrome C
L-cysteine
Lipoic acid
N-acetylcysteine
Selegeline
Selenium
Vitamin C
Vitamin E (oral, intravenous,
   and intramuscular)

Cholinergic agents
Neostigmine
Physostigmine
Priscoline
3,4-diaminopyridine

"Neurotrophic" agents
Brain-derived neurotrophic factor,
   (subcutaneous; intrathecal
   administration now in clinical trials)
Ciliary neurotrophic factor
Insulin-like growth factor (IGF-1,
   myotrophin)
SR57746A (currently in
   clinical trials)

Antimicrobial agents
Ceftriaxone
Tilerone hydrochloride
Trypan blue
Trypan red

Antiviral agents
Amantadine
Isoprinosine
Transfer factor
Zidovudine

**Nutritional supplements
   and vitamins**
Crude liver extract
Intravenous amino acids
Octacosanol
Vitamin B1 (thiamine)
Vitamin B6 (pyridoxine)
Vitamin B12
   "Vitamin B" in yeast preparation

**Calcium channel blockers and
   chelating agents**
Calcium disodium edetate
Dantrolene
Penicillamine

Other
"Adrenal cortex"
Antihistaminic agents
Balneotherapy (natural mineral
   water baths)
Bovine gangliosides
Bromocriptine
Cervicodorsal electroshock therapy
Guanidine
5-hydroxytrytophan
Phthalazinol
Snake venom (modified neurotoxin)
Toluloxy propanediol

in ALS (49). Currently riluzole is the only medication approved by the U.S. Food and Drug Administration for the treatment of ALS. But riluzole is not the last word in ALS treatment. More effective therapies are necessary, and every suggestion for a potential treatment is considered seriously. The ease of electronic communication is impacting ALS treatment. The recent trial of gabapentin, which was developed as an antiepileptic agent, was initiated in part because of a patient's report of beneficial response to this medication on an electronic bulletin board (50). Active clinical trials at this time include oxandrolone, creatine, topiramate, and coenzyme Q10 (see Chapter 16).

Nondrug Therapies

In 1955 Schwarz and King reported that "present treatment is basically a matter of supportive treatment and good medical art" (51). Good medical care remains the cornerstone of ALS treatment in 2001 and includes attention to both the physical and the emotional effects of this disorder. There also is increasing recognition of the importance of quality of life and end-of-life issues. Only in the past several years has systematic investigation of nondrug therapies been undertaken in an attempt to better define what "good medical art" means for ALS. For example, a recent study demonstrated that noninvasive assisted ventilation prolongs survival in ALS (52). However, the optimal time for initiation of such treatment is not yet known. More clinical studies are now under way to assess such therapies as the utility of early feeding tube placements and early noninvasive ventilatory support in ALS.

CLASSIFICATION OF ALS

One can approach the classification of ALS in several ways, based on (1) clinical syndromes, (2) mode of acquisition, and (3) degree of diagnostic certainty.

ALS belongs to a large family of inherited and acquired disorders that constitute the motor neuron diseases. The family of motor neuron diseases, which includes such diverse disorders as botulism, tetanus, poliomyelitis, and spinal muscular atrophy, as well as ALS, should not be confused with motor neuron disease, a term that often is used interchangeably with ALS. Motor neuron diseases are disorders that affect anterior horn cells, neurons in the spinal cord that control voluntary movements. Classic ALS also affects the motor neurons in the brain and brain stem. Clinical history, physical signs and symptoms, and laboratory testing allow for distinction among the various motor neuron diseases.

Clinical ALS Syndromes

The various ALS syndromes differ according to clinical signs and symptoms, as well as prognosis. To better understand the classification schemes for ALS, one must have a rudimentary understanding of neuroanatomy. Motor neurons are those cells in the brain, brain stem, and spinal cord that control voluntary movements of muscles. There are two types of motor neurons: upper motor neurons and lower motor neurons (also called anterior horn cells). Both sets of motor neurons are required for optimal control of skeletal muscles. Upper motor neurons reside in the brain in a region called the motor cortex. The upper motor neurons send out processes, called axons, that connect (synapse) with lower motor neurons in the brain stem and spinal cord. In turn, the lower motor neurons send out axons that synapse on muscles in the face, pharynx, chest, and limbs. Upper motor neurons are involved in initiation of voluntary movements and in the maintenance of appropriate muscle tone. When upper motor neurons are damaged, the limbs become spastic and the reflexes are exaggerated. When lower motor neurons are lost, the muscles become weak and wasted, or atrophic, and the reflexes may disappear. The combination of symptoms and signs of damage to both upper and lower motor neurons in several body regions allows the neurologist to make a diagnosis of definite ALS. Classic ALS is marked by exaggerated reflexes, or spasticity, along with weakness and wasting of the facial, limb, and respiratory muscles.

Sometimes, however, there may be signs of either upper motor neuron or lower motor neuron loss, but not both. At other times the symptoms and signs of disease may be present in only one region, such as the speech and swallowing, or bulbar, apparatus. This leads to some confusion about the diagnosis for patients, as physicians may use other terms to describe the clinical syndrome: primary lateral sclerosis, progressive muscular atrophy, or progressive bulbar palsy.

In *primary lateral sclerosis* only the upper motor neurons degenerate, leaving the lower motor neurons intact. The limbs become stiff and spastic, without the development of significant weakness or atrophy. This is a rare syndrome and should be considered an entity distinct from ALS. In some instances, patients with pure upper motor neuron findings initially will later develop more typical features of ALS. This is called upper motor neuron onset–ALS, or the primary lateral sclerosis form of ALS.

When only the lower motor neurons are affected, leading to severe wasting and weakness in the muscles with loss of reflexes, the disorder is known as *progressive muscular atrophy*. The signs of upper motor neuron dysfunction are not noted. This is called lower motor neuron onset–ALS, or the progressive muscular atrophy form of ALS.

With *progressive bulbar palsy,* the disorder starts in the muscles of speech and swallowing, causing slurred speech and choking. Patients eventually lose all ability to speak and swallow. Pure progressive bulbar palsy is also extremely rare; most patients later develop classic ALS.

Mode of Acquisition

People acquire ALS in one of two ways, sporadically or genetically. The vast majority of patients (90 percent to 95 percent) have sporadic ALS, in which there is no family history of the disorder. A small percentage (5 percent to 10 percent) of patients have an inherited form of ALS called familial ALS, or FALS. Some people with FALS have a defect in the gene for superoxide dismutase, but for most people with FALS the genetic abnormalities are not known at this time.

Certainty of Diagnosis

Perhaps most confusing and frustrating for patients is the classification of ALS based on degree of diagnostic certainty. At the present time there is no single laboratory test that allows one to make a diagnosis of ALS with 100 percent certainty, particularly in its early stages. The diagnosis is based on a constellation of physical symptoms and signs and laboratory data that are consistent with ALS and the exclusion of other diagnostic entities that may mimic ALS. In the very earliest stages of the disease, when its signs and symptoms are limited to a single body region, the clinical features may suggest another neurologic disorder. It is the progression of disease to involve multiple body regions that allows for a diagnosis of definite ALS. The following diagnostic categories have been defined by the World Federation of Neurology Research Group on Motor Neuron Diseases: Clinically Possible ALS; Clinically Probable–Laboratory Supported ALS; Clinically Probable ALS; and Clinically Definite ALS (Table 1-3) (53,54). Diagnostic criteria for each category have been established (and refined in 1998) to increase the degree of likelihood that the disease is really ALS and serve to alert the physician to search for disorders that may mimic ALS, particularly in its early stages. Although the use of these terms is sometimes distressing to patients because they are uncer-

Table 1-3: Diagnostic Categories for ALS: (UMN = Upper Motor Neuron; LMN = Lower Motor Neuron) (54)

---

1. **Clinically Definite ALS** is defined on clinical evidence alone by the presence of UMN, as well as LMN signs in three regions.

2. **Clinically Probable ALS** is defined on clinical evidence alone by UMN and LMN signs in at least two regions with some UMN necessarily rostral to (above) the LMN signs.

3. **Clinically Probable — Laboratory-supported ALS** is defined when clinical signs of UMN and LMN dysfunction are in only one region, or when UMN signs alone are present in one region, and LMN signs defined by EMG criteria are present in at least two limbs, with proper application of neuroimaging and clinical laboratory protocols to exclude other causes.

4. **Clinically Possible ALS** is defined when clinical signs of UMN and LMN dysfunction are found together in only one region or UMN signs are found alone in two or more regions; or LMN signs are found rostral to UMN signs and the diagnosis of Clinically Probable — Laboratory-supported ALS cannot be proven by evidence on clinical grounds in conjunction with electrodiagnostic, neurophysiologic, neuroimaging, or clinical laboratory studies. Other diagnoses must have been excluded to accept a diagnosis of Clinically Possible ALS.

---

tain of their diagnosis when told they have "possible" or "probable" ALS, the criteria are in place to protect the patient from an improper diagnosis.

Conclusions and Future Directions

The twentieth century has seen tremendous scientific discoveries and technologic advances (Figure 1-2). Unraveling of the DNA molecule by Watson and Crick, elimination of smallpox and a significant reduction in poliomyelitis by the devel-

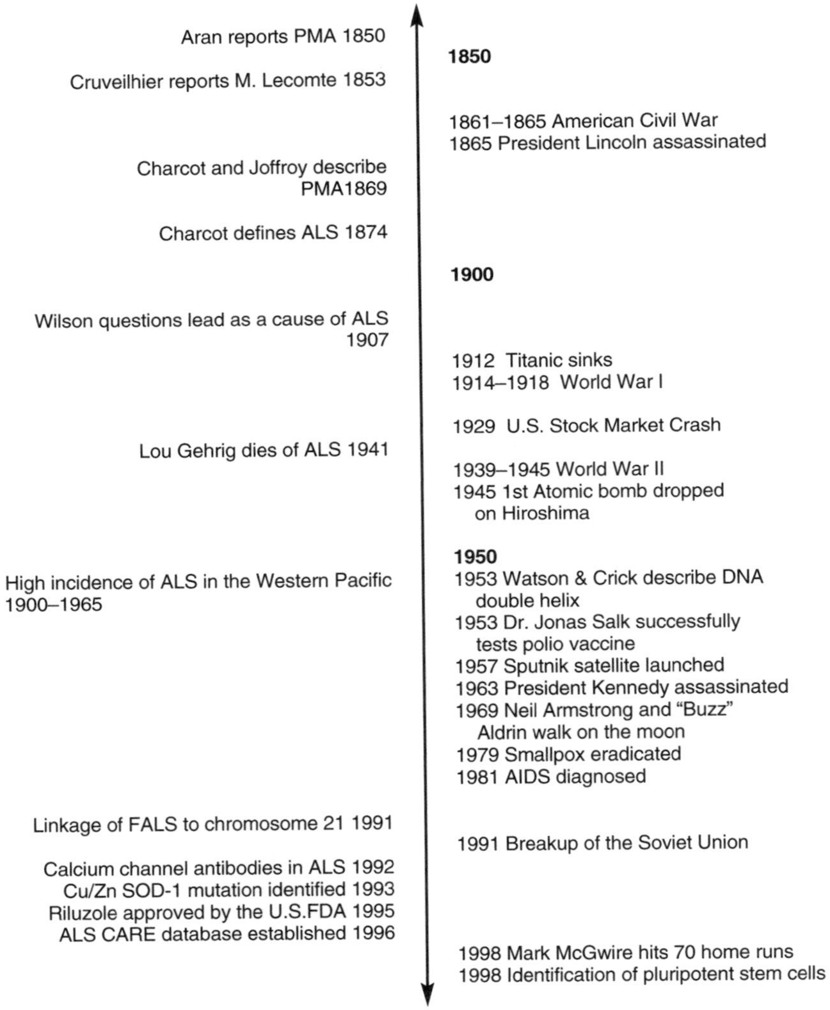

Aran reports PMA 1850	**1850**
Cruveilhier reports M. Lecomte 1853	
	1861–1865 American Civil War
	1865 President Lincoln assassinated
Charcot and Joffroy describe PMA1869	
Charcot defines ALS 1874	
	1900
Wilson questions lead as a cause of ALS 1907	
	1912 Titanic sinks
	1914–1918 World War I
	1929 U.S. Stock Market Crash
Lou Gehrig dies of ALS 1941	
	1939–1945 World War II
	1945 1st Atomic bomb dropped on Hiroshima
	1950
High incidence of ALS in the Western Pacific 1900–1965	1953 Watson & Crick describe DNA double helix
	1953 Dr. Jonas Salk successfully tests polio vaccine
	1957 Sputnik satellite launched
	1963 President Kennedy assassinated
	1969 Neil Armstrong and "Buzz" Aldrin walk on the moon
	1979 Smallpox eradicated
	1981 AIDS diagnosed
Linkage of FALS to chromosome 21 1991	1991 Breakup of the Soviet Union
Calcium channel antibodies in ALS 1992	
Cu/Zn SOD-1 mutation identified 1993	
Riluzole approved by the U.S.FDA 1995	
ALS CARE database established 1996	
	1998 Mark McGwire hits 70 home runs
	1998 Identification of pluripotent stem cells

Figure 1-2: Selected notable events in ALS and world history, 1850–1999

opment of viral-specific vaccines, and the walk on the moon by Neil Armstrong and Buzz Aldrin are but a few examples. However, despite the tremendous strides in scientific knowledge and technology, the cause and treatment of ALS remain elusive. Inroads have been made, but much work remains to find the cause and develop truly effective therapies for this devastating disorder. The last decade has seen a concerted, multinational effort to achieve these goals, an effort that will continue into this new century. To date, this effort has included:

1. The organization of regional consortia to coordinate research efforts in North America and Europe.

2. Significant participation by pharmaceutical companies in developing and testing treatments for ALS.

3. The development and implementation of the North American ALS Patient C.A.R.E. database (55). The purpose of this project is to develop a better understanding of the physical, emotional, and financial impact of this disease on patients, as well as to track information about diagnostic methods, treatments, and symptom management across different regions in North America. As part of this effort, the impact of ALS on caregivers is being assessed for the first time (see Chapter 17).

4. Attention to ethical, psychosocial, and quality of life issues that affect people with ALS and their families.

5. Yearly international scientific meetings devoted solely to ALS, along with an increase in the number of courses about ALS that are offered at annual neurologic meetings.

6. Attempts to identify specific objective "markers" for ALS that may allow for earlier and more definitive diagnosis, and which may potentially be used to monitor disease progression and response to therapies.

In addition, two exciting scientific discoveries suggest the potential for the development of novel therapeutic strategies for ALS and other neurodegenerative disorders. The first was the recognition that neurons may regenerate, a process long thought impossible [56]. The second is the report in November 1998 that embryonic stem cells, the precursors of all human tissues, can be stimulated to differentiate and produce neural tissues, which are capable of forming functional connections [57,58]. These efforts and discoveries provide hope that someday not only will there be a way to stop this devastating disease called ALS, but also perhaps a way to even reverse it.

References

1. Bak Richard. *Lou Gehrig: An American classic.* Dallas: Taylor Publishing Co., 1995:160–161.

2. Bell C. *The nervous system of the human body.* London: Longman, 1830:132–136, 160–161.
3. Aran FA. Recherches sur une maladie non encore decrite du systeme musculaire (atrophie musculaire progressive). *Arch Gen Med* 1850; 24:15–35.
4. Duchenne G. Paralysie musculaire progressive de la langue, du voile du palais et des levres. *Arch Gen Med* 1860;16:283–296,431–445.
5. Veltema AN. The case of the saltimbanque Prosper Lecomte. A contribution to the study of the history of progressive muscular atrophy (Aran-Duchenne) and amyotrophic lateral sclerosis (Charcot). *Clin Neurol Neurosurg* 1975; 78:204–209.
6. Charcot J-M. De la sclerose laterale amyotrophique: Symptomatologie. *Progres Med* 1874; 2:453–455.
7. Jean M. Charcot. In: Beighton P, Beighton G (eds). *The man behind the syndrome.* Berlin Heidelberg: Springer-Verlag, 198:27.
8. Guillain G. Amyotrophic lateral sclerosis. In: Bailey P (ed. and trans.). *J.-M. Charcot. 1825–1893 His life—his work.* Paul B. Hoeber, Inc. 1959:106–108.
9. Kimura K, Yase Y, Higashi Y, et al. Epidemiological and geomedical studies on amyotrophic lateral sclerosis. *Dis Nerv Syst* 1963; 24:155–159.
10. Reed DM, Brody JA. Amyotrophic lateral sclerosis and parkinsonism—dementia on Guam, 1945–1972. *Am J Epidemiol* 1975; 101:287–301.
11. Gajdusek DC. Motor-neuron disease in natives of New Guinea. *N Engl J Med* 1963; 268:474–476.
12. Kurland LT. Amyotrophic lateral sclerosis and Parkinson's disease complex on Guam linked to an environmental neurotoxin. *Trends Neurosci* 1988; 11:51–54.
13. Yase Y. The pathogenesis of amyotrophic lateral sclerosis. *Lancet* 1972; 2:292–296.
14. Chad D, Mitsumoto H, Adelman LS, et al. Conjugal motor neuron disease. *Neurology* 1982; 32:306–307.
15. Cornblath DR, Kurland LT, Boylan KB, et al. Conjugal amyotrophic lateral sclerosis: Report of a young married couple. *Neurology* 1993; 43:2378–2380.
16. Paolino E, Granieri E, Tola MR, Rosati G. Conjugal amyotrophic lateral sclerosis [letter]. *Ann Neurol* 1983; 14:699
17. Camu W, Cadilhac J, Billiard M. Amyotrophic lateral sclerosis: A report on two couples from southern France. *Neurology* 1994; 44:547–548.
18. Estrin WJ. Amyotrophic lateral sclerosis in dizygotic twins. *Neurology* 1977; 27:692–694.
19. Sienko DG, Davis JP, Taylor JA, Brooks BJ. Amyotrophic lateral sclerosis: A case-control study following detection of a cluster in a small Wisconsin community. *Arch Neurol* 1990; 47:38–41.
20. Melmed C, Krieger C. A cluster of amyotrophic lateral sclerosis. *Arch Neurol* 1982; 39:595–596.
21. Hochberg FH, Bryan JA, Whelan MA. Clustering of amyotrophic lateral sclerosis. *Lancet* 1974; 1:34.
22. Kilnes AW, Hochberg FH. Amyotrophic lateral sclerosis in a high selenium environment. *JAMA* 1977; 237:2843–2844.
23. Olivares L, Esteban ES, Alter M. Mexican "resistance" to amyotrophic lateral sclerosis. *Arch Neurol* 1972; 27:397–402.
24. Cendrowski W, Wender W, Owsianowski M. Analyse epidemiologique de la sclerose laterale amyotrophique sur le territoire de la Grand-Pologne. *Acta Neurol Scand* 1970; 46:609–617.
25. Rosati G, Pinna L, Granieri E, et al. Studies on epidemiological, clinical and etiological aspects of ALS disease in Sardinia, Southern Italy. *Acta Neurol Scand* 1977; 55:231–244.

26. Salemi G, Fierro B, Arcara A, et al. Amyotrophic lateral sclerosis in Palermo, Italy: An epidemiologic study. *Ital J Neurol Sci* 1989; 10:505–509.
27. Charcot JM. Observation communique en 1875. a la Societe de Biologie par M. Raymond. Paralysie essentielle de l'Enfance: Atrophie musculaire consecutive. *Gaz Med* (Paris) 1875:225–226.
28. Cremer NE, Oshiro LS, Norris FH, Lennette EH. Cultures of tissues from patients with amyotrophic lateral sclerosis. *Arch Neurol* 1973; 29:331–333.
29. Roos RP, Viola MV, Wollmann R, Hatch MH, Antel JP. Amyotrophic lateral sclerosis with antecedent poliomyelitis. *Arch Neurol* 1980; 37:312–313.
30. Weiner LP, Stohlman SA, Davis RL. Attempts to demonstrate virus in amyotrophic lateral sclerosis. *Neurology* 1980; 30:1319–1322.
31. Wilson SAK. The amyotrophy of chronic lead poisoning: amyotrophic lateral sclerosis of toxic origin. *Rev Neurol Psychiatr* 1907; 5:441–445.
32. Currier RD, Haerer AF. Amyotrophic lateral sclerosis and metallic toxins. *Arch Environ Health* 1968; 17:712–719.
33. Roelofs-Iverson RA, Mulder DW, Elveback LR, Kurland LT, Molgaard CA. ALS and heavy metals: A pilot case-control study. *Neurology* 1984; 34:393–395.
34. Boothby JA, deJesus PV, Rowland LP. Reversible forms of motor neuron disease. *Arch Neurol* 1974; 31:18–23.
35. Adams CR, Ziegler DK, Lin JT. Mercury intoxication simulating amyotrophic lateral sclerosis. *JAMA* 1983; 250:642–643.
36. Wechsler IS, Sapirstein MR, Stein A. Primary and symptomatic amyotrophic lateral sclerosis: A clinical study of 81 cases. *Am J Med Sci* 1944; 208:70–71.
37. Ask-Upmark E. Amyotrophic lateral sclerosis observed in 5 persons after gastric resection. *Gastroenterology* 1950; 15:257–259.
38. Ask-Upmark E. Precipitating factors in the pathogenesis of amyotrophic lateral sclerosis. *Acta Med Scand* 1961; 170:717–723.
39. Siddique T, Figlewicz DA, Pericak-Vance MA, et al. Linkage of a gene causing familial amyotrophic lateral sclerosis to chromosome 21 and evidence of genetic-locus heterogeneity. *N Engl J Med* 1991; 324:1381–1384.
40. Rosen DR, Siddique T, Patterson D, et al. Mutations in Cu/Zn superoxide dismutase gene are associated with familial amyotrophic lateral sclerosis. *Nature* 1993; 362:59–62.
41. Rothstein JD, Van Kammen M, Levey AI, Martin LJ, Kuncl RW. Selective loss of glial glutamate transporter GLT-1 in amyotrophic lateral sclerosis. *Ann Neurol* 1995; 38:73–84.
42. Smith RG, Hamilton S, Hofmann F, et al. Serum antibodies to L-type calcium channels in patients with amyotrophic lateral sclerosis. *N Engl J Med* 1992; 327:1721–1728.
43. Bak R. *Lou Gehrig: An American classic.* Dallas: Taylor Publishing Co., 1995: 164.
44. Wechsler IS. The treatment of amyotrophic lateral sclerosis with vitamin E (tocopherols). *Am J Med Sci* 1940; 200:765–778.
45. Eaton LM, Woltman HW, Butt HR. Vitamins E and B6 in the treatment of neuromuscular diseases. *Mayo Clin Proc* 1941; 16:523–527.
46. Denker PG, Scheinman L. Treatment of amyotrophic lateral sclerosiswith vitamin E (alpha-tocopherol). *JAMA* 1941; 116:1895.
47. Ferrebee JW, Klingman WO, Frantz AM. Vitamin E and vitamin B6. Clinical experience in the treatment of muscular dystrophy and amyotrophic lateral sclerosis. *JAMA* 1941; 116:1895–1896.
48. Gurney ME, Cutting FB, Zhai P, et al. Benefit of vitamin E, riluzole, and gabapentin in a transgenic model of familial amyotrophic lateral sclerosis. *Ann Neurol* 1996; 39:147–157.
49. Bensimon G, Lacomblez L, Meininger V. A controlled trial of riluzole in amyotrophic lateral sclerosis. ALS/Riluzole Study Group. *N Engl J Med* 1994; 330:585–591.

50. Miller RG, Moore D, Young LA, et al., and the WALS Study Group. Placebo-controlled trial of gabapentin in patients with amyotrophic lateral sclerosis. *Neurology* 1996; 47:1383–1388.

51. Schwarz GA, King G. Neuromuscular diseases of later maturity. Part I. *Geriatrics* 1955; 10:197–207.

52. Aboussouan LS, Khan SU, Meeker DP, Stelmach K, Mitsumoto H. Effect of noninvasive positive pressure ventilation on survival in amyotrophic lateral sclerosis. *Ann Intern Med* 1997; 127:450–453.

53. Brooks BR. El Escorial World Federation of Neurology criteria for the diagnosis of amyotrophic lateral sclerosis. *J Neurol Sci* 1994; 124 (Suppl):96–107.

54. Brooks BR, Miller RG, Swash M, Munsat TL, and the Airlie House "Current Issues in ALS Therapeutic Trials" Workshop Contributors. El Escorial Revisited: Revised criteria for the diagnosis of amyotrophic lateral sclerosis. A consensus conference held at Airlie House, Warrenton, Virginia, April 2–4, 1998.

55. Miller RG, Anderson F, on behalf of ALS C.A.R.E. Study Group. The ALS patient care database: A resource for measuring and improving ALS outcomes. *Neurology* 1998; 50:A245.

56. Lowenstein DH, Parent JM. Brain, heal thyself. *Science* 1999; 283:1126–1127.

57. Thomson JA, Itskovitz-Eldor J, Shapiro SS, et al. Embryonic stem cell lines derived from human blastocytes. *Science* 1998; 282:1145–1147.

58. Shamblott MJ, Axelman J, Wang S, et al. Derivation of pluripotent stem cells from cultured human primordial germ cells. *Proc Natl Acad Sci* 1998; 95:13726–13731.

2

The Clinical Features and Prognosis of ALS

Hiroshi Mitsumoto, M.D.

The human brain has billions of nerve cells, or neurons. There are more than 80 different types of these nerve cells, and some are highly specialized. Diseases that cause neuron loss or impair neuron function, such as Alzheimer's disease, Parkinson's disease, and amyotrophic lateral sclerosis (ALS), are a group of neurodegenerative disorders that affect specific types of neurons. For example, Alzheimer's disease affects neurons that control memory and intelligence, whereas in Parkinson's disease, the neurons that control the complex performance of body movements are diseased. ALS is familiar to many people as Lou Gehrig's disease, named for the baseball legend who suffered from it. It is a disorder of the motor neurons, which are responsible for contracting the skeletal muscles. To varying degrees, it affects two groups of motor neurons, the upper and lower motor neurons. In ALS the motor neurons gradually lose their ability to function, and the symptoms that are characteristic of ALS eventually appear. This chapter reviews the clinical signs and symptoms of ALS, their neuroanatomic and physiologic bases, the initial (presenting) symptoms, and the prognosis of the disease.

The Preclinical Stages of ALS

The important question as to when ALS really begins remains unanswered. It is generally agreed that the disease is probably already well along in its course when patients first notice muscle weakness. A well-documented record of this "preclinical" course in ALS is Lou Gehrig's batting average—his batting average and number of home runs started deteriorating one year before he recognized the symptoms of the disease that forced him to retire from baseball. An extensive autopsy study done many years ago in patients who died of acute poliomyelitis (rapid paralysis caused by poliovirus infection) showed that as many as 50 percent of the motor neurons in the spinal cord had been depleted even when the muscles controlled by those neurons had normal strength. In a similar study in patients with ALS, as many as 80 percent of these cells had been lost before muscle weakness was detected. These studies suggest that by the time motor neuron disease is diagnosed, a significant proportion of motor neurons may have already been lost.

To understand the mechanisms of how the disease progresses so insidiously during the preclinical stage and how normal muscle strength is maintained while motor neurons are progressively lost, some knowledge is needed about the anatomic and physiologic relationship between the motor neuron and the muscle fibers (Figure 2-1). Each skeletal muscle is composed of numerous muscle fibers, and each motor neuron in the spinal cord controls a number of muscle fibers. In large muscles, such as those of the trunk, buttock, or calf, one motor neuron controls more than 1,000 muscle fibers, whereas in the much smaller hand muscles, one motor neuron controls (innervates) only about 100 muscle fibers. The nerve fiber, or axon, that emerges from the motor neuron branches extensively after it enters the muscle so that each small nerve branch innervates a single muscle fiber. The entire group of muscle fibers innervated by one motor neuron is called the *motor unit*. The muscle fibers in one motor unit are not grouped together in the muscle. Instead they are scattered widely and intermixed with other muscle fibers that belong to many other motor units.

When a motor neuron is diseased, it no longer can control its motor unit (Figure 2-2). This process is called *denervation*. Muscle fibers that are denervated lose their ability to contract and thus waste and shrink, a process called *denervation atrophy*. Once muscle fibers are denervated, nerve fibers that belong to healthy motor neurons develop "sprouts" and take over the neural control of denervated muscle fibers. In this way denervated muscle fibers are reinnervated by healthy motor neurons so that muscle contraction is maintained. On the other hand, healthy motor neurons expand the size of their motor units. As long as the balance between denervation and reinnervation is maintained, muscle weakness may not become clinically apparent. However, as the disease progresses, the speed of neuronal degeneration exceeds that of reinnervation; moreover, once-healthy motor neurons may be affected. The process seems to be initially undetectable because patients have no symptoms that they or their physician notice. It is not known how long this preclinical stage lasts before muscle weakness becomes clinically apparent. It depends on the rate of motor neuron degeneration and reinnervation.

When detailed electrodiagnostic tests that measure the electrical activity of nerves and muscles are performed, neurologists may find evidence of extensive reinnervation, even when ALS is in a very early stage.

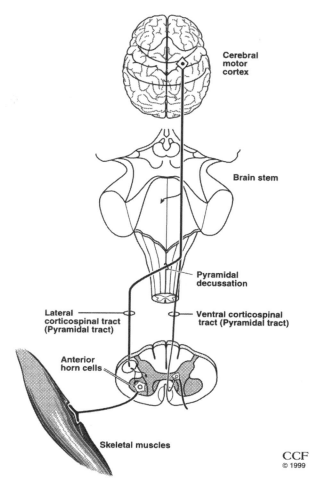

Cerebral
motor
cortex

Brain stem

Pyramidal
decussation

Lateral
corticospinal tract
(Pyramidal tract)

Ventral corticospinal
tract (Pyramidal tract)

Anterior
horn cells

Skeletal muscles

CCF
© 1999

Figure 2-1. As described in the text, two types of motor neurons control muscle contraction. One is the upper motor neuron system. The upper motor neurons are found mainly in the cerebral motor cortex and exert superior control over the lower motor neurons, often called anterior horn cells. Nerve fibers arising from the upper motor neurons descend from the cerebral cortex to the lower brain stem, where the majority of nerve fibers cross over, reach the opposite side, and further descend through the spinal cord finally to reach lower motor neurons. These descending bundles of fibers are called the *pyramidal tracts*. The tracts transmit the muscle contraction signal arising from the upper motor neurons. When this signal reaches and stimulates lower motor neurons, a new signal is generated within the lower motor neurons, which transmit the signal beyond the spinal cord to ultimately reach individual muscle fibers and directly contract these fibers.

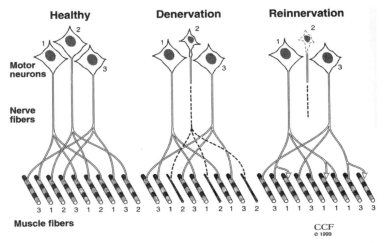

Figure 2-2. In the healthy motor neuron system, each lower motor neuron (anterior horn cell) controls (innervates) a number of muscle fibers (the motor unit). This relationship is depicted in the left panel. The middle panel shows the events that occur in motor neuron disease. When a motor neuron (neuron 2) is diseased, it no longer can control the muscle fibers it innervates, and the fibers undergo denervation (dotted lines in middle panel). Denervated muscle fibers shrink and become unable to contract (muscle fibers 2 in the middle panel). If surrounding lower motor neurons (neurons 1 and 3) are still healthy, these motor neurons can activate regeneration of nerve fibers to take over the control of the denervated muscle fibers. When this takeover process, called reinnervation, is completed, the denervated muscle fibers are controlled by different motor neurons. As shown in right panel, the end result is that neurons 1 and 3 expand their motor unit territory—motor neuron 1 now controls five muscle fibers instead of three and motor neuron 3 now controls four muscle fibers. As long as this process is maintained, normal muscle strength can be sustained while the number of motor neurons are slowly reduced.

Presenting Symptoms

ALS is one of several progressive wasting and weakening diseases of the skeletal muscle. Approximately 60 percent of patients notice weakness as the first symptom. The weakness typically occurs in the arm or leg muscles or in the muscles that control speech and swallowing (the bulbar muscles). In general, in one-third of patients the weakness begins in the arm; in another one-third it begins in the leg. Approximately one-fourth of patients first develop weakness in the bulbar muscles. The few remaining patients experience a generalized onset, with simultaneous involvement of the arms, legs, and bulbar muscles. On rare occasions weakness affects only one side of the body in the initial stages or resembles a nerve palsy (paralysis) that occurs in nerves of the forearm (radial or ulnar nerves) or a nerve at the shin (peroneal nerve). Other unusual initial symptoms include weakness that first involves muscles at the back of the neck or respiratory difficulty because muscles that assist in breathing have been affected. When the initial symptoms begin in such unusual locations, the diagnosis of ALS is difficult to make and is often delayed for some time.

Other presenting symptoms that lead patients to consult a physician are pain or muscle cramps. In our experience, pain and cramps are relatively rare as initial symptoms. However, muscle cramping is one of most common symptoms in the early stages of the disease and occurs in more than 80 percent or 90 percent of patients. Muscle twitching (fasciculations) and weight loss may be the first symptoms in a small percentage of patients. Muscle stiffness, difficulty walking, or excessive fatigue may be presenting symptoms in other patients. Muscle twitches and muscle cramps occur in completely healthy people, so it is important to understand that there is absolutely no reason to suspect ALS when these symptoms occur alone.

Neuroanatomic and Physiologic Bases of the Clinical Symptoms

Motor neurons are located in the brain, brain stem (a structure at the base of the brain that is inside the skull and connects the brain to the spinal cord), and spinal cord. The hallmark of ALS is muscle weakness that is caused by dysfunction of lower motor neurons. ALS also affects the upper motor neurons, and the involvement of these two motor neuron groups produces the features that are characteristic of ALS. A brief overview of the upper and lower motor neuron anatomy is helpful to understand how the specific signs and symptoms develop in ALS.

Upper Motor Neurons

The upper motor neurons are responsible for both voluntary and involuntary control over lower motor neurons. Upper motor neurons reside anatomically above the level of lower motor neurons and are found in the brain and brain stem. The brain's cerebral cortex is divided into individual areas that specialize in particular function. The cerebral motor cortex is specialized in motor control and constitutes several different cortical areas, consisting of the *primary motor cortex,* the *supplementary motor cortex,* and the *premotor area,* all of which work together to execute the most complex human body movements. Upper motor neurons that are located in the primary motor cortex can directly contract individual muscles. For example, the principle motor neurons in the primary motor cortex, called *giant pyramidal neurons* or *Betz cells,* contract individual skeletal muscles, working with a greater number of surrounding smaller motor neurons.

Nerve fibers coming from the motor neurons in the motor cortex form the largest descending nerve fiber groups of the brain and are called the *corticospinal* and *corticobulbar tracts*. Nerve fibers arising from neurons in the primary motor cortex constitute approximately one-third of these tracts. Another one-third are derived from the areas that plan and program motor performance. The remaining one-third are derived from the somatic sensory cortex and the adjacent temporal lobe region. This arrangement indicates that lower motor neurons receive broad control from the cerebral cortex, including the frontal lobes (the primary and supplementary motor cortices, and premotor areas), parietal lobe (the primary sensory cortex), and the temporal lobe.

The corticobulbar tracts descend with the corticospinal tracts but then branch away in the brain stem. They provide upper motor neuron control over brain stem lower motor neurons that belong to cranial nerves V (jaw movement), VII (face and lip movements), IX and X (throat and vocal cord movements), and XII (tongue movements).

The main corticospinal tracts (called pyramidal tracts) descend from the brain through the brain stem. Most corticospinal fibers (75 percent to 90 percent), however, cross to the opposite side in the brain stem and form the lateral corticospinal tract in the spinal cord. The fibers that do not cross continue to descend on the same side and form the ventral or anterior corticospinal tracts. The lateral corticospinal tract sends fibers to lower motor neurons that control arm and leg muscles that require independent, unilateral control. For example, these motor neurons allow the right hand to move independently of the left hand. In contrast, the anterior corticospinal tract sends fibers bilaterally to motor neurons that control postural muscles near the center of the trunk, which must have bilateral control so they can act together to hold the body upright and straight.

Brain Stem Motor Control

Motor neurons of the spinal cord are also controlled by special neurons in the brain stem (such as vestibular nuclei and the reticular formation) that modulate the sensitivity of muscle reflexes, muscle tone, and balance between the flexor and extensor muscle groups of the upper and lower extremities, trunk, and neck. When we stand, sit, or position our bodies in virtually any way, we have continuous automatic (involuntary) control of muscle tone; otherwise, our body could not maintain postures. This system is complex, controlling many reflexes and involuntary body postures. The neurons that belong to these brain stem nuclei are considered upper motor neurons in a broad sense because they strongly influence skeletal muscle tone. These brain stem upper motor neurons send nerve fibers in the form of several descending tracts to lower motor neurons in the spinal cord.

Limbic Motor Control

The limbic system consists of a number of brain structures that together are closely involved in emotional experience and expression. The system is closely associated with a wide variety of autonomic, visceral, and endocrine functions. (Autonomic function refers to functions regulated by the autonomic nervous system, such as sweating or heart rate; they may also be affected by one's emotional state and "visceral" pertains to the gastrointestinal organs.) Recent studies clearly indicate that the limbic system strongly influences lower motor neurons in the brain stem and spinal cord. Thus the emotional status and experience of an individual affects the overall spinal cord motor neuron activity. Of particular importance, several brain stem nuclei belonging to the limbic system influence basic, instinctive behaviors, such as respiration, vomiting, swallowing, chewing, and licking, and emotional expression, including crying and laughing.

Lower Motor Neurons

The lower motor neurons are located in the brain stem and spinal cord and send out nerve fibers to directly innervate skeletal muscle fibers. These motor neurons are lowest in the hierarchy of motor control. They are clustered in pools, forming columns. Because lower motor neurons are located in the anterior gray matter, or anterior horn, of the spinal cord, they are also known as *anterior horn cells.* The anterior horn contains neurons associated with the motor system, whereas the posterior horn contains neurons associated with the sensory system. Anterior horn cells vary in size. Large motor neurons are the most common and often are called *alpha-motoneurons;* they are the principal motor neurons that innervate muscle fibers.

The alpha-motoneuron is among the largest neurons of the nervous system. It has a single nerve fiber (axon) that extends to innervate its muscles, and it has a number of large extensions called *dendrites,* which branch like a tree and receive signals extensively from other neurons, including upper motor neurons and the sensory feedback system. One alpha-motoneuron innervates one group of muscle fibers, or motor unit, as briefly discussed previously.

Interneurons

Interneurons are small neurons in the anterior horn or in the brain stem motor neuron groups. They are of paramount importance in determining how the lower motor neurons control muscle contraction. The interneurons receive extensive upper motor neuron control from the brain stem descending tracts, corticospinal tracts, and limbic system. They also receive sensory feedback information from the skeletal muscles. Interneurons form intricate neuronal circuits to program numerous basic leg, arm, or body movements. For example, the quick reflex to a sudden sting to your arm is programmed in the interneurons. These circuits are a basic component of complex, fine motor movements.

Signs and Symptoms of Upper Motor Neuron Dysfunction

Slowly progressive dysfunction and impairment of upper motor neurons causes the characteristic clinical signs and symptoms discussed here.

Loss of Dexterity

Voluntary movements that require fine dexterity are the product of the integrated activation of complex lower motor neuron/interneuron circuits of the spinal cord that control fine muscle contractions; however, the upper motor neurons—through the corticospinal tracts—ultimately control such actions. Thus a prominent and early sign of upper motor neuron dysfunction is loss of dexterity. When dexterity is impaired, voluntary and even reflex motions become awkward. This loss may be expressed as stiffness, slowness, and clumsiness in any motion that requires fine movement, such as any rapid repetitive motion of the fingers, feet, or even the lips or tongue.

Loss of Muscle Strength (Weakness)

Another sign of upper motor neuron dysfunction is loss of muscle strength. Because the motor units are preserved, muscle weakness resulting from upper motor neuron dysfunction generally is mild and not as severe as that seen in lower motor neuron involvement. In patients with severe upper motor neuron syndrome, accurately assessing muscle strength becomes difficult because spasticity and loss of dexterity prevent effective activation of the motor units.

Spasticity

Spasticity is an abnormal state of sustained increase in muscle tension that occurs when the muscle is lengthened. When spasticity exists, passively stretching or actively shortening a muscle spontaneously elicits a reflex that increases muscle tone. This reflex occurs because motor neurons are generally more excitable. Thus muscle relaxation is delayed, making smooth muscle contraction difficult when antagonist muscles—the opposite muscles that normally relax and elongate when the other muscles contract—also increase their muscle tone.

Passive movement becomes nearly impossible when muscles are severely spastic. Sometimes muscles lose their normal smooth action during passive movement, suddenly increase their resistance, and then resist further passive movement. This particular type of muscle resistance is referred to as a "catch." However, when a sustained passive stretch is applied to spastic muscles, they quickly release the tension and relax, an event often described as the "clasp-knife phenomenon."

Although spasticity is the central feature of upper motor neuron dysfunction, how this dysfunction leads to spasticity is not fully understood. There are several likely explanations. Upper motor neurons in the cerebral cortex have superior control over some brain stem upper motor neurons that control muscle tone. When this superior control is lost, the brain stem upper motor neurons become overactive and signal to increase muscle tone in extremity muscles; upper motor neuron dysfunction also increases muscle fiber spindle (receptors in the muscle) sensitivity, so muscles become more sensitive to passive stretching. Moreover, upper motor neuron dysfunction reduces the available amount of an excitatory signaling chemical called glutamate. Lower motor neurons and interneurons become hypersensitive to glutamate, so that a small amount of glutamate can easily and force-fully contract muscles.

Pathologic Hyperreflexia

Pathologic hyperreflexia (exaggerated muscle stretch reflexes) is another crucial manifestation of upper motor neuron dysfunction in ALS. When the muscle tendon is tapped, the muscle spindle (a receptor) stretches and sends an excitatory impulse. In healthy people this impulse produces a typical reflex with quick muscle contraction called a *monosynaptic muscle stretch reflex*. When upper motor neuron control is disrupted, stretch reflexes become abnormally exaggerated because the inhibition exerted by the upper motor neuron circuit is impaired. In pathologic hyperreflexia, only a slight or distant stimulus is needed to elicit the reflex response. For example, an ordinary tendon tap elicits reflexes in neighboring muscles (spreading), and manual stretching of the muscle induces repeated, rhythmic muscle contraction called *clonus*. Such responses indicate that upper motor neurons are disrupted or dysfunctional.

Pathologic Reflexes

A pathologic reflex is a reflex whose presence is abnormal; in healthy individuals these reflexes are inhibited and thus are not seen. These are primitive reflexes; that is, they are normally present early in development but then disappear. When upper motor neurons and their tracts are dysfunctional, these reflexes are no longer inhibited and can be easily elicited. The Babinski sign (extensor plantar response) is one of the most important signs in clinical neurology. It is characterized by an upward extension of the great toe, often accompanied by fanning of the other toes, that occurs when one strokes the outer edge of the sole upward from the heel with a blunt object. In healthy adults the great toe flexes (curls down) in response to this stimulation. If present, the Babinski sign is a definitive sign of upper motor neuron dysfunction. Other pathologic reflexes also may be present, most of which are variations of the Babinski sign.

In the upper extremities, Hoffmann's sign may indicate abnormality. This reflex is triggered by the quick release that occurs after the forceful flexion of the joint at the tip of the middle finger. A reflex inward flexing of the thumb on the same hand is a positive response. Tapping the belly of the middle finger tip can also elicit a similar thumb flexion (the Trömner sign). When these reflexes appear only on the one side, they are always abnormal. However, bilateral positive reflexes may not be abnormal because they are not unusual in healthy young individuals.

Spastic Bulbar Palsy

When upper motor neurons and the corticobulbar fibers that control speaking, chewing, and swallowing are affected, a unique upper motor neuron syndrome appears, called *spastic bulbar palsy*. The term *spastic* indicates that the dysfunction is located in the upper motor neurons. The actual weakness in muscles participating in bulbar function (see below) is milder than that found in *paretic* or *flaccid bulbar palsy,* terms that are used to describe the effects of lower motor neuron dysfunction in these muscles. The voice may sound forced because much effort is needed to force air through the upper airway. Repetitive movements of the lips, tongue, and pharynx become particularly slow because of reduced dexterity. The term *pseudobulbar palsy* is often used to distinguish spastic palsy from paretic bulbar palsy, which occurs when the lower motor neurons of the brain stem are affected.

Symptoms include difficulties in speaking, chewing, and swallowing because the highly coordinated bulbar muscle movements are slowed and stiffened. Patients with spastic bulbar palsy also appear to have poor emotional control, as characterized by spontaneous or unmotivated crying and laughter. In daily life discussions or questions about subjects with emotional content often trigger crying or laughter that is embarrassing to patients. The underlying mechanism may be caused by rhythmic contractions of muscles involved in speech and respiration. This phenomenon occurs because they have lost inhibition of the limbic motor neurons, which control muscles producing "primitive" vocalization (crying and laughing).

Signs and Symptoms of Lower Motor Neuron Dysfunction

Loss of Muscle Strength (Weakness)

The loss of a motor neuron means the loss of its motor unit. In contrast, impaired motor neuron function leads to abnormal or impaired activation of the motor unit. In either case a progressive reduction in the number of functional motor units decreases muscle strength. In ALS weakness caused by lower motor neuron dysfunction is much more significant than that caused by upper motor neuron dysfunction.

Muscle weakness is the cardinal sign and symptom of ALS. It almost always occurs in isolated muscle areas at onset and is followed by progressive weakness. Weakness in ALS usually is not associated with pain.

Muscle weakness in the hand muscles causes difficulty in performing fine movements with the fingers, such as pinching, turning keys, buttoning, using a zipper, or writing. When it occurs in the arms, people may be unable to carry an object, throw a ball, or raise an object above shoulder level. When weakness develops in the foot, the foot commonly slaps the floor. Such "foot drop" makes climbing stairs difficult, and patients may trip and fall.

Muscle Atrophy

The muscle fiber volume decreases markedly when muscle fibers are denervated, a process called *denervation atrophy.* Motor neuron death leads to atrophy of all muscle fibers belonging to the motor unit; partial damage to a motor unit causes atrophy in a limited number of its muscle fibers. In ALS the progressive loss of motor neurons results in atrophy that is clinically observed as a wasting of the affected skeletal muscles. Atrophy of the hand muscles, one of most common sites of muscle atrophy in ALS, is easily recognized by patients and physicians, even in the early stages of the disease. Muscle atrophy can affect any skeletal muscles, but muscles in the forearms or hands and lower leg and foot muscles (called distal muscles) generally atrophy more often than muscles near the body trunk (called *proximal muscles*).

Hyporeflexia

If the disease involves only the lower motor neurons, muscle stretch reflexes are reduced or even absent. This is in contrast to the hyperreflexia that occurs in upper motor neuron dysfunction. Hyporeflexia results from the loss of active motor units and insufficient muscle contraction. When muscles become totally paralyzed or atrophied, hyperreflexia that may have developed earlier in the course of the disease may disappear.

Muscle Hypotonicity or Flaccidity

Hypotonicity or flaccidity refers to the decrease or complete loss of normal muscle resistance to passive movements. In contrast to spasticity, the muscle lies inert and floppy when passively manipulated.

Fasciculations

Fasciculations are fine, rapid, flickering, and sometimes vermicular (wormlike) twitchings of a portion of the muscle. They occur irregularly in time and location. Fasciculations are believed to result from spontaneous electrical discharges at the membrane of the motor neuron nerve fiber. The cause is not known. In general, the larger the muscle, the greater the size of the fasciculations. In tongue muscles, for example, the fasciculations are small movements on the tongue surface. Fasciculations are found in almost all patients with ALS, but rarely are they an initial symptom. When their presence cannot be confirmed by clinical examination, needle electromyographic examination may be helpful to identify fasciculations. It is important to remember that fasciculations are common and occur in healthy persons, a condition that is termed *benign fasciculation.* In the absence of neurologic findings, such as weakness or atrophy, benign fasciculations usually have no serious clinical implications.

Muscle Cramps

Muscle cramps (or charley horse) are another common symptom of lower motor neuron dysfunction. The cause of muscle cramps is poorly understood, although cramps and fasciculations are likely to share a similar mechanism, that is, hyperexcitability of motor axons—in hyperexcitability, the electrical discharge from the cell membrane is continuous. A muscle cramp is a sudden, involuntary, sustained muscle contraction with severe pain that interrupts activity or sleep. In a true cramp the abrupt, involuntary, and painful shortening of the muscle is accompanied by visible or palpable knotting and often shifts the affected joint into an abnormal position; stretching or massaging relieves it. Sudden muscle pains often described as "muscle spasms" are not associated with severe muscle contraction, so they are not true muscle cramps.

As with fasciculations, muscle cramps (especially in the calves) are common in healthy people. In ALS, however, muscle cramps occur not only in the usual sites, such as the calf, but also in the thighs, arms, hands, abdomen, neck, jaw, or even the tongue. They are one of the most frequently encountered symptoms in ALS.

Truncal Muscle Weakness

Weakness in cervical and thoracic extensor muscles, which keep the body and head erect and straight, often occur in ALS. Such weakness allows the head to fall forward (head droop). In advanced stages the neck becomes completely flexed so that the head drops forward and patients cannot see farther than several feet away. Consequently, walking, eating, and even breathing are seriously impaired. Muscle pain in the overstretched neck extensors is common. To compensate, patients may bend the body backward in an attempt to maintain distant view while walking.

Bulbar Signs and Symptoms

Muscles controlling speaking, chewing, and swallowing are innervated by the cranial nerves VII (facial), IX (glossopharyngeal), X (vagus), and XII (hypoglossal). The neurons that control these muscles are located in a brain structure called the *medulla*. Because the medulla is also known as the "bulb," neurologic signs and symptoms resulting from the loss of medullary neurons and their axons are referred to as *bulbar palsy*. Although not controlled in the medulla, cranial nerve V (trigeminal) usually is also implicated because it controls jaw movement. When the medullary lower motor neurons are primarily affected, the condition is called *flaccid* or *paretic bulbar palsy*. In contrast, when upper motor neurons and their descending tracts (the corticobulbar tracts) are affected, spastic ("spastic" indicating the upper motor neuron dysfunction) bulbar palsy develops, as discussed in the section on upper motor neuron dysfunction. A mixed bulbar palsy that consists of a varying mixture of flaccid and spastic components is usually seen in ALS.

When the bulbar muscles are affected, examination may reveal weakness in the facial muscles. Patients may not be able to close their eyes tightly or may have difficulty opening and closing their mouth. Puckering the lips and puffing the cheeks out while holding air in the mouth also is difficult, as is smiling broadly or naturally. The tongue surface may be wavy and irregular because of wasting of the tongue muscle. The fasciculations can be observed only when the tongue is in a resting position. Tongue movement may be impaired and moving the tongue to either side may be difficult, indicating weakness. The soft palate raises when one speaks, but in ALS this elevation may be limited if the palate muscle is weakened.

Dysarthria

Dysarthria refers to difficulty in speaking because the muscles involved in producing sound and speech are impaired. Initial problems include an inability to shout or sing, a weakened voice, and difficulty with enunciation. Speech sometimes becomes slurred and slowed. When paralysis of the vocal cords starts, the voice takes on either a hoarse or a whispering quality. When the muscles acting as a valve between mouth and nasal cavity become weak, air may leak from the mouth into the nose during enunciation, which results in a nasal tone. In either case, enunciation becomes progressively more difficult, and in the advanced stages of ALS speech becomes hard to understand and finally nonexistent (anarthria).

Dysphagia

Dysphagia means that chewing and swallowing are impaired; it usually is accompanied by dysarthria. Manipulating food inside the mouth is difficult, and food can become trapped between the gum and the cheek. Patients may be unable to form a small ball of food or push food down into the throat, and they may experience weak or uncoordinated movements when swallowing. Small pieces of dry, crumbly food are more difficult to handle than food with a soft, smooth consistency. Patients with dysphagia caused by neural dysfunction generally also have more difficulty swallowing liquids than solids because liquids move quickly into the throat before the epiglottis—the valve that closes the airway to the lungs—can fully close. Liquids sometimes regurgitate into the nose if the valve between the mouth and nose does not close properly. Swallowing eventually may trigger reflex coughing, a warning that dysphagia is serious and has led to food or liquid entering the airway, called *aspiration*. At this stage patients require increasingly more time to finish a meal, and eating becomes a great chore. Talking while eating, a bulbar function that requires skillful coordination, eventually becomes impossible. The risk of aspiration becomes significant when the cough reflex is weakened by paralysis of vocal, swallowing, and respiratory muscles. Speech pathologists should be consulted to evaluate swallowing dysfunction in detail; a modified barium swallowing test may be useful to analyze dysphagia and train suitable swallowing techniques (see Chapter 10).

Sialorrhea

Patients with ALS frequently report sialorrhea (drooling) that is both disabling and embarrassing. It occurs because the spontaneous automatic swallowing that normally clears excessive saliva is reduced and the lower facial muscles have become too weak to close both lips tightly to prevent leakage. It is aggravated by the drooping head posture discussed previously.

Aspiration and Laryngospasm

In normal individuals the epiglottis closes automatically upon swallowing. Incomplete or uncoordinated closure may allow liquid, saliva, or food to pass into the larynx. This aspiration usually triggers the cough reflex or choking. Aspiration can be a life-threatening event and may result in aspiration pneumonia. However, no signs of aspiration may be apparent when the amount aspirated is small. A modified barium swallowing test, which should be attended by an experienced speech pathologist, is required to investigate possible aspiration.

Cough attacks, an exaggerated gag reflex, or aspiration to the larynx may trigger a sudden narrowing of upper air way (laryngospasm), which is characterized by loud breathing during inhalation. Laryngospasm is generally considered not to be life threatening.

Respiratory Symptoms

Weakness in the respiratory muscles causes the respiratory symptoms seen in ALS. Three sets of muscles are used during respiration: the diaphragm, which is the sole respiratory muscle used actively during inhalation; those between the ribs (intercostals); and abdominal muscles, which function during exhalation. During inhalation the diaphragm moves downward, pushing the abdominal contents downward. This action creates a negative pressure in the chest cavity, so the air flows into the lungs. When a person is upright, gravity also acts to pull the abdominal contents downward. However, when a person is lying down, gravity does not have this effect when a person is lying down, so that only the diaphragm acts on the abdominal contents. Consequently, people with ALS may sleep poorly or breathe with difficulty when sleeping on their back. Although poor sleep can have many causes, when respiratory problems occur only at night, the cause must be identified. In the early stages of respiratory muscle weakness, people with ALS often prefer lying on their side or using extra pillows to prop the body partially upright. In later stages, patients may be unable to lie flat on their back because of respiratory difficulty. Some patients experience a condition called sleep apnea, which is caused by upper airway obstruction and, on rare occasions, by abnormalities in the respiratory center in the brain stem. Dull headaches upon awakening in the morning may be a sign of poor respiration during the night.

Respiratory difficulty during exercise is common, and frequent sighs at rest may represent respiratory symptoms at an early stage in the disease. A severe decrease in the depth and rate of breathing may develop during sleep, primarily because of diaphragmatic weakness. In patients with moderately advanced respiratory distress, contraction of accessory muscles is visible in the anterior neck, along with shoulder movements during respiration. Measurements of a pulmonary characteristic called the *forced vital capacity* are useful to identify early respiratory problems and are indispensable to follow changes in the respiratory condition.

On rare occasions, muscle weakness first affects the respiratory muscles, leading to impending respiratory failure. This presentation is associated with a poor prognosis. These patients often need immediate respiratory support in the intensive care unit, and it is not unusual for them to become completely ventilator dependent. In such cases the cause of respiratory failure initially is not known, and the correct diagnosis of ALS can often be significantly delayed.

Generalized Signs and Symptoms

Weight Loss

Ongoing muscle wasting and reduced caloric intake caused by difficulty in eating or loss of appetite can lead to progressive weight loss in people with ALS. Occasionally, however, the weight loss is far more pronounced than would be expected in those with little or only mild muscle wasting. This unusual weight loss, called *ALS cachexia,* primarily involves loss of fat below the skin and in the abdominal cavity. Weight loss exceeding 20 percent of body weight within six months from the onset of weakness is not unusual in this form of cachexia. The body weight in all ALS patients should be checked at every office visit because the rate of weight loss is a useful indicator of nutritional management.

Fatigue

Fatigue is common in many neuromuscular diseases. In ALS excessive fatigue may occur early and is identical to that which occurs in myasthenia gravis (a disease that produces severe fatigue because of dysfunction at the nerve and muscle junction). The physiologic basis for the fatigue is not well understood. Recent studies of fatigue in people with ALS showed that its source is not dysfunction at the nerve and muscle junction or within the muscle membrane. Rather the activation of contraction is impaired, in part because of changes within the muscle cells themselves.

Musculoskeletal Signs

Foot and Hand Contractures

Foot and hand deformities can occur in ALS. Patients who experience a relatively slow course of upper motor neuron dysfunction develop stiffness in the extensor muscles of the lower legs. This stiffness results in Achilles tendon shortening. Claw hand is a fairly common hand deformity seen with ALS. It occurs because of weakness in certain deep muscles of the hand and muscles between the hand bones. The metacarpophalangeal joints (the base joint between hand bones and fingers) consequently become overextended, whereas the distal finger joints become flexed. Almost invariably, joint contracture then develops and further complicates the hand deformity.

Shoulder Subluxation

Skeletal muscles not only move two bones at their joint but also hold the bones tightly together at the joint. When these muscles weaken, the joint loosens and sometimes partially separates, a process called *subluxation* or *partial dislocation*. Shoulder subluxation is common in patients with ALS, who usually have weak shoulder girdle muscles. The arm then feels heavy and constantly sags from the should joint. This process usually is painless.

Joint Contracture

Contracture (abnormal muscle shortening) develops relatively quickly in joints that have little mobility or are immobile because of paralysis. Joint contracture and a condition called *pericapsulitis* can cause severe pain and discomfort when the joint is voluntarily or passively moved. Pericapsulitis often affects the shoulder joints. Because of the pain, patients tend to not move the affected joints, which further aggravates the contracture. Aggressive physical therapy and range-of-motion exercise is crucial to prevent painful contracture.

Rare Manifestations of ALS

Clinically, ALS is a "pure" motor neuron syndrome; however, other systems, such as the sensory system and autonomic systems, the external ocular (eye) muscles, or higher cortical function (memory and intelligence), are not completely spared. Instead, these systems appear to be affected in the late stages of the disease or the impairment is evident only if highly sophisticated techniques are used. Generally, however, when impairment of the sensory system, ocular muscles, or higher cortical function is identified, neurologists must be cautious in their diagnosis of ALS.

Sensory Impairment

A small proportion of patients with ALS report "numbness" or ill-defined pain in the lower legs or arms. The use of the word *numbness* does not necessarily imply sensory impairment; patients may even be describing muscle weakness. Sensory impairment has not been found in ALS patients, but sensory complaints are not unusual. In our studies nearly 20 percent of patients with motor neuron disease (180 with ALS and 36 with progressive muscular atrophy) had ill-defined sensory symptoms of paresthesia (burning, prickling sensation) or focal pain. However, sensory examination showed no abnormalities except a decreased sensitivity to vibration in the toes, which is not unusual in healthy elderly people.

Although a routine neurologic examination reveals no sensory abnormalities in most patients with ALS, more sophisticated quantitative sensory testing may reveal clear abnormalities. These patients have abnormally elevated sensory thresholds, particularly to vibratory stimuli, but sensitivity to touch and changes in temperature is normal. Electrophysiologic tests, including somatosensory evoked potentials, are abnormal in some people with typical ALS. Pathologic studies reveal that the number of myelinated fibers in the peripheral sensory nerves is lower in these individuals. These findings support the opinion that ALS is not a pure motor neuron syndrome but rather a generalized neuronal disease primarily involving the motor neurons.

Dementia

Although rare, dementia may occur in patients who have otherwise typical ALS. Epidemiologic data on dementia in ALS are scarce, but its frequency is reported as less than 5 percent. Mild dementia may not be detected, particularly in patients with bulbar palsy whose impaired ability to speak makes the assessment of mental function particularly difficult. In addition, the dementia in ALS seems to be more common in those with bulbar palsy than in those with predominantly extremity involvement; consequently, dementia may not have been detected in some of these latter patients.

Confusion, forgetfulness, personality change, and poor memory retention are usual early symptoms of dementia in ALS. Behavioral and psychotic changes are rare. The Mini-Mental Status Examination should be given to everyone who is being evaluated for ALS. Depression is one of the most common psychological processes in patients with ALS, and it may mimic dementia. Therefore, neurologists must be careful to distinguish depression from dementia.

The cause of dementia in ALS is complex and may have several explanations. For example, dementia is a part of the parkinsonism-dementia complex seen in the western Pacific. Patients with this condition have symptoms of Parkinson's disease plus dementia. Clinically, about 5 percent of the patients in the western Pacific who have parkinsonism-dementia develop ALS, but 38 percent of patients with ALS in this region develop parkinsonism-dementia. However, detailed autopsy studies of the brain in these patients revealed that the ALS and the parkinsonism-dementia complex of the western Pacific are the same disease process. Although the complex of ALS and parkinsonism-dementia most commonly occurs in the western Pacific as an endemic form, both familial and sporadic cases of a clinically identical syndrome have been reported outside this region. To further complicate matters, the dementia in ALS and in Alzheimer's disease can be identical clinically. However, non-Alzheimer's dementia, which is characterized by neuronal degeneration in the frontal and temporal lobes, is perhaps the most common form of dementia in ALS. Further investigation, including autopsy studies, is crucial to understanding the mechanisms of dementia in ALS.

Extrapyramidal (Parkinsonian) Signs

Parkinsonism is a key feature of the parkinsonism-dementia complex in the western Pacific. Although parkinsonian signs are rare in patients with classic ALS outside this region, some cases have been reported in the United States and other countries. Parkinsonian features include slow body movements, increased muscle tone, diminished facial expression, stooped posture, and postural instability. In ALS, however, these features may be masked by marked spasticity and dominated or replaced by progressive lower motor neuron signs, such as muscle atrophy and weakness, even if parkinsonian features may be present,

Ocular Palsy

The eye muscles typically are spared in ALS. When ocular motility is tested in depth, however, the velocity of smooth pursuit movement (how fast both eyes move simultaneously) is lower in approximately 50 percent of patients with typical ALS. Such ocular abnormalities are thought to be caused by dysfunction in the neural system (the upper motor neuron) that controls motor performance and planning. Patients who have been on a ventilator for long periods may have a high frequency of ocular abnormalities, such as the inability to voluntarily close the eyes or complete ocular paralysis (ophthalmoplegia). Therefore, ocular motor control may be affected in the later stages of ALS.

Bladder and Bowel Dysfunction

A group of motor neurons located near the end of spinal cord called the *Onufrowicz nucleus* controls the pelvic floor muscles and the muscles for emptying urine from the bladder and emptying stool at the anus. However, a detailed analysis of bladder function in 38 patients with ALS revealed that almost one-third had abnormal bladder function. Because bladder and bowel control involves not only skeletal muscles but also involuntary autonomic neurons, these data suggest that supranuclear control over sympathetic, parasympathetic, and somatic neurons may be abnormal in ALS. Although bowel function in ALS has not been systematically studied, in our experience abnormal bowel function is very rare.

Bed Sores

Sensory perception and cutaneous autonomic function remain normal in people with ALS; thus they may help prevent bedsores (decubiti). However, bed sores occasionally do occur, particularly in patients who require prolonged ventilatory support.

Prognosis in ALS

It is important to understand that the prognosis of ALS varies greatly from patient to patient. Patients rarely may die within several months after the onset, whereas others may live more than 30 years. A slowing in progression and even improvement in patients have been reported, but these reports are rare. The prognosis of ALS is usually expressed in terms of the duration of the disease. The duration of disease in ALS is defined as the interval between the onset of symptoms and death. Recent studies indicate that the average duration of disease in ALS ranges from 27 to 43 months. However, the median duration ranges from 23 to 52 months. The median is important to consider because it is a measure that eliminates the extreme cases—those with a very short duration such as several months or a very long duration of 20 or more years. Compared to the duration of disease, the survival rate may be a better indicator of prognosis because it gives the probability of survival at the time of study (or diagnosis). In ALS, the 5-year survival rate ranges from 9 percent to 40 percent, with an average of 25 percent; the 10-year-survival rate ranges from 8 percent to 16 percent.

Factors That Influence Prognosis

Epidemiologic studies suggest some factors that are related to prognosis. Age probably has the strongest relationship to prognosis: usually the younger the patients, the longer the duration of the disease. In general, severe clinical involvement at diagnosis reliably predicts a rapidly progressive clinical course. A short interval between symptom onset and diagnosis is also associated with increased disability scores and poor prognosis, whereas a longer delay from onset of symptoms to diagnosis is associated with less disability and longer survival. However, this factor should be viewed with caution because ALS is now diagnosed much earlier since public awareness and medical diagnostic approaches have improved in recent years.

One of the most intriguing and important studies in recent years indicates that the better the patient's psychological well-being, the longer the survival. Other factors associated with better prognosis include presence of either a purely upper motor neuron or a purely lower motor neuron form, and extremity-onset compared with bulbar-onset ALS. A poorer prognosis also is linked to impaired respiratory function at diagnosis or respiratory failure at the onset of disease. Low serum chloride levels are associated with poorer prognosis.

Patients with a Prolonged Course

It is well known to ALS experts that occasional patients who appear to have typical ALS may either cease to progress or progress very slowly. A good proportion of patients with ALS are long survivors, living beyond 5 years after diagnosis, and 8 percent to 16 percent of patients live up to 10 years. The duration of illness alone does not distinguish between typical and protracted forms of ALS. In fact, people who survive for more than 10 years may not be all that rare. We have followed up patients who had a protracted course, but we were not certain about the diagnosis of ALS; we designated their condition "atypical" ALS. Such patients require further investigation to characterize this aspect of ALS.

The two longest documented durations of ALS are 32 years and 39 years. In fact, one of the leading ALS experts (the late Forbes H. Norris, M.D.) even used the term *benign ALS* because the course of ALS in such cases was not the typical progressive course. In these patients, the annual decline in function is minimal. Although the disease progresses very slowly, overall functional impairment is still severe. In 28 male patients of 613 patients with sporadic ALS, progression ceased for at least five years. Others have suggested that a patient's disease "resistance" might influence the course of ALS. Determining whether patients with a more benign course have more reinnervation activity or experience other moderating influences is particularly important to improving our understanding of prognosis in ALS.

"Reversible" ALS

People have been described who presented with ALS-like features and subsequently improved. In one such patient, ALS developed but progressed minimally over six years; however, the patient then suddenly grew worse, developed generalized fasciculations, and died within two years. Mulder and Howard reported a 49-year-old surgeon who developed weakness in the left arm followed by weakness in the left leg along with fasciculations. Examination showed features typical of ALS. The muscle strength in his extremities gradually improved over several months, and reexamination after six years showed nearly normal muscle strength.

Similar cases of recovery or improvement from other motor neuron diseases also have been reported. It is interesting that all cases reported to date are characterized by predominantly lower motor neuron signs, although in some patients, reflexes are abnormal but not pathologic. No patient had spasticity or bulbar symptoms. Based on the El Escorial World Federation of Neurology diagnostic criteria, these cases probably are not classic ALS. Identifying and understanding similar cases of this "reversible" ALS syndrome is an important task for neurologists.

Acknowledgment: I express my gratitude to the many patients with ALS and their families who visited our ALS Clinic and candidly discussed so many issues with us. We are very indebted to our patients for teaching us about this difficult disease. I also am personally grateful for the support, dedication, and excellent work provided by the health care team at the Cleveland Clinic ALS Center. Cassandra Talerico, M.A., Department of Anesthesiology, provided a substantive editing.

Suggested Reading

1. Mitsumoto H, Chad DA, Pioro EP. *Amyotrophic lateral sclerosis.* New York: Oxford University Press, 1997.

2. Belsh JM, Schiffman PL (eds.). *Amyotrophic lateral sclerosis.* Armonk, NY: Futura, 1996.

3

The Diagnosis of Amyotrophic Lateral Sclerosis

David A. Chad, M.D.

You—or a loved one—probably were first referred to a neurologist for assistance in establishing a diagnosis because of an unexplained weakness or clumsiness in the hand or foot, muscle cramping associated with weakness, or difficulties speaking or swallowing. The neurologist's task was to review all prior records, take a careful history, and perform a detailed and meticulous physical examination. He or she was then in a position to arrive at the most likely "clinical diagnosis" (a diagnosis grounded in clinical evidence) and "differential diagnoses" (possible alternative considerations). Laboratory studies probably were recommended, including radiologic or imaging studies of the brain and spinal cord, electrodiagnostic testing (nerve conduction studies and electromyographic needle examination), and a variety of blood tests. When this testing—a process that may take a couple of weeks—was complete, the neurologist probably met with you to discuss the clinical and laboratory findings and to present his or her diagnostic impression.

History of the Illness—Listening to Your Concerns

An important first step in the diagnostic process is for the neurologist to listen to what the patient and family say about new symptoms experienced by the patient. After the patient and family relate their observations and describe changes in how the patient feels and how he or she has been functioning, the neurologist generally asks specific questions in an effort to understand the nature of the problem as fully as possible. Although your main complaint may appear to involve

37

only one or two regions of the body, the neurologist's questions typically will be designed to evaluate neurologic regions literally from "head to toe." He asks about speaking, chewing, swallowing; the facility with which the patient feels he or she can maintain the head erect; strength and dexterity in the arms; and the ease of rising from a seated position, walking a distance, or climbing a flight of stairs. There are questions about the ease of breathing, particularly at night and during exercise. Patients are asked about the state of their muscles—if there has been loss of muscle bulk, twitching, or cramping.

The neurologist also asks about neurologic functions controlled by nervous system structures outside the motor system (recall that ALS is almost always strictly a disease of motor function), although such functions generally are not affected by ALS per se. The reason for asking these questions is to look for clues that suggest the motor complaints to be part of a neurologic disorder other than ALS. For example, the neurologist asks about memory loss; visual changes; and the presence of numbness, tingling, or prickling. There also will be inquiries as to the presence of pain, particularly in the neck spreading into the arms or in the back spreading into the legs, and whether the patient has any difficulties controlling the bladder or bowel. Questions such as these are asked because some nervous system disorders involve the motor system and one or more of the following systems: cognitive, visual, sensory, and autonomic. Unless the answers to these questions are sought, a disease masquerading as ALS could be missed or its diagnosis delayed. The neurologist typically also asks about the patient's general health. Although certain changes are expected in ALS, such as fatigue, difficulty sleeping, weight loss, and depression (the latter often as a reaction to the presence of unexplained symptoms), other symptoms might indicate an unexpected medical condition that might be associated with features of ALS. For example, the neurologist will probe the patient's past and recent history for signs of an infectious disease, thyroid abnormalities, an underlying tumor, or exposure to toxic agents, each of which could cause at least some of the motor changes found in ALS.

The neurologist also asks questions about family history. Up to 10 percent of all people with ALS carry a genetic mutation that is passed on to their children. In 20 percent of these "familial" cases, a mutation involves the gene coding for copper/zinc superoxide dismutase (SOD1), an enzyme whose normal function is to limit the production of potentially toxic intracellular free radicals. More than 80 different mutations have now been identified. The precise mechanism by which the mutated SOD1 enzyme causes the neuron loss in ALS is not certain, but it is likely that the mutation confers on the enzyme an unwanted neurotoxic property. The familial disease is clinically very similar to the more common "sporadic" (arising spontaneously) form.

When the history taking is completed, the patient, family, and neurologist should feel that the neurologist has heard an up-to-date and complete account of the patient's medical and neurologic history.

The Neurologic Examination

The neurologist approaches the examination in an orderly fashion, beginning with the evaluation of behavior, mood, language, and memory. Most people with ALS have a normal "mental status" examination, and another diagnosis is considered if abnormalities are detected in one or more areas of mental or cognitive function.

The next part of the neurologic examination focuses on cranial nerve function. We are especially interested in those nerves that supply the muscles of the head and neck, which are commonly affected in ALS. These nerves are responsible for the normal appearance and function of facial, tongue, jaw, pharyngeal, and laryngeal (throat) muscles. The neurologist inspects these muscles looking for signs of muscle atrophy and spontaneous twitching (fasciculations) and tests their strength. Other functions controlled by the cranial nerves are assessed, including vision, eye movements, and hearing, but these typically are preserved in ALS; if they are affected, the involvement may be a clue to the presence of another disease.

In the third portion of the neurologic examination, muscle bulk and strength are assessed in the upper extremities, chest, and abdomen, and in the lower extremities. The neurologist examines the muscles for evidence of atrophy; scans the facial muscles, tongue, limb, and trunk musculature for tremors; and evaluates muscle strength. Muscle strength typically is graded on a scale [called the Medical Research Council (MRC) scale ranging from 5 (normal) to 0 (representing complete paralysis)]. A grade of MRC 4 indicates mild to moderate muscle weakness; a grade of MRC 3 indicates that a muscle is so weak it can only oppose the effects of gravity; and a muscle graded MRC 2 is weaker still, active only if gravity can be eliminated. A muscle graded MRC 1 has sufficient strength to generate only a flicker of movement and does not quite move around a joint. Although a person may be complaining of weakness in only one area, such as an arm or a leg, the neurologist typically explores all areas, even those that are not symptomatic, and often finds abnormalities of which the patient has perhaps not yet become aware.

The next step during the course of the examination is to assess muscle tone and reflexes. Normally there is no notable resistance to movement when a portion of a limb is flexed or extended around a joint. Because of the degeneration of the upper motor neuron that occurs in ALS, there is mild to moderate resistance to passive extension of a limb around its joint, followed by a sudden giving way during extension, a deviation from normal tone called spasticity. Because of this increased muscle tone, repetitive motions such as finger and foot tapping cannot be performed quickly but rather are done in a slow and effortful fashion. In ALS the activity of reflexes is increased; tapping the tendon of one joint often leads to activation not only of the expected reflex but also of adjacent reflexes, a phenomenon known as spread of reflex activity, which is indicative of upper motor neuron loss. Tendon reflexes are expected to be active or hyperactive in ALS. It is not uncommon for reflexes to be normal in the early stages of the illness and increase in activity as the disease progresses. If reflexes are persistently reduced or absent, an alternative diagnosis might be explored.

Ambulation or gait is the next function to be tested. If the disease has affected the lumbosacral region, leg muscles may be weakened or spastic, and walking will accordingly be abnormal. A common initial manifestation of ALS is weakness of the foot and toe dorsiflexor muscles, leading to footdrop. The wide-based, staggering gait characteristic of diseases that involve the cerebellum or sensory loss is not a part of ALS unless an additional disease complicates it.

Sensation—the ability to detect pin prick, cold, light touch, tuning fork vibration, movements of a joint up or down—usually is evaluated last. Sensory function is typically normal in ALS. Elderly people may have some reduction in the acuity of their sensation, but more pronounced degrees of sensory loss raise the possibility of an alternative diagnosis.

Clinical Diagnosis

As we have seen in earlier chapters, two major categories of neurologic findings are required to establish the clinical diagnosis of ALS: (1) evidence on clinical examination of muscle weakness, atrophy, and fasciculation (tremor); these are known as lower motor neuron signs and are caused by the degeneration or loss of motor nerve cells in the brain stem or spinal cord; and (2) increased muscle tone with slow and difficult movements associated with heightened reflexes (hyperreflexia) and the spread of reflex activity; these are upper motor neuron signs caused by degeneration or loss of motor nerve cells in the brain (motor cortex).

Because a variety of neurologic disorders produce lower motor neuron signs, upper motor neuron signs, or both, criteria have been proposed to increase the level of certainty about the diagnosis of ALS. Neurologists experienced in the diagnosis, management, and care of ALS patients met in April 1998 at Airlie House for the World Federation of Neurology ALS Conference to revise the diagnostic criteria for ALS. The group stated that the diagnosis of ALS be considered probable on clinical grounds when the combination of upper motor neuron and lower motor neuron signs are found in at least two regions, with some upper motor neuron signs being found above some lower motor neuron signs. The diagnosis of clinically definite ALS is made when there is evidence on clinical grounds of the presence of combined upper motor neuron and lower motor neuron signs in the bulbar region and at least two spinal regions, or when upper motor neuron signs are present in two spinal regions and lower motor neuron signs are present in three spinal regions.

There are four defined regions for these signs: the bulbar region of the brain and three spinal regions—cervical, thoracic, and lumbosacral. Each region encompasses specific muscle groups. The designation *bulbar* indicates that we are referring to the jaw, face, palate, tongue, and laryngeal muscles. The cervical region includes the neck, arm, hand, and diaphragm muscles. The thoracic region includes the back and abdominal muscles. The lumbosacral region refers to the back, abdominal, leg, and foot muscles.

The clinical findings of upper motor neuron or lower motor neuron signs or both often are restricted to a single region, or the findings may be in multiple regions but are only upper motor neuron or only lower motor neuron in type. In these cases the diagnosis of ALS cannot be established with certainty, and the neurologist will want to repeat the examination in several months to determine if there has been progressive spread of signs to other regions or the development of UMN and LMN signs combined. Only in these instances is it possible to make the diagnosis of ALS clinically with a greater degree of certainty.

Differential Diagnoses

In our experience, if the clinical evidence points to either probable or definite ALS, the diagnosis is most often correct. Because a variety of neurologic disorders present with features similar to those of ALS, however, we need to ask whether our patient might have a more benign disorder. This is termed a differential diagnosis because we must distinguish the disease from other diseases whose symptoms may be similar.

Diseases that affect the brain stem may produce combined upper motor neuron and lower motor neuron signs in cranial nerve–supplied muscles (the bulbar region). These conditions include neoplasms of the brain stem, most commonly brain stem glioma; multiple small strokes of the brain stem; and multiple sclerosis. They usually can be readily identified on a magnetic resonance imaging (MRI) scan of the brain that includes brain stem structures. In all three conditions, the MRI would be abnormal. In contrast, the MRI usually is normal in ALS.

Another group of conditions whose symptoms can mimic ALS involve the spinal cord. Perhaps the most common is osteoarthritis of the cervical spine (spondylotic myelopathy) that leads to compression of the cervical spinal cord and nerve roots. Its symptoms include lower motor neuron signs in the arms (sometimes with coexisting upper motor neuron signs) and upper motor neuron signs in the legs, features that certainly are consistent with ALS. However, spondylotic myelopathy is often painful, and, in addition to the motor abnormalities, sensory symptoms and signs are usually quite prominent, and there may be a disturbance in the control of urination and bowel function. The latter are simply not seen in ALS. Magnetic resonance imaging of the cervical spine can determine whether there is a significant degree of spondylotic myelopathy. Although arthritic changes of the cervical spine are common in the age group of patients who develop ALS, clinically significant spondylotic myelopathy rarely occurs without an accompanying radiologic picture of rather advanced disease. In ALS cervical cord and adjacent nerve roots are typically normal or at the most only mildly compromised by arthritic change; hence spondylotic myelopathy can usually be excluded by the combination of clinical and radiologic features.

Another disease that affects the cervical spinal cord is syringomyelia, a condition in which a fluid-filled cavity develops in the central portion of the cord and gradually expands to cause injury to both lower motor neurons and descending corticospinal tracts, as well as the ascending sensory pathways that convey sensations of pain and temperature. The clinical result is a combination of lower motor neuron signs in the arms and sometimes upper motor neuron signs in the legs, which alone suggest ALS except that there also is typically rather pronounced loss of feeling to pain and temperature in the hands. The disease is recognized radiologically by MRI studies that disclose the central cord cavity.

Some diseases of the peripheral nerves may produce fairly widespread lower motor neuron signs and hence simulate at least lower motor neuron involvement of ALS. Specific electrodiagnostic testing (see subsequent section), however, can assess the function of the peripheral nerves. Focal regions of demyelination (loss of the thick, lipid-rich insulation that surrounds motor axons) along upper extremity motor nerve fibers underlie a condition called multifocal motor neuropathy, with a block in nerve conduction that simulates ALS. This condition can almost always be recognized with careful electrodiagnostic testing. Apart from mild to moderate reduction in motor amplitudes because of a loss of motor neurons, people with ALS per se are expected to have essentially normal nerve conduction studies

Some diseases of muscle may suggest ALS, especially those that involve muscle wasting and weakness. Electromyography is a powerful diagnostic tool in distinguishing this condition from ALS.

Laboratory Investigations

We recommend a variety of investigations to confirm or disprove a diagnosis of ALS, including electromyography, neuroimaging of the brain and spinal cord, and clinical laboratory (blood test) studies. Testing is needed to confirm the diagnosis. In addition, because a variety of neurologic disorders present with features similar to those of ALS, it is important to search for test abnormalities that are characteristic of these conditions.

Electrophysiologic testing, known as electromyography or EMG, is done to confirm lower motor neuron dysfunction in clinically affected regions and to detect electrophysiologic evidence of lower motor neuron dysfunction in areas that do not yet appear to be involved clinically. There are two parts to the EMG examination. The first involves the evaluation of peripheral nerve function—determining whether motor and sensory nerve conduction velocities and motor and sensory elicited responses are normal. In ALS the speed of nerve conduction velocity should be within the normal range or only mildly reduced. Slowed velocities suggest that the patient's problem might stem from a peripheral neuropathy. We look for a difference between the amplitudes of the motor responses when the nerve is stimulated at different sites. Only minor differences should be found in ALS, so the detection of major differences points to an alternative diagnosis.

In the second part of the study a needle electrode is inserted into various muscles from different anatomic regions. There is no spontaneous electrical activity when the needle is inserted into healthy muscle. As the normal muscle begins to contract, the electrical signatures of motor unit potentials can be observed, and they have expected "normal" firing rates. In contrast, when the electrode is inserted into a muscle affected by ALS, there is abnormal spontaneous activity that indicates loss of innervation by individual muscle fibers, which is called acute denervation. During the voluntary muscle contraction portion of the test, many fewer units than normal fire and the surviving motor unit potentials fire at rapid rates. Additionally, instead of the normal waveform, higher amplitude waveforms of longer duration than normal are seen. If the needle EMG examination is normal, it suggests that either the disease process has not yet involved the area being studied or that the diagnosis of ALS is mistaken and the clinical problem should be carefully reevaluated.

Although the EMG is sometimes associated with transitory discomfort, we strongly believe that it is an essential component of the diagnostic process and should be performed by an experienced practitioner on every patient in whom the diagnosis of ALS is being considered. Neuroimaging studies (MRI) are done to confirm normal anatomy and examine for motor pathway abnormalities occasionally seen in ALS. Another major purpose of the test is to look for structural pathology in the brain, brain stem, or cervical spinal cord that may cause upper motor neuron and/or lower motor neuron signs and may simulate ALS.

Blood testing is done primarily to confirm that results are normal. In most patients with ALS, we do not expect to find abnormalities in blood count or in the various blood chemistry tests used to indirectly assess the function of the bone marrow, liver, kidney, and other major organ systems. Although no blood test abnormalities are specifically diagnostic of ALS, we are looking for evidence of treatable or reversible disorders of an autoimmune, metabolic, endocrine, neoplastic, infectious, or toxic nature that may on occasion alter the nervous system in such a way as to produce upper motor neuron and lower motor neuron signs, thereby simulating ALS.

In addition to blood test studies, we examine the cerebrospinal fluid (CSF) in some patients when features of the clinical presentation are atypical. This includes people with clinical evidence of ALS who are younger than the age range typically encountered for the disease (usually < 40 years), when there is evidence of a systemic or nervous system infection, or when we suspect an underlying systemic malignancy. Tests performed on the CSF include measurement and analysis of protein, sugar, and total number of white blood cells.

In a few cases, we recommend bone marrow evaluation, a procedure that is indicated to look for an underlying neoplasm (usually a lymphoma or Hodgkin's disease), which is on rare occasion associated with clinical features of ALS.

Other special tests include evaluation for the presence of an antibody called anti-Hu. A neurologist might be prompted to test for anti-Hu when abnormal signs in nonmotor areas such as cognitive functioning, coordination, and sensation accompany clinical features of ALS. Such a constellation of findings suggests a more diffuse CNS disorder—possibly a paraneoplastic syndrome in which neurologic findings are immune-mediated and triggered by the presence of a tumor (typically small-cell lung carcinoma). Another test that may be ordered is the leukocyte hexosaminodase-A assay. Patients recommended for this test typically are much younger than the usual age range of onset of ALS and have associated mental changes, incoordination, and sensory abnormalities.

We recommend the DNA test for the cytosine-adenosine-guanidine (CAG) expanded trinucleotide repeat in the androgen receptor gene on the X chromosome in men who are younger than the usual age of onset for ALS (< 40 years) and have associated enlargement of breast tissue (gynecomastia), sensory changes, and abnormalities of coordination. Patients who test positive have the disease known as bulbospinal neuronopathy, or Kennedy's syndrome.

Presentation of the Diagnosis

The diagnosis of ALS requires a process of clinical evaluation, neuroimaging and electrodiagnostic testing, and laboratory studies. Because of the varied nature and complexity of testing procedures, it simply takes time for the full investigation to be completed, usually two to three weeks. During that time, you and your family will understandably be anxious for the neurologist to share his or her thoughts on the nature of the ailment. Before coming to the neurologist, you probably were concerned that the underlying problem was serious and may have already considered ALS as a possibility. Even before all the laboratory data are gathered together, therefore, you will want at least some preliminary opinion from the neurologist. In these circumstances many of us share our thoughts with our patients. Although the laboratory tests may not yet have been completed, if there is strong clinical evidence of ALS and the patient suspects the diagnosis, we would indicate that findings detected on the examination are indeed compatible with ALS but that further testing is needed for confirmation. We also point out that we will explore the laboratory tests carefully and leave no stone unturned as we search for clues for remediable or treatable conditions.

Neurologists experienced in ALS diagnosis and care present the diagnosis frankly, with honesty and hope and only after careful evaluation and testing. We prefer to provide information to you and your family gradually so that you will have time to adjust. Facts should not be thrust on you until you are ready for them. Patients report that disclosure is best when they are not overwhelmed with too much information too soon. Written materials are useful because they can be read at your own pace after the initial shock of the diagnosis has lessened. We also often ask a nurse to contact patients weekly for a period of several weeks immediately after diagnosis to provide support and information and to schedule physician appointments if warranted.

At the time of diagnosis we attempt to provide hope in several ways.

- We emphasize that you will not face the disease alone and will never be ignored or abandoned. A team of health professionals will provide multidisciplinary care every step along the journey, helping you to cope with new physical and psychosocial realities and adapt to the ongoing changes and challenges of the disease.

- We point out that the conventional wisdom of rapid deterioration does not necessarily apply to everyone and that slower progression is well documented, with some patients having 5, 10, 15, or more years ahead of them after diagnosis.

- We find that engaging in short straightforward lessons about normal nervous system anatomy, the structures that are affected, and, importantly, the structures that are spared also fosters hope. Although the course of ALS is one of progressive weakness, it is important to emphasize that cognitive clarity and psychic energy are totally preserved and that they can compensate for loss of strength and movement by maintaining an ever-increasing social interaction.

- Presenting the current state of knowledge of the pathogenesis of ALS is helpful to some people. We inform them that no one yet fully understands ALS, that we are uncertain about the cause and pathogenesis, but that we are entering a new era of therapies based on evidence from research in the basis sciences. We repeat Dr. Lewis Rowland's "fifth level of hope," which to paraphrase, is that one day, a very bright scientist or researcher is going to get lucky and unravel the mysterious biology of ALS so that we have an effective treatment.

- We attempt to involve patients in clinical trials, which provide additional hope.

- We indicate that there is now one FDA-approved drug for ALS, riluzole, that has a modest effect on the course of the disease and that other drugs with promise are in clinical trial.

- Finally, we fully expect those patients and family members will have doubts that the diagnosis is correct and will request a second opinion, a request we fully support and facilitate.

4

Treating the Symptoms of ALS

Deborah Gelinas, M.D.

Amyotrophic lateral sclerosis (ALS) is a disease that strikes fear in the hearts of patient, family, and physician alike. In addition to progressive weakening of the arms and legs, ALS can rob a person of the ability to speak and swallow. Because ALS is an incurable disease, people often feel powerless in the face of it. This chapter stresses informed management decision making for people with ALS and their families. By introducing strategies for coping with decreasing physical abilities, we hope to empower them to lessen the impact of the disease on their daily quality of life.

Amyotrophic lateral sclerosis is an uncommon disease that affects both men and women in middle adulthood. It results in a progressive paralysis of voluntary muscles while intellect and personality remain largely intact. Many people have never heard of this disease until they are diagnosed with it. The diagnosis of ALS challenges a person to find ways to cope with the progressive weakening of the body and forces him or her to become slowly and increasingly dependent on others to carry out a need or desire. Knowing the disability that lies ahead, it is not surprising that many people feel powerless to adequately cope with this disease. The task may appear overwhelming. However, many people have successfully coped with this disease and have succeeded in living full lives.

The man or woman with ALS must struggle to live each day well—even while being forced to let go of many capabilities that in the past made life worth living.

People with ALS frequently complain that their physicians don't want to see them, don't want to talk to them, and don't know how to comfort them. This is often true, as the physician also may feel powerless over ALS. However, once the physician accepts that ALS cannot be cured, he or she can focus on the fact that many of the most bothersome symptoms associated with the disease can be treated. Patients do not necessarily expect their physicians to be experts in ALS. They do, however, expect them to take the time to become informed about their specific problems with ALS. At each visit the patient will teach the physician more about ALS as it affects him today, and the physician must help prepare the patient for tomorrow.

General Management Principles

Periodic evaluations that include tests of breathing function should take place every two to three months, depending on disease progression (3). At each visit you and your family members should guide the physician as to his or her choices for how the disease should be managed. Although varying treatment options may be presented, they may not all be acceptable to you. You are the one who decides the course of disease treatment—*when and if* to accept various interventions. The physician should serve as your advisor, informing you of various options and the consequences of those options. This entails an ongoing discussion and ongoing reevaluation of patient desires. These issues often cannot be resolved in one session. A Statement of Patient Autonomy—an advance directive—that clearly states your desires is an important document and helps your physician manage the disease. These advance directives should be revisited periodically and revised as the circumstances dictate. People change during the course of ALS, and sometimes life becomes so precious that conditions that would have once been considered intolerable are not so any longer.

Disease-Specific Treatment

Once the diagnosis of ALS has been established, patients are primarily interested in pursuing treatment. The only disease-specific treatment for ALS that is approved by the U.S. Food and Drug Administration (FDA) at this time is riluzole, which functions as an inhibitor of glutamate, a substance involved in nervous system function. Two placebo-controlled double blind trials (see Chapter 16) demonstrated that riluzole modestly extended survival for patients with ALS by an average of two to three months (6). The pros and cons of treatment with riluzole should be discussed, and the drug should be offered (where available) with the hope of slowing the progress of the disease. Patients often will be interested in pursuing treatment with drugs that are not yet approved by the FDA but are being actively investigated. You should become informed of ongoing research. Both the ALS Association and the Muscular Dystrophy Association publish periodic newsletters announcing research trials in ALS. This information is also available unofficially through various Internet locations such as the ALS Digest (www.brunel.ack.uk~hssrsdn/alsig/alsig.htm) or (http://www.flash.net/~gnichola).

Alternative Treatment

People with ALS are often dissatisfied—as are their physicians—with the disease-specific treatment offered by conventional medicine. Many patients therefore seek alternative solutions to their disease. These holistic approaches may benefit the patient greatly in affording a sense of mastery over the disease. Nutritional regimens that stress the role of antioxidant vitamins in postponing symptom manifestation have some experimental basis, although they are still not of proven value. These and other approaches (such as therapeutic massage, visual imagery, etc.) may offer support, encouragement, and hope (7). You should be encouraged to share the exploration into alternative treatments with your physician. The physician should serve as an advisor, steering you away from exploitative and harmful therapies and toward those where the provider is doing no harm and seeking to do good. If you desire such a holistic approach, it is important to ask your physician to listen with an open mind, to seek to understand, and to accept your decision. With such support, you should also feel free to ask for more conventional therapies. Conventional medicine and holistic medicine can work hand in hand to provide benefit.

Symptom-Specific Treatments

Table 4-1 summarizes the commonly used medications to treat the symptoms of ALS, which are described here in detail.

Table 4-1. Commonly Used Medications for Symptomatic ALS Treatments

Symptoms	Treatment
Muscle cramps and spasms	Lioresal
	Zanaflex
	Intrathecal baclofen
Excessive crying or laughter	Amitriptyline
	Fluoxetine
	Paroxetine
Urinary urgency or frequency	Oxybutynin
Excessive saliva	Amitriptyline
	Glycopyrrolate
	Scopolamine
Thick phlegm/post nasal drip	Guaifenesin

Table 4-1. Commonly Used Medications for Symptomatic ALS Treatments
(cont.)

Symptoms	Treatment
	Propranolol
	Nebulized acetylcysteine solution
Jaw quivering/clenching	Clonazepam
	Diazepam
	Lorazepam
Laryngospasm	Clonazepam
	Diazepam
	Lorazepam
Acid reflux	Omeprazole
	Famotidine
	Ranitidine
	Cimetidine
	Cisapride
	Metoclopromide
Nasal congestion	OTC nasal spray
	Beclomethasone dipropionate nasal spray
	Diphenhydiamine
	Pseudoephedrine sulfate
Sleep disturbance	Amitriptyline
	Trazodone
	Zolpidem
	Temazepam
	Sertraline
	Bupropion
Depression/anxiety	Fluoxetine
	Paroxetine
	Sertraline
	Buproprion
Shortness of breath	Morphine sulfate elixir
Pain	Various analgesics
	Ibuprofen
	Morphine sulfate elixir
Nausea	Prochlorperazine
Agitation/anxiety	Lorazepam
	Diazepam
Terminal management	Lorazepam
	Morphine sulfate elixir
	Morphine subcutaneous pump

Weakness

Although the progressive muscle weakness of ALS cannot be reversed, there are alternative ways to compensate for it. People with ALS should be evaluated by rehabilitation specialists in order to maximize their function at all stages of disease. Occupational therapists can provide numerous assistive devices to maintain independence with activities of daily living such as feeding, dressing, and methods of maintaining hygiene (see Chapter 8). Physical therapists can teach stretching exercises to maintain range of motion and minimize joint pain, and they can provide devices such as ankle-foot orthoses to compensate for footdrop, knee sleeves for buckling of the legs, and abdominal binders for paraspinal weakness (see Chapter 7). Wheeled walkers can compensate for weakened trunks and leg muscles and permit continued ambulation. A variety of lifts are available to assist with transfers, and there is adaptive equipment for the bathroom. When ambulation is no longer an option, a manual or motorized wheelchair permits continued mobility. Certain pieces of equipment may no longer be useful as a person's needs change. When possible, you should prepare in advance for equipment needs (9). However, some people are simply not ready and refuse canes, walkers, and wheelchairs until very late in the course of the disease. The reluctance to use adaptive equipment can be overcome through continued education as to how they can improve mobility and independence. The myriad of insurance plans available today pose serious challenges to obtaining the correct equipment. People often become exhausted and demoralized trying to obtain insurance approval for a piece of necessary equipment. Those who have the will to persist in their demands usually obtain what they ask for. Keep asking. Advocating for the patient by health care professionals can be a time-consuming project.

Cramps, Spasms, and Myalgias

A muscle cramp is a sudden unintended muscle contraction that may be triggered by exertion of any muscle group in the arms, legs, chest, back, abdomen, jaw, or throat. Cramps are caused by a brief contraction of a weakened muscle due to an explosive overactivity of motor nerves. These contractions may be extremely painful and prolonged. You may notice visible knotting in the muscle and abnormal posture until the cramp passes.

Cramps can be effectively managed through several strategies, including proper hydration and diet, as well as avoiding overexertion of weakened muscles. Manual stretching of a muscle cramp is very effective. When cramps and muscle spasms are particularly frequent and severe, medications such as quinine sulfate, baclofen, dantrolene, clonazepam, lorazepam, diphenylhdantoin, and gabapentin can be prescribed. When spasticity is extremely severe and not adequately controlled by oral medication, you should discuss with your physician the option of an indwelling pump to administer medication directly to the spinal fluid (11). This entails a minor surgical procedure, but it may be very helpful.

Certain musculoskeletal problems are particularly troublesome in ALS. Patients with shoulder weakness may develop a frozen shoulder that limits range of motion and causes excruciating pain. Neck weakness may result in painful muscles and stiffness. The best treatment is prevention with joint stabilization and a daily home exercise program consisting of stretching and range of motion exercises. Manuals on appropriate therapeutic exercise for people with ALS are available through the Amyotrophic Lateral Sclerosis Association at (800) 340-7500 and are recommended.

Fatigue

General muscle fatigue and exhaustion are common features of ALS. As nerve cells die, remaining ones send signals to activate the otherwise unused muscle, and a single surviving nerve cell may be doing a hundred times its normal workload. This may result in temporary exhaustion of overburdened nerve cells. Thus there may be times when you can perform a task such as climbing stairs only when you have rested beforehand. You should pace yourself wisely in terms of energy expenditure throughout the day and the week. Various medications have been tried for fatigue with little success and are therefore not recommended (12). When persistent overwhelming fatigue is a problem, your quality of sleep should be evaluated because ineffective nighttime sleep is a common cause of daytime fatigue (13).

Sleep Disturbance

Sleep disturbance can lead to many quality of life consequences such as depression and fatigue (14). Many factors can contribute to an inability to sleep. Sleep disorders in ALS include depression and anxiety, as well as nighttime breathing disturbances due to sleep apnea or weakened respiratory muscles (15). A sleep study known as a polysomnogram is the best method to investigate sleep difficulties. A simpler and less expensive way to evaluate sleep is by monitoring heart rate and oxygen saturation of the blood with a home nocturnal oximetry (13). Drops in oxygen may continuously awaken you from sleep throughout the night. These breathing disturbances may be difficult to diagnose in people with ALS, as they may occur only at night and only with certain stages of sleep (16). Repeated awakenings may also occur due to excess secretions or spasm of vocal cord muscles. These micro-arousals disrupt sleep and may result in daytime fatigue (17–19).

Nighttime breathing difficulties may respond to noninvasive ventilatory support with positive pressure devices, such as pressure ventilators or volume ventilators (17,18). These ventilators deliver room air through a mask over the nose or mouth and guarantee deep breathing throughout the night. Success in using noninvasive ventilatory support depends on the patient's motivation and the adequate control of saliva (21). Simpler measures of relieving nighttime breathing difficulties include elevation of the head of the bed and sleeping on the side instead of on the back. The antidepressant protriptyline hydrochloride has been used with some success in sleep problems, as it may lessen nighttime breathing abnormalities (18).

All antidepressants decrease time spent in dream sleep, the period of greatest breathing disturbance, and thus may be helpful (22).

Periodic leg movements caused by spasticity or muscle spasms can be relieved through the use of such medications as levodopa, baclofen, and codeine. Anxiety and depression respond well to antidepressants. Respiratory muscle fatigue has been reported to respond favorably to theophylline (20). "Sleeping pills" should be avoided. However, if other options have failed and care and comfort are the main concern, short-acting sedative sleeping pills may be effective.

Uncontrollable Laughter or Crying

People with ALS sometimes develop difficulty controlling emotions, crying or laughing inappropriately or excessively. This is thought to be caused by the loss of nerve cell inhibition over the brain centers involved in laughing and crying. Antidepressants such as amitriptyline are effective in treating these unwanted emotional displays (12,23,24).

Dementia

Dementia is rare in ALS—occurring in only 5 percent to 10 percent of cases (25). However, more subtle changes relating to mental inflexibility or stubbornness may be present in as many as 25 percent of all people with ALS. These changes are more prevalent in those who have speech and swallowing difficulties and may include features such as apathy, altered social skills, and personality changes. In those very rare cases in which frank dementia is present, it is important that the patient be encouraged to pursue conservatorship so that appropriate medical decisions can be made (see Chapter 25).

Urinary Urgency and Frequency

Although ALS is not thought to involve the bladder muscles, people with ALS frequently develop an irritable bladder with urinary urgency and frequency. This may be due to the lack of nerve cell inhibition over brain centers for urination. In addition, urinary tract infections increase bladder spasms and frequency of urination. Therefore, a urinalysis should be performed, and any infection should be treated with antibiotics. In men the prostate gland may be enlarged, resulting in the need to urinate frequently. If no infection is present, oxybutynin may be helpful to relax the bladder and lessen urinary symptoms.

Swelling of Hands and Feet

Swelling frequently occurs in a very weak limb due to the failure of muscle pumping action to increase blood return to the heart. Passive range of motion, elevation of paralyzed limbs, and compression hose are helpful. When swelling is painful or fails to decrease after overnight elevation, a blood clot or deep vein thrombosis (DVT) should be ruled out immediately because of the risk of the clot traveling to the lungs (pulmonary embolism). You should discuss DVT prophylaxis with your physician before prolonged periods of inactivity, such as airplane travel.

Excess Saliva

Excess saliva is a common feature of ALS and results in increased drooling, choking, or coughing. The problem is not believed to be due to overproduction of saliva but to decreased swallowing (26). In ALS saliva is not swallowed automatically, and repetitive volitional swallowing is needed to compensate for this. Excess saliva may be further increased by anxiety, hunger, and acid reflux (27). Medications that may decrease saliva include glycopyrrolate, amitriptyline, diphenhydramine, oxybutynin, and scopolamine, and should be requested from your physician (12,28,29). Surgery and radiotherapy have both been tried for excess secretions but often result in excessively thickened secretions and are therefore not recommended (30).

Thick Phlegm and Postnasal Drip

People with ALS may develop a habit of mouth-breathing because of fatigue of jaw muscles or nasal congestion. Mouth-breathing causes saliva to dry out and thicken. Furthermore, medications taken to reduce drooling can cause excessive dryness and thick secretions, which can result in a bothersome sensation of postnasal drip, chronic cough, or a need to clear the throat. Medications such as metoprolol or propranolol have been reported to thin secretions when added to anti-saliva regimens (29). Over-the-counter cough syrups, such as guaifenescin, or even homeopathic treatments, such as papaya juice, may be helpful in thinning saliva. Chicken broth and hot tea, as well as the use of room humidifiers, oral suction machines, and aerosolized breathing treatments with acetylcysteine solutions, can also help. When allergies contribute to postnasal drip, antihistamines and steroid nasal inhalers may also be useful. Many noninvasive breathing machines provide an excellent way of clearing thick upper airway secretions (such as cofflators and IPVs) (31).

Jaw Quivering, Jaw Clenching

Some people with ALS may experience an uncomfortable tightening or chattering of the jaw due to noxious stimuli such as cold, anxiety, or pain. Medications such as clonazepam, diazepam, and lorazepam may be helpful in relieving these symptoms.

Laryngospasm

Laryngospasm, or tightening of the throat, is an abrupt and prolonged closure of the vocal cords that results in sudden gasping for breath and an expiratory wheeze. This phenomenon can cause panic because of airway constriction and the fear of suffocation (32). Laryngospasm may also occur with exposure to increased emotion, smoke, strong smells, alcohol, cold or rapid bursts of air, and even spicy foods. It can also occur with aspirated liquids or saliva as well as acid reflux disease (33). Laryngospasm normally clears spontaneously in a few seconds but may be more immediately relieved by breathing through the nose and repetitive swallowing. Possible precipitants of laryngospasm should be eliminated, and a trial of antacids should be instituted.

Acid Reflux

Acid reflux, also known as gastroesophageal reflux disease (GERD), is a common condition in people with ALS. It is due to weakness of the diaphragm muscles involved in breathing, which normally form a tight band around the opening to the stomach to keep the acids down. The signs and symptoms may include heartburn, acid taste, throat irritation, chest pain, hoarseness, shortness of breath, nausea, and insomnia (32). These symptoms are thought to be caused by the reflux of stomach acid into the lower esophagus (33). Caffeine, spicy foods, overeating, and diaphragm weakness all increase acid reflux into the esophagus. Particular care in managing this problem is necessary if a feeding tube is in place because the stomach may be easily overfed. Medications to increase clearance of foods from the stomach such as cisapride and metoclopramide, as well as antacids such as ranitidine hydrochloride, cimetidine, famotidine, and omeprazole are quite effective (34).

Nasal Congestion

The tone of the muscles in the nose and mouth may be weakened, resulting in a failure to elevate and open the nostrils, upper airways, and eustachian tubes. The nasal airways can be opened effectively by nasal tape, as used by athletes. Antihistamines and nasal sprays also may be used to bring relief.

Constipation

Constipation is common in ALS and can be difficult to manage. It can result in hours spent on the toilet with abdominal pain and bloating. The causes include decreased fluid, inadequate diet, lack of exercise, and a reduced ability to bear down with abdominal muscles. Proper management is essential because hospitalization for bowel obstruction may be necessary if the condition persists. Medications taken to control excessive saliva and pain can contribute to constipation and should be decreased if possible or discontinued when necessary. An excellent dietary recipe to normalize bowel movement is "power pudding," which consists of equal parts of prunes, prune juice, apple sauce, and bran. Two tablespoons with each meal and at bedtime, along with adequate fluid intake and fruits and vegetables in the diet, helps in maintaining a bowel regimen. Stool softeners, laxatives, and periodic enemas should be used liberally when necessary.

Depression and Anxiety

Depression is common in anyone who has increasing physical disability, and it should be treated (35). Depression is dramatically underdiagnosed in people with a wide variety of medical diseases and has a negative effect on the quality of life of both patients and their families (36). Newer antidepressants such as fluoxetine, sertraline, and paroxetine are preferable to older antidepressants such as amitriptyline because of their greater efficacy and lesser incidence of side effects. When effective, antidepressants should be continued for at least six months to one year and then slowly tapered as indicated (37). When anxiety and agitation are the main problems, buspirone and benzodiazepines can be used on as as-needed basis. Buspirone is preferable because it does not suppress the muscles involved in breathing.

Difficulty in Swallowing

Weakness and incoordination of mouth and throat muscles can result in swallowing problems. A swallowing evaluation by a speech therapist can be helpful in determining which foods cause the greatest difficulty (see Chapter 11). For mild swallowing problems, patients should (1) tuck their chin down while swallowing, (2) swallow two to three times per mouthful of food, (3) avoid foods that cause the greatest difficulty, and (4) perform a clearing cough after each swallow (39). When dysphagia results in weight loss or when a patient becomes fatigued in his or her attempts to consume a meal, a percutaneous gastrostomy (PEG) should be considered (see Chapter 11). Ideally, the procedure should be performed before weight loss occurs and while the patient has good breathing function, as the risk of complications increases in weaker patients (40). Patients should be fed only in an upright position and should avoid bending or lying flat for at least one hour after feeding. In many instances, medicines such as metoclopramide should be added to aid stomach emptying (34). Most people with a PEG prefer feedings at regular mealtimes to leave many hours for other activities. A variety of feeding formulas are available. In general, concentrated formulas with high fat and sugar content are harder to digest and may result in cramping and diarrhea. Less concentrated solutions are preferable and may be specifically selected to meet individual needs (i.e., high-fiber formulas for constipation, high protein and lipid, low-carbohydrate formulas for patients with shortness of breath) (41).

Slurred Speech

Slurred, slow, or strangulated speech is caused by incoordination and weakness of the lips, tongue, and throat muscles. Patients with speech problems should be evaluated by a speech therapist, and alternative communication methods should be offered (see Chapter 10). Some form of communication can usually be established and must be sought (38). It is essential that the family members recognize the patient's need to communicate, even when it is time-consuming.

Shortness of Breath

Breathing problems may arise from many different causes in ALS. For this reason, breathing difficulties should be evaluated by a physician who is familiar with both pulmonary problems and ALS (see Chapter 12). Reversible causes of breathing difficulties must always be sought and treated where appropriate. These include infections, excess saliva, and pulmonary emboli. When shortness of breath is due to progression of ALS and respiratory muscle weakness, it typically occurs initially during sleep, especially dream sleep (14,15). People may complain of frequent arousal, bad dreams, attacks of anxiety, and daytime sleepiness (18). Later they often complain of headaches, confusion, and hallucinations. Weakness of breathing muscles may be successfully treated with noninvasive ventilators, which increase patient well-being and survival (21). If you are unable to tolerate nasal ventilators due to excessive saliva or other factors, a tracheostomy (surgical procedure to bypass the mouth and provide an opening to the airways) should be discussed. A ventilator can then be connected to the tracheostomy opening. Although the financial and emotional costs of tracheostomy ventilation are high, the majority of people who choose this option report a satisfactory quality of life (43,44).

Pain and Pressure Sores

Although pain is not generally thought to be a feature of ALS, it is extremely common late in the course of disease (48,49). Pain may be due to muscle cramping or to joint changes such as hip dislocation. Pain can also occur when there is prolonged immobility of paralyzed limbs or pressure sores. Pressure sores are particularly apt to develop over bony prominences, such as the tip of the spine. When needed, specialized mattresses and seating cushions, such as alternating air flow mattresses and air and gel cushions, can reduce pressure over these tender spots. Mild pain associated with pressure sores may be relieved by medications such as ibuprofen or acetaminophen. In the case of more severe pain, narcotic medications may be needed (12) (see Chapter 28). Side effects from narcotics may result in nausea and constipation, which can be treated with antinausea medications such as prochlorperazine and the liberal use of laxatives. If you cannot take medication by mouth and do not have a PEG, medications may be given through an indwelling venous line or a subcutaneous pump. Transdermal patches for pain control are often erratic in drug absorption and therefore are not recommended. We also discourage injections, which may be painful, especially when given repeatedly.

Modes of Mechanical Ventilation

Patients with respiratory muscle weakness may choose to use mechanical ventilators to treat shortness of breath and increase survival. Ventilators may be either invasive (administered via a tracheostomy or tube down the throat) or noninvasive (applied directly to the face or body). Patient survival can be extended indefinitely through ventilator use, although the disease course will progress unabated, with the eventual loss of all patient communication and independence. Invasive ventilation has a number of major drawbacks, including the exorbitant costs involved, the need for 24-hour nursing care, and its significant negative impact on the quality of life of both the patient and his or her caregiver. Indeed, in many countries invasive ventilation is not available to patients with ALS. Even in countries where it is available, patients seldom choose invasive ventilator support (43,45). Noninvasive mechanical ventilators are easy to use and much less expensive. They are available in many varieties, most commonly ventilating the lungs through a nasal mask or an oral mask. For patients who cannot tolerate nasal ventilators, devices such as the chest shell, also known as the cuirass, may be of benefit. The cuirass is a rigid shell that is applied to the chest from the neck down to the bottom of the rib cage and adheres to the chest by negative pressure suction. As air is pumped out from under the shell, the lungs expand. Since the patient's face and limbs are outside the cuirass, greater mobility is possible. Nasal ventilators tend to be more effective in restoring air exchange, but patients who cannot use a nasal ventilator have occasionally used the cuirass with success. Nasal ventilators administer pressurized air to the lungs, thereby allowing greater air volumes to enter the lungs. There are many varieties of ventilators, but not all are appropriate for people with ALS. One type of ventilator known as a CPAP (continuous positive airway pressure) is commonly used for otherwise healthy patients with sleep apnea, but it is entirely inappropriate for patients with ALS because it offers no breathing support. In contrast, Bi-PAP (bi-level positive airway pressure) applies a differential pressure with expiration than inspiration, thus reducing the work of breathing. The Bi-PAP nasal ventilator is typically used for six to eight continuous hours during sleep, although it can be used for longer periods according to patient needs. It is a very effective method of treating the signs and symptoms of air hunger in ALS patients. The major limitation to Bi-PAP is that patients with considerable mouth and throat weakness may have difficulty learning how to use the device (46). Other positive pressure ventilation methods include the IPV (intermittent positive vibration) and cofflator. Intermittent positive vibration delivers vibrating nebulized saline or medicines under pressure through the mouth for 10- to 15-minute periods in order to help clear airway secretions. The cofflator also delivers air under pressure and then sucks the air back out, thereby helping the patient to cough and clear the airways. For patients who may have an upper respiratory tract infection, this device can be very effective in preventing more serious pneumonia. When mechanical ventilation is started, a contract should be made between patient, family, and physician, agreeing on terms for eventually withdrawing the ventilator support. This is especially important in invasive ventilation involving tracheostomy. People with ALS have the right to refuse to start or continue ventilator support (47). This is important because although ventilators may prolong survival, they do not stop the progressive weakness of ALS (48,49). For this reason, an agreement should be reached that ventilator support may be discontinued if the patient is too weak to be able to communicate. A patient who so chooses to discontinue ventilator support should be reassured that his or her physical and emotional comfort will be maintained. A combination of medications such as narcotic analgesics and/or lorazepam or diazepam eliminate anxiety and shortness of breath (50,51).

Terminal Management

At some point in the progression of ALS, a patient may become tired of the struggle to remain living. Many people with ALS ultimately reach a level where they feel they can no longer maintain a satisfactory quality of life. At this point the emphasis shifts from extending life to making the remaining days more comfortable (see Chapter 28). Home nursing agencies can arrange home visits when patients find it more difficult to go to the clinic for periodic evaluation. Hospice may be indicated, especially when the disease is advanced and help is needed in the home. Hospice typically is instituted when life expectancy is approximately six months. Hospice and home nursing agencies are able to mediate between patient and physician to ensure that all needs are addressed in a timely fashion. It is crucial that lines of communication between patient, hospice, and physician remain open so that care can be seamlessly coordinated. At this stage of the disease, patients typically desire to be pain-free, to be as alert as possible during the day, and to have a comfortable uninterrupted night's sleep. The patient should be given whatever treatment is necessary to relieve suffering, even if it shortens life (53). Antianxiety medications such as lorazepam, sleeping pills such as temazepam, and pain relievers including morphine should be available as needed. Patients sometimes may require antinausea medications such as prochlorperazene, as both shortness of breath and the medications to relieve it may cause stomach upset. In this advanced stage the family should play a more active role in communicating with the physician so that the patient's needs and comforts are ensured. As a family, you will need a lot of support because everyone dealing with the situation will feel frightened and isolated. While home nursing care may be preferable, other settings (hospice, nursing facilities, etc.) can and should be explored, especially if the primary caregiver is frail or in poor health. Clergymen can often provide comfort to both patient and family. Toward the end, the patient will become progressively less attentive to the demands of the outside world and will be more focused on preparing for death. Death often can and should occur in the bosom of family and friends, with the patient drifting into a deepening sleep. Most people are reassured by the knowledge that their death will be peaceful without struggle, air hunger, or pain.

Quality of Life

Although no one would ever choose to have ALS, many people with the disease affirm that ALS has brought blessings as well as sufferings. They report new appreciation of family, friends, the beauty of nature, and life itself. Many patients find the capacity to enjoy life each and every day. Morrie Schwartz, who had ALS, wrote, "After you have wept and grieved for your physical losses, cherish the functions and life that you have left (54)." As a physician, I consider it a privilege to be included in this intimate celebration of living, to witness how ordinary people summon extraordinary faith and courage to overcome the hardships imposed by ALS and continue to live full lives.

References

1. El Escorial World Federation of Neurology criteria for the diagnosis of amyotrophic lateral sclerosis. *J Neurol Sci* 1994; 124(Suppl):96–104.
2. Louwerse ES, Visser CE, Bossuyt, Weverling GJ. Amyotrophic lateral sclerosis: Mortality risk during the course of disease and prognostic factors. *J Neurol Sci* 1997; 152 (Suppl):510–517.
3. Fallat RJ, Norris FH, Holden D, et al. Respiratory monitoring and treatment: Objective treatments using noninvasive measurements. *Adv Exp Med Biol* 1987; 209:191–200.
4. Cedarbaum JM, Stamblers N. Performance of the amyotrophic lateral sclerosis functional rating scale in multicenter clinical trials. *J Neurol Sci* 1997; 152(Suppl): 51–59.
5. Gay P, Westbrook PR, Daube JR, et al. Effects of alterations in pulmonary function and sleep variables on survival in patients with amyotrophic lateral sclerosis. *Mayo Clin Proc* 1991; 66:686–694.
6. Bensimon G, LaComblez L. Meininger V. ALS/Riluzole Study Group: A controlled trial of riluzole in amyotrophic lateral sclerosis. *N Engl J Med* 1994; 330:585–591.
7. Gurney ME, Cutting FB, Zhai P, et al. Benefit of vitamin E, riluzole and gabapentin in a trangenic model of familial amyotrophic lateral sclerosis. *Ann Neurol* 1996; 39: 147–157.
8. "Functioning When Your Mobility Is Affected." Living with ALS Manual 1994, #4. ALS Association, p. 25 (table).
9. Mendoza M, Rafter E. "Functioning When Your Mobility Is Affected." Living with ALS Manual 1997, #4. ALS Association, p. 13–25.
10. Davidoff RA. Pharmacology of spasticity. *Neurology* 1978; 29(2):46–51.
11. Coffey RJ, Cahill D, Steers W, et al. Intrathecal baclofen for intractable spasticity of spinal origin: Results of a long term, multicenter study. *J Neurosurg* 1993; 78: 226–232.
12. Norris FH, Smith RA, Denys EH. Motor neurone disease: Towards better care. *Br Med J* 1985; 291:259–262.
13. Marcello N. Ortaggio F. Detection of sleep respiratory disturbances by transcutaneous PCO2 and PO2 monitoring in advanced cases of Duchenne muscular dystrophy. *Acta Cardiomiologica* 1990 II N.I.:55–66.
14. Flemons WW, Tsai W. Quality of life consequences of sleep disordered breathing. *J Allergy Clin Immunol* 1997; 99:750–756.
15. DeWester JN. Recognizing and treating the patient with somatic manifestations of depression. *J Fam Pract* 1996; 43(Suppl):513–515.
16. Fergusson KA, Ono T, Lowe AA, Ryan CF, Fleetham JA. The relationship between obesity and craniofacial structure in obstructive sleep apnea. *Chest* 1995; 108(2):375–381.
17. Guilleminault C, Stooks R, Clerk A, et al. From obstructive sleep apnea syndrome to upper airway resistance syndrome. Consistency of daytime somnolence. *Sleep* 1992; 15:513–516.
18. Guilleminault C, Stooks R, Quera-Salva MA. Sleep related obstructive and nonobstructive apneas and neurologic disorders. *Neurology* 1992; 42(Suppl 6):53–60.
19. Glesson K, Zwillich CW, White DP. The influence of increasing ventilatory effort on arousal from sleep. *Am Rev Respir Dis* 1990; 142:205–300.

20. Schiffman PL, Belsh JM. Effect of respiratory resistance and theophylline on respiratory muscle strength in patients with amyotrophic lateral sclerosis. *Am J Respir Dis* 1989; 139:1418–1423.
21. Aboussouan LS, Khan SU, Meeker DP< et al. Effects of noninvasive positive-pressure ventilation on survival in amyotrophic lateral sclerosis. *Ann Int Med* 1997; 127(6):450–453.
22. George CFP. Principles and practices of sleep medicine. *Neuromuscular Disorders.* Chapter 74.
23. Iannaccone S, Ferrini-Strambi L. Pharmacologic treatment of emotional lability. *Clin Neuropharmacol* 1996; 19(6):532–535.
24. Schiffer RB, Cash J, Herndon RM. Treatment of emotional lability with low dose tricyclic antidepressants. *Psychosomatics* 1983; 24:1094–1096.
25. Neary D, Snowden JS, Mann DMA, et al. Frontal lobe dementia and motor neuron disease. *J Neurol Neurosurg* 1990; 53:23–32.
26. Charchafflie RJ, Fernandez LB, Perec CJ, et al. Functional studies of the parotid and pancrease glands in amyotrophic lateral sclerosis. *J Neurol Neurosurg Psychiatry* 1974; 37:863–867.
27. Mandel L. Tamai K. Sialorrhea and gastroesophageal reflux. *JADA* 1995;126:1537–1541.
28. Stern LM. Preliminary study of glycopyrrolate in the management of drooling. *J Pediatr Child Health* 1997; 33:52–54.
29. Newall AR, Orser R, Hunt M. The control of oral secretions in bulbar ALS/MND. *J Neurol Sci* 1996; 139(Suppl):43–44.
30. Webb K, Raddihough DS, Johnson DH, Bennett CS. Long term outcome of salivary control surgery. *Dev Med Child Neurol* 1995; 37:755–762.
31. Hanayama K, Ishikawa Y, Bach JR. Amyotrophic lateral sclerosis: Successful treatment of mucous plugging by mechanical insufflation-exsufflation. *Am J Phys Med Rehab* 1997; 76(4):338–339.
32. Bortolotti M. Laryngospasm and reflex central apnea caused by aspiration of refluxed gastric content in adults. *Gut* 1989; 30:233–238.
33. Bauman N, Sandler AD, Schmidt C, Maher J, Smith RJH. Reflex laryngospasm induced by stimulation of distal esophageal afferents. *Laryngoscope* 1994; 104:209–214.
34. Sartori RB, Trevisian L, Tassinari D, et al. Prevention of aspiration pneumonia during long term feeding by percutaneous endoscopy: Might cisapride play a role? An open pilot study. *Support Care Cancer* 1994; 2:188–190.
35. Bruce ML, Seeman TE, Merrill SS, Blazer DG. The impact of depressive symptomatology on physical disability: MacArthur studies of successful aging. *J Public Health* 1994; 84(II):1796–1799.
36. Cunningham LA. Depression and anxiety in the primary care setting. *Comp Ther* 1997; 23(6):400406.
37. De Wester JN. Recognizing and treating the patient with somatic manifestations of depression. *J Fam Prac* 1996; 43(Suppl 6):S3–S15.
38. Kazandjian MS. *Communication intervention communication and swallowing solutions for the ALS/MND community.* Singular Publishing Group, 1997:7–40.
39. Carter G, Miller RG. Comprehensive management of amyotrophic lateral sclerosis. *Rehabil Neuromusc Dis* 1997; 9(1):271–284.
40. Matthus-Vligeen LMH, Louwerse LS, Markus MP, et al. Percutaneous endoscopic gastrostomy in patients with amyotrophic lateral sclerosis and impaired pulmonary function. *Gastrointest Endosc* 1994; 40:463–469.
41. Drickamer MA, Cooney LM. A geriatrician's guide to enteral feeding. *JAGS* 1993; 41:672–679.

42. Louizou LA, Small M, Dalton GA. Cricopharyngeal myotomy in motor neurone disease. *J Neurol Neurosurg Psychiatry* 1980; 43:42–45.

43. Moss AH, Casey P, Stocking CB, et al. Home ventilation for amyotrophic lateral sclerosis patients: Outcomes, costs, and patient, family and physician attitudes. *Neurology* 1993; 43:438–443.

44. Cazzoli P. Oppenheimer EA. Home mechanical ventilation for amyotrophic lateral sclerosis: Nasal compared to tracheostomy–intermittent positive pressure ventilation. *J Neurol Sci* 1996; 139(Suppl):123–128.

45. Moss AH, Casey P, Stocking CB, et al. Home ventilation for amyotrophic lateral sclerosis patients: Outcomes, costs, and patient, family and physician attitudes. *Neurology* 1993; 43:438–443.

46. Aboussuan LS, Khan SU, Meeker DP, Stelmach L, Mitsumoto H. Effect of noninvasive positive pressure ventilation on survival in amyotrophic lateral sclerosis. *Ann Int Med* 1997; 127:450–453.

47. Goldblatt D,. Greenlaw J. Starting and stopping the ventilator for patients with amyotrophic lateral sclerosis. Neurol Clin 1989; 7(4):789–805.

48. Oliver D. The quality and care and symptom control: The effects of the terminal phase of ALS/MND. *J Neurol Sci* 1996; 139:134–136.

49. Newrick PG, Langton-Hewer R. Pain in motor neuron disease. *J Neurol Neurosurg Psychiatry* 1985; 48:838–840.

50. Campbell MJ, Endersby P. Management of motor neurone disease. *J Neurol Sci* 1984; 64:65–71.

51. Wilson WC, Smedira NG, Fink C. McDowell JA, Luce JM. Ordering and administration of sedatives and analgesics during the withholding and withdrawal of life support from critically ill patients. *JAMA* 1992; 267:949–963.

52. Truog RD, Burns JP. To breathe or not to breathe. *J Clin Ethics* 1994; 5:39–41.

53. Moss AH, Oppenheimer EA, Casey P, et al. Patients with amyotrophic lateral sclerosis receiving long term mechanical ventilation. *Chest* 1996; 110:249–255.

54. *Tuesdays with Morrie: An old man, a young man, and the last great lesson.* New York: Doubleday, 1997.

5

A Comprehensive Approach to Managing Amyotrophic Lateral Sclerosis

**Rhoda R. Jacobs, R.N., B.S.N., and
Hiroshi Mitsumoto, M.D., D.Sc.**

Patients with amyotrophic lateral sclerosis (ALS) may receive care in a variety of clinical settings. When such care is provided in a comprehensive clinic that specializes in ALS (and possible other neuromuscular disorders), all of the relevant specialists needed to manage the disease are brought together in one location. When patients are seen in many other types of clinics and practice settings, they will often receive care from these same specialists but in a slightly different rehabilitation setting, often managed within a department of Physical Medicine and Rehabilitation.

We strongly believe in the interdisciplinary or multidisciplinary approach for the most effective management and care for people ALS. At the weekly ALS Clinic at the Cleveland Clinic Foundation, patients are seen by a multidisciplinary team consisting of a neurologist, a nurse coordinator, a physical therapist, an occupational therapist, a speech pathologist, a dietitian, and a social worker. Other disciplines, such as pulmonology, gastroenterology, home health care, hospice, or orthotics, are called upon by the neurologist or nurse coordinator on an individual basis. This chapter discusses the responsibility of each of these specialists.

If you are not receiving care in an ALS clinic, the organization of your care may be more similar to that discussed in the next chapter, which considers the provision of care in a rehabilitation medicine setting.

The Team Approach

People living with ALS, their family members, and their caregivers all benefit from a comprehensive multidisciplinary approach to care and management because the needs of people with ALS are ever-changing. This approach has a positive impact on the ability of people with ALS to function and manage their symptoms (1). Until a curative treatment is found, this holistic and comprehensive approach offers the best physical and emotional support for the patient and the family. "A commitment on the part of the patient, family and health care providers to collaborate in a way that can bring meaning and hope to circumstances that make no sense and a sense of wholeness in the face of relentless physical disintegration" (2). "Those who provide health care to patients with ALS need to combine their resources creatively to continue care . . . The benefits of four independent resources that are used in combination: the ALS clinic, home care, alternate care sites, and hospice care . . . for effective management" (3). Ongoing comprehensive evaluation in the clinic setting as well as in the home by the home health care or hospice team provides timely management of the patient's needs.

Advantages of a Team Approach

The team plays an important role in education and advocacy, makes referrals, and acts as liaisons as needed. To the team as described in Table 5-1, the patient and family may wish to add their clergyman and the local ALS support group.

It is vitally important for the successful management and care of the ALS patient that the team have experience with ALS patient care. At our center the multidisciplinary approach is provided in a clinic setting that includes evaluations by the neurologist and various other members of the team. This saves time for the patient because varied expertise in the many facets of care are available at one location during the prescheduled clinic. Repeat visits to see other specialists are avoided, and the patient receives comprehensive care for multiple problems at one place and time. A block of time is set aside for each patient to be seen both individually and privately by each member of the team. The members of the team communicate with each other both during the clinic and subsequently regarding the various needs of the patient. During the session the team members confer about the findings and recommendations. A team meeting takes place after the open clinic to review each patient's status and needs.

When a comprehensive team is not available, an office visit with a neurologist who has experience in managing ALS, possibly including a nurse coordinator, is an alternative. They will refer you to other therapists and disciplines when specific needs are identified.

Disadvantages of the Team Approach

One disadvantage of our approach is that the appointment may last three to four hours and may become tiring for the person with ALS. Also, the cost of a visit may

Table 5-1. The Multidisciplinary Team

- •• Neurologist
- •• Nurse coordinator
- •• Physical therapist
- •• Occupational therapist
- •• Speech pathologist
- •• Dietitian
- •• Social worker
- •• Prosthordontist
- •• Orthotist
- •• Pulmonologist
- •• Respiratory therapist
- •• Gastroenterologist
- •• General surgeon
- •• Psychologist or psychiatrist
- •• Alternate site coordinator
- •• Research nurse coordinator
- •• Research physical therapist

be high if multiple team members are seen. The time allocated for each team member may not be sufficient if you have multiple issues to discuss, and follow-up appointments may be necessary.

The Team Members

The Person with ALS

The patient is central to the ALS team. Decision making requires that you thoroughly understand the disease process and treatment options. Members of the health care team should work with you to set goals for treatment, but the final decisions regarding care issues rest with you. The ALS Association has drafted a Patient Bill of Rights for People Living with ALS (Table 5-2) (4). Its purpose is to inform people living with ALS of their rights as they relate to their health care and health plan (insurance coverage).

Caregivers

Although he or she may have some symptoms, the person with ALS is usually independent with regard to mobility and personal care in the early stages of the

Table 5-2. The Amyotrophic Lateral Sclerosis Association's Patient Bill of Rights for People Living with ALS

As a person living with ALS, you have a right to:

1. Receive comprehensive information about ALS, including treatment options and resources for your health care needs. This includes the right to communicate with your government representatives regarding policies of the FDA, NIH—and other agencies—that relate to ALS.

2. Participate in decisions about your health care with the highest level of decision-making possible. This includes the right to discontinue or refuse treatments and therapy.

3. Receive ALS specialty care in a timely manner.

4. Receive health care that is coordinated and individualized for you across the spectrum of home, hospice, hospital, nursing home, outpatient, and work-place and throughout all the phases of your illness.

5. Access health care benefit coverage and life insurance coverage without discrimination based on your ALS diagnosis or disability.

6. Obtain clear, timely information regarding your health plan including benefits, exclusions and appeal procedures.

7. Review your medical records and have the information in your records explained to you.

8. Prepare an advance directive to state your wishes regarding emergency and end-of-life treatment choices.

9. Receive care that is considerate, respects your dignity, and holds information confidential. You have this right no matter what choices you make about treatments and therapy, what your disabilities related to ALS might be, or what your financial circumstances are.

10. Receive maximum support to enhance the quality of your life and have your family involved in all aspects of your health care.

disease. As symptoms progress, more assistance with day-to-day care will be needed. Family and friends will begin to provide assistance as the ability to function independently decreases, with family members providing most of the support. The person with ALS is usually not considered in need of "skilled care" as defined by Medicare and the insurance industry. The term *skilled care* implies either a return to a baseline medical status that existed before the illness or to an expected response to rehabilitation. Insurance and Medicare do not cover long-term care in the home if no further improvement is expected. Home care visits are terminated after instruction regarding care is provided to the patient and caregivers.

The role of caregiver can be both rewarding and overwhelming. Caregivers become important members of the team because physical and emotional care is provided in the home. A caregiver's participation in the ALS Clinic helps to provide an important link between the health care professionals and the continuity of care. It is important to be aware of the challenge and increased responsibility placed on caregivers. They are called upon to provide an increasing level of physical and emotional care as the disease progresses. These increasing demands, in addition to demands such as children and a job outside the home, result in stress and strain and may lead to burnout.

The Core Team

The following specialists are core members of the ALS team at our center and are always available as resources.

Neurologist

Neurologists are physicians who specialize in the evaluation and treatment of diseases of the nervous system. They are responsible for making the diagnosis of ALS, as well as any underlying disease process. An ALS Clinic is directed or led by neurologists who specialize in ALS. They refer or arrange for those who have an established diagnosis of ALS to be seen in the ALS Clinic. At the Cleveland Clinic Foundation (CCF) ALS Clinic, neurologists usually divulge the diagnosis of ALS and discuss the diagnosis before referring the patient to the Clinic. Neurologists prescribe and order symptomatic treatment, often based on the recommendations made by other members of the team. They explain how the disease progresses and the purpose and side effects of symptomatic treatments or specific treatments for ALS such as riluzole (Rilutek). Currently riluzole is the only treatment approved by the U.S. Food and Drug Administration (FDA) for the treatment of ALS. They conduct an ongoing evaluation of the patient's response to drug treatment and other therapies.

Neurologists also discuss future treatment alternatives such as percutaneous endoscopic gastrostomy (PEG) tubes for receiving nutrition if the patient develops difficulty taking food by mouth (see Chapter 11). They explain noninvasive ventilatory support (external ventilator or Bi-PAP) and the availability of tracheostomy for the person experiencing impending respiratory difficulty or difficulty managing secretions (see Chapter 12). The decision to pursue these options is made by the patient after a detailed explanation and upon the recommendation of various members of the team. In addition, neurologists discuss advance directives such as a Living Will and Durable Power of Attorney for Health Care. They identify patients who qualify for research protocols and often act as investigators of these studies. Those who are involved in research and the evaluation of data collected from ALS patients monitor their responses to current methods of treatment and supportive care in their search for new insight into the cause of ALS and possible future treatment.

A potential conflict of interest exists when the treating neurologist is also a research investigator. Clinicians are required to provide the best symptomatic treatment and offer new therapies that may be potentially beneficial. New therapies are studied and proven effective within the context of controlled clinical trials. Clinical trials help develop new effective treatments and help to increase our understanding of ALS. Once a clinical trial is begun, no deviation from the original research plan may occur unless the protocol is formally changed. In some cases this may mean that a patient is given a placebo rather than the drug being tested. All events related to patient care must be recorded in the patient record, and all major adverse effects must be reported.

Nurse Coordinator

The availability of an experienced, compassionate nurse coordinator is essential for the success of the team approach. The nurse coordinators act as liaison between the various members of the ALS team, the patient, and the family or caregivers, as well as community resources. The nurse coordinator practices under the direction of the neurologist and plays a critical role as a patient advocate.

The patient or family member is referred to the nurse coordinator by the physician once the diagnosis has been made. The nurse coordinator is responsible for providing information to the patient and family. She acts as liaison, coordinating appointments and consultations with the ALS Clinic or with individual members of the team when necessary. She provides literature and answers questions about the disease, the ALS Clinic, and overall medical care. Because much of the information may be overwhelming at first, the nurse coordinator is available at future clinic visits or by phone to address needs and concerns and make appropriate referrals. The person with ALS must not feel abandoned even when he can no longer come to the Clinic. Care may be coordinated through communication with a home care or hospice agency even if the patient can no longer come to the clinic, and they continue to be available for psychological support to the patient and family.

The nurse coordinator also discusses issues such as the necessity for a feeding tube (PEG) placement or assistance with breathing (noninvasive vs. tracheostomy). At some point she should initiate a discussion of advance directives—Durable Power of Attorney for Health Care and the Living Will. The nurse coordinator is a resource for other nurses, health care providers, and home care agencies, and monitors the patient's response to treatment. In addition, she coordinates contact with research trials by either referring the patient to a research coordinator for participation in a clinical trial or by overseeing participation in the trial.

Physical Therapist

Physical therapists evaluate people who have experienced an injury or a disease that has affected their functional status. They assess motion of joints, muscle strength, and endurance. Physical therapists evaluate leg strength and the ability to walk and transfer safely. They can prescribe a program of range of motion exercises to prevent contractures of the muscles, which cause pain and loss of function of the joints.

Physical therapists may recommend stretching exercises and teach the proper method for either active exercises performed by the patient or passive exercises performed by the caregiver. In the earlier stages of the disease, some mild resistance exercises may be used for the unaffected muscles. Physical therapists also encourage walking, swimming, or performance of usual activities around the house as long as they do not produce fatigue. Patients may be fitted with equipment to ensure safety and/or braces to provide support for weak muscles, such as a cervical (neck) collar or an ankle-foot orthosis for weak ankles (see Chapter 7).

Occupational Therapist

Occupational therapists help people to live as fully and as normally as possible within their environment. Occupational therapists in the ALS clinic evaluate arm and hand function and make suggestions to conserve energy. Adaptive skills are taught to help increase or maintain the performance of daily tasks. They also may recommend splints to support weakened muscles and joints. Splints limit or prevent painful and debilitating contractures that would limit the function of weakened arms and hands. Other adaptive devices may also be recommended to make daily activities such as feeding and dressing easier. Occupational therapists teach people with ALS how to conserve energy and thus prevent fatigue. When wheelchairs become advisable, an occupational therapy evaluation provides the proper dimensions and adaptations (see Chapter 8).

Speech Pathologist

Most people with ALS will develop problems with speech and swallowing at some time. The muscles that control the functions of speech and swallowing are controlled by nerves that originate in an area of the brain called the medulla, or "bulb" because of its shape. These problems are therefore called bulbar and result from weak muscles of the face, throat, and neck. Since the speech and language areas of the brain are not affected, constructing and understanding language and the desire to communicate are not affected by the disease. Speech pathologists evaluate the patient's speech and ability to communicate and recommend speech and communication devices to assist or replace speech weakened or lost as the ALS progresses. They also evaluate the ability to chew and swallow, noting the presence of extra saliva, choking and coughing on food and saliva, and the need for extra time to complete a meal. Patients are then taught methods to eat safely and to conserve energy during meals (see Chapter 10).

Dietitian

Weight loss may occur as muscles of the mouth and throat weaken because the quantity of food and liquid taken by mouth may not be adequate for proper nutrition and energy requirements. The dietitian assesses the nutritional status of the patient and makes recommendations that prevent aspiration (swallowing down the "wrong tube"); prevent weight loss; and maintain appropriate fluid, calorie, and protein requirements. Recommendations may begin with appropriate posture during meals and changes in food consistency, such as a softer diet to make chewing and swallowing easier. Fatigue causes the patient to stop eating before adequate nutrients have been taken in. Eating smaller amounts during more frequent meals and snacks may prevent fatigue during mealtime, and nutritional supplements may be recommended. Eventually she will discuss a PEG (feeding) tube as an alternative to taking food by mouth (see Chapter 11).

Social Worker

The social worker is available to assess the emotional status of the person with ALS and the family and to determine how they are coping with living with ALS. Living arrangements and home care needs will be discussed. Advance directives such as a Living Will and Durable Power of Attorney for Health Care will be reviewed at the appropriate time. The social worker is also available to guide the patient and family members if assistance with financial resources needs to be explored.

The person with ALS may be referred to the Medicaid program that provides health care insurance for those who lack financial resources. Medicaid may also be available to those with private insurance. Medicaid Passport provides home care for people 60 years old and older. This home care does not necessarily have to be skilled or performed by a nurse or a physical therapist. The patient may just need assistance with daily activities such as feeding, bathing, and transfers. Medicaid Waiver is the same as Passport, but it is for patients under the age of 60 years. Guidance may be given to apply for Social Security Disability. The social worker can also make a referral if the patient and/or family members need an outside counselor. Coverage for counseling depends on the specifics of each person's insurance coverage.

The Extended Team

The following specialists are available individually by recommendation of the neurologist as specific needs arise.

Pulmonologist

A pulmonologist is a physician who specializes in and manages respiratory or breathing problems. Amyotrophic lateral sclerosis does not affect the lungs directly, but it does affect the muscles that control breathing, and shortness of breath or respiratory distress may occur. During each visit at our ALS clinic, we measure the forced vital capacity (FVC)—the amount of air that can be moved in and out of the lungs. The percentage of what is considered normal for each patient is determined. The pulmonologist is consulted as early as possible after ALS is diagnosed to establish a baseline respiratory function. If the person with ALS has a history of smoking or respiratory problems such as asthma or chronic obstructive lung disease, the pulmonologist can provide the necessary evaluation. The rate of change of respiratory function can be measured, and interventions or treatments can be prescribed sooner. The pulmonologist will discuss options, including assisted cough, tracheostomy, invasive or permanent ventilator support (breathing machine), and noninvasive or external ventilator, and will manage or oversee the care involving these options (see Chapter 12).

Gastroenterologist or General Surgeon

A consultation with a gastroenterologist, a physician who manages medical problems related to the stomach and intestines, or a general surgeon is recommended when the person with ALS has agreed to have a PEG or feeding tube placed. The decision to have a PEG tube placed is made if chewing and swallowing begin to result in unusual fatigue, if choking frequently occurs, and/or if weight loss is present. Ideally, the PEG tube should be placed while the patient has an adequate forced expiratory capacity. The PEG tube is placed with minimal sedation under local anesthetic. After an overnight stay for observation, the dietitian will discuss general nutrition and delivery of nutrition by PEG tube with the patient and caregivers (see Chapter 11).

Prosthoordontist

A prosthoordontist is a dentist who may be consulted in the presence of dysarthria, or impaired speech. A dental prosthesis may be designed to lift the soft palate, thus increasing the clarity of speech. In some patients, this prosthesis may be particularly useful.

Research Nurse Coordinator

Patients frequently qualify to participate in clinical trials in the search for new treatments in ALS. The neurologist may act as the chief investigator, and a research nurse coordinator oversees the study. The coordinator evaluates patient records to make certain that each participant meets the criteria established by the pharmaceutical company conducting the study and to ensure good clinical practice as determined by the FDA. The coordinator makes certain that all the required information is collected and that patients are followed up at the appropriate time intervals. The data must be carefully stored and submitted to the pharmaceutical company. Information is kept confidential. Under the guidance of the neurologist, the research nurse coordinator often acts in a clinical capacity regarding medical problems.

Research Physical Therapist

The effectiveness of a study or investigational drug must be measured at specific intervals throughout the course of the study or the period of time the patient participates. The pharmaceutical company outlines and describes specific areas to be measured. Strength, daily function, and respiratory function are measured by the research physical therapist. The measurements are performed in a uniform manner with all patients to ensure consistency during data collection. This ensures a higher degree of accuracy at the end of the study, when the effectiveness of the drug is evaluated.

Psychiatrist and Psychologist

Depression is a natural psychological process when one faces a serious illness such as ALS. It may affect every aspect of a person's life, including his or her personal relationships, work status, and financial status. Marital relationships and other social issues and relationships may be affected. Because physical changes are ongoing, the situation may at times seem overwhelming. Emotional and social adjustment become necessary as the role of each member of the family changes in response to the physical changes of ALS. Members of the ALS team make every effort to provide ongoing support to the patient and family. Antidepressants often provide relief from depression, and a psychologist or psychiatrist may be consulted to assist with adjusting to the disease process or to help work out family issues.

Orthotist

Deformity of the joints can occur as muscle weakness progresses. This leads to a loss of the ability to function effectively. Orthoses, or orthopedic appliances, will be recommended by the physical therapist or the occupational therapist. The physical therapist typically addresses issues concerning the neck and arms, whereas the occupational therapist is concerned with the legs and addresses such issues as the ability to function at home or on the job as well as mobility.

Orthopedic appliances are used to support or properly align the joints, the movable parts of the body. Orthoses help to prevent and/or correct deformities or contractures of the joints. Proper support and alignment of the joints relieves the pain that may occur as a result of weakness and deformity.

A referral is made to the orthotist by the physical therapist or occupational therapist, and a prescription for the necessary appliance is provided by the neurologist. The orthotist then designs and builds the orthopedic appliance. One example is a neck brace, or cervical collar, used to support weakened neck muscles. Posture is improved, which makes eating, sitting, standing, and walking easier, and neck pain that results from from overworked muscles is relieved. Similarly, an ankle brace or ankle-foot orthosis (AFO) provides support to a weakened ankle, and the ability to walk is improved because the risk of tripping is decreased.

Home Health Team

Issues about caring for the patient at home usually arise. As care issues become more challenging, the nurse coordinator may arrange for a home health care nurse. Care must be taken to choose a home care team that is knowledgeable about the disease because the needs of a person with ALS are unique. The team makes recommendations that will provide increased safety for the patient and caregivers. During a home visit the home care nurse will evaluate the extent of the patient's disability and ability to function in the home; the need for adaptive equipment such as a hospital bed, equipment for bathing, or a lift; and lifestyle adaptation. The home health care nurse will work with the ALS clinic nurse coordinator. A referral may be made for home visits by a physical therapist, occupational therapist, respiratory therapist, social worker, or home health aid. The nurse, patient, and family members may address emotional and psychological concerns. The responsibility of caring for the person with ALS often falls to the family members because of variations in coverage or reimbursement by health care plans. There typically is a limit to the amount of care that is covered, making careful planning and use of home care resources necessary. Once the patient and caregiver demonstrate the ability to provide care, insurance no longer covers visits to the home. Should new issues arise, the patient or caregiver may request further services in the home by contacting the nurse coordinator. A referral will again be made to the home care agency by the nurse coordinator. Families with greater financial means may be able to afford more help in the home (see Chapter 26).

Hospice Care

Hospice care was developed to provide support and care for people who are in the last phases of an incurable disease. Patients are referred to hospice by their neurologists or primary care physicians. A recommendation for hospice care may be made by the home care nurse or the nurse coordinator. Patients are either transferred to hospice care from the home health care team or enter hospice care directly. Hospice care requires a team approach and may take place at home or in a nursing facility. Caregivers must be available, such as family, friends, or the staff of a nursing facility. The emphasis of hospice care is to provide physical and emotional comfort. Comfort is provided to the family as well as the patient, with a focus on quality of life. Patients who have a tracheostomy and are permanently ventilated may not receive hospice care. Should the patient change his mind and receive a tracheostomy after entering hospice, he is no longer eligible for hospice.

The hospice team is led by a nurse case manager who develops a plan of care for the patient. Other members of the team include:

- the medical director who manages the patient care and provides medical services
- the social worker who provides assistance with financial issues, coordinates community services, and provides emotional support
- pastoral care to meet the spiritual needs of the patient and caregivers
- the home health aide who helps to provide personal services for the patient
- the hospice volunteer

Bereavement support is provided by the hospice team. Care is coordinated with the neurologist and the ALS Clinic nurse coordinator. Reports regarding the patient's status are provided by the nurse case manager to the neurologist and the ALS Clinic nurse coordinator. Medicare and insurance policies generally provide coverage for hospice care (see Chapter 29).

Patient Advocacy Groups

The ALS Association (ALSA) and the Muscular Dystrophy Association (MDA) are the primary advocacy groups for ALS. Certification for ALS centers is provided by the ALS Association and separately by MDA at the national level and is based on standards of excellence in the diagnosis of ALS and the delivery of care to the ALS patient. Table 5-3 describes the standards and requirements for certification under the ALSA Center Program (5).

Varying degrees of financial support are provided to ALS centers at the local level by the local ALS chapter for patient services. Services available to patients include provision of education regarding ALS, support groups, home care consultants, and loan banks for equipment in the home. The ALSA and the MDA are considered to be an important part of the team in the multidisciplinary approach to management of ALS.

"The ALS Association (ALSA) is the only not-for-profit voluntary health agency in the United States dedicated solely to Amyotrophic Lateral Sclerosis. The mission of the organization is . . . to raise funds to support cutting edge research, to increase public and governmental awareness, and to assist patients and families in coping with the day-to-day challenges they face living with ALS" (6). ALSA and MDA not only provide funds for research and work to increase public awareness about ALS, but also provide direct service to patients and their families.

Database

Critical to the understanding of the disease process is the collection of data or information. Information is stored and shared with health professionals, providing insight into the disease process as well as response to treatment. Currently there is a national database, ALSCARE, where data from multiple ALS centers, individual neurologists, patients, and caregivers is stored. The data reflect the effect— physically, emotionally, and financially—on the patient and caregivers living with ALS. Data, which are provided by patients and their caregivers, provide insight into the relationship between a patient's financial status and health outcomes. The data are kept confidential.

We at the Cleveland Clinic Foundation have developed a database that promotes "outcome-based management" of the patient (7). The information is collected at specific intervals during patient visits to the ALS Clinic. The relationship between medical interventions, or recommendations, and health outcomes, or the patient's response to treatment, is outlined. The interventions are recommended by

TABLE 5-3. The ALSA Center Program

Mission of the ALSA Center Program

To define, establish and support a national standard of care in the management of amyotrophic lateral sclerosis (ALS), sponsored by The Amyotrophic Lateral Sclerosis Association (ALSA).

Objectives of the ALSA Center Program

To encourage and provide state of the art, multidisciplinary and interdisciplinary care and clinical management of ALS through:

- •• The involvement of all necessary health care disciplines in the care of the ALS patient and family;
- •• The offering of multidisciplinary and interdisciplinary care regardless of the ability to pay;
- •• Collaborative work among Centers to enhance ALS patient care techniques.

To select, certify and support distinguished regional institutions recognized as the best in the field with regard to knowledge of and experience with ALS; and which have neurological diagnostics and imaging, and available on-site licensed and certified ancillary services on clinic days including (but not limited to):

- •• physical therapy
- •• occupational therapy
- •• respiratory therapy
- •• nursing
- •• registered dietitian services
- •• Ph.D. psychology or psychiatry
- •• speech and language pathology
- •• MSW social work services
- •• To establish a cohesive relationship among ALSA Centers, ALSA Chapters, and ALSA Free Standing Support Groups and the ALSA national organization to fulfill the mission of The ALS Association and its ALSA Center program.

the neurologist and the other members of the team under the guidance of the neurologist. All members of the team have access to the data collected, which enables them to make further recommendations for patient care based on previous response to care. When such data are used collectively, it allows for higher standards of care by reducing the chance for variability by individual health care professionals as they evaluate the patient and manage their care. The data are also used for medical record documentation as well as outcome-based research.

Data are collected for the CCF ALS Clinic Patient Care Database by the neurologist, nurse coordinator, physical therapist, occupational therapist, speech pathologist, nutritionist, and social worker.

Information that is collected is specific to the concerns of each member of the team as it applies to the evaluation of the patient and the decision-making process. Information collected by the neurologist and the nurse coordinator would include patient age and gender, onset of symptoms, and the level of diagnostic certainty in the clinical diagnosis of ALS according to the El Escorial World Federation of Neurology criteria. Levels of certainty progress from Suspected ALS to Possible ALS, Probable ALS, and Definite ALS. Differentiation is made between Sporadic ALS (SALS) and Familial ALS (FALS). A score is given based on the ALS Functional Rating Scale (ALSFRS), which quantifies the severity of the ALS based on motor function in the arms and legs and respiratory function. The forced vital capacity (FVC) is measured. Current symptoms and medications are listed, as is involvement in clinical trials.

The physical therapist evaluates the patient's living arrangement and the need for home equipment. The ability of the joints to move, muscle strength in the legs, balance, and any deviation in the ability to walk is described and in some cases rated on a scale. Function of the legs, such as the ability to climb stairs or rise from a chair independently or with help, is rated. Based on previous and current evaluations, recommendations are made in such areas as gait training to increase safety when walking, exercises, family instruction, and energy conservation. Adaptive equipment may be selected, and outpatient or home physical therapy may be ordered.

Living arrangements and the need for home equipment are also evaluated and documented by the occupational therapist. Muscle strength is rated, and range of motion in the joints is described, with a focus on the arms. The ability to perform activities of daily living (ADLs) such as bathing and dressing as well as the ability to transfer oneself from one place to another is documented. The presence of shoulder pain is noted, along with the degree of discomfort. Recommendations are again based on previous response to intervention and current evaluation and include equipment needs and exercise.

Recommendations for increased safety from choking when swallowing food, liquids, and saliva are made by the speech pathologist after an evaluation of swallowing ability is made. Documented changes may include posture changes during meals; changes in food texture, consistency, and temperature; and feeding techniques such as the use of a cup or straw or the placement of a PEG tube. Speed of tongue and lip movements is timed, and the ability to communicate is evaluated. Changes in the voice and speech are noted. Recommendations are noted in the database for improving articulation and the use of augmentative aides for communication.

The nutritionist documents the current diet in the database, and the patient's weight is tracked, noting weight loss or gain. Documentation is made of the time needed to complete a meal and whether the time is increasing. Based on documented weight loss and difficulty swallowing, calorie and protein needs are recommended and the presence of risk for malnutrition is established.

The social worker also contributes information to the database by documenting the source of income in the home and the type of insurance coverage. Primary caregivers are noted, and those who provide a support system for the patient and primary caregiver are identified. The presence of other health problems of the patient and caregivers are listed because they may affect patient care. Advance directives are discussed if they are not already in place. The appropriateness of home care versus an extended care facility or hospice care is noted and discussed. Mental health issues are assessed, and counseling recommendations are made if appropriateness is determined.

There are pros and cons to maintaining a database. The database provides a focused evaluation by health care professionals, which helps reduce variability in the care provided. Medical record documentation is consistent. Research is promoted. In contrast, the collection of data may be tiring for the patient. The evaluation process may become time-consuming for the health care professionals.

References

1. Carter GT. Rehabilitation management in neuromuscular disease. *J Neuro Rehab* 1997; 11(2):69–80.
2. Thompson B. Amyotrophic lateral sclerosis: Integrating care for patients and their families. *Am J Hosp Pall Care* 1990; 7:27–32.
3. Mitsumoto H, Chad DA, Pioro EP. *Comprehensive care: Amyotrophic lateral sclerosis.* Philadelphia: FA Davis, 1998:305–320.
4. "Patient Bill of Rights for People Living with ALS," The Amyotrophic Lateral Sclerosis Association, National Office, 21021 Ventura Blvd., Suite 321, Woodland Hills, CA 91364.
5. "The ALSA Center Program," The Amyotrophic Lateral Sclerosis Association, National Office, 21021 Ventura Blvd., Suite 321, Woodland Hills, CA 91364.
6. Klein LM. The role of the national voluntary agency in ALS. In: Mitsumoto H, Norris FH (eds.). *Amyotrophic lateral sclerosis.* New York: Demos, 1994:317.
7. Mitsumoto H, et al. Cleveland Clinic ALS Database for Care and Management for Patients with ALS, Presented at International Alliance of ALS/MND Associations–9th International Symposium on ALS/MND, Munich, Germany, 16–18 November 1998.

Suggested Reading

1. Miller RG, Rosenberg JA, Gelinas DF, Mitsumoto H, et al., and the ALS Practice Parameters Task Force. Practice parameter: The care of the patient with amyotrophic lateral sclerosis: An evidence-based review. *Neurology* 1999;52: 1311–1323.

2. Mitsumoto H (section editor). *Continuum. Motor Neuron Disease.* American Academy of Neurology. Baltimore: Williams & Wilkins, 1997.

6

Rehabilitation Issues

Lisa S. Krivickas, M.D.

Unless you are receiving care in a comprehensive ALS center, much of the management of the disease will take place under the auspices of rehabilitation medicine. This chapter provides an overview of how care is provided in this setting.

Amyotrophic lateral sclerosis (ALS) is a disease that is now helped by rehabilitation techniques. As defined in one of the major medical textbooks for the specialty of physical medicine and rehabilitation (also known as physiatry):

"Rehabilitation is defined as the development of a person to the fullest physical, psychological, social, vocational, avocational, and educational potential consistent with his or her physiologic or anatomic impairment and environmental limitations. Realistic goals are determined by the person and those concerned with his or her care. Thus, one is working to obtain optimal function despite residual disability, even if the impairment is caused by a pathological process that cannot be reversed" (1).

As researchers develop additional drugs to slow disease progression in ALS, life expectancy will increase and rehabilitation strategies will become even more important.

To fully appreciate the concept of rehabilitation, it is helpful to understand the distinction between the terms *impairment, disability,* and *handicap.*

- Impairment is a disruption in one's health status.

- Disability refers to the way impairment affects a person's life, such as losing the ability to meet personal, social, or occupational demands.

- Handicap is the impact of the disability on a person's normal role in society.

Having an impairment does not necessarily mean that a person has a disability or a handicap, and the goal of rehabilitation is to prevent impairments from producing disability or handicap. For example, a person with ALS may have leg weakness or limited range of motion, and these are impairments. The disability associated with them may be a loss of independent mobility because of an inability to walk. However, using a self-propelling wheelchair removes the disability without altering the impairment. This same person may have the handicap of not being able to perform his job as a bank manager, but if his worksite is made wheelchair-accessible, he loses his handicap.

Comprehensive ALS medical care should include rehabilitation to restore the person with ALS to optimal functioning in his or her normal environment and to allow as high a quality of life as possible. For a healthy individual, the highest quality of life attainable is defined as achieving optimal function and the use of all of the assets that he or she has (2). For the person with ALS, this means rehabilitation to the optimal functional performance that is achievable given the stage of the disease.

For people with ALS, rehabilitation is a constantly changing process because of changing physical status. For the rehabilitation professional, rehabilitation of the person with ALS is more challenging than it is for patients with static functional deficits produced by events such as a stroke. One of the most difficult tasks for the rehabilitation team is to predict how quickly the patient's ALS will progress; it is crucial to attempt to do this to stay ahead of the disease. By looking at the course of disease progression, health professionals can help you to avoid purchasing equipment that may not be useful for any length of time. For example, a person who has only moderate leg weakness but whose disease seems to be progressing rapidly should not order a manual wheelchair that takes 10 weeks for customization and delivery; by the time the chair arrives, he may need a power chair.

There are two broad approaches to rehabilitation, one focusing on changing the individual with a disability (restoring function) and the other focusing on altering the environment. These approaches are depicted in Figure 6-1. When a person acquires physical disabilities as a result of ALS, his environment shrinks. To return him to a more balanced relationship with his environment, we can either remove his impairment or we can expand his environment so that it is no longer too small for him. Unfortunately, we can not at the present time get rid of the ALS. Thus we must use rehabilitation techniques, including adaptive equipment, assistive devices, and environmental controls, to enlarge the environment of the person with ALS so that he can once again function within it.

This chapter is an overview of the concept of rehabilitation as it applies to ALS. Subsequent chapters (Chapters 10–15) provide more specific information regarding various aspects of rehabilitation.

Conceptual Overview of Enabling/ Disabling Processes

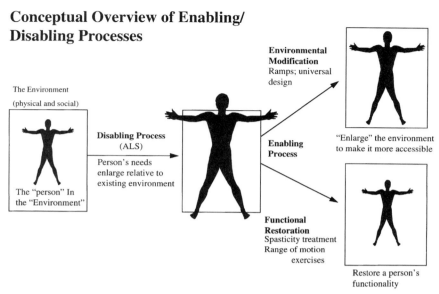

Figure 6-1. Conceptual overview of enabling–disabling processes. The environment, depicted as a square, represents both physical space and social structures (family, community, society). A person who does not manifest any disability is fully integrated into society and "fits within the square." A person with ALS has increased needs (expressed by the size of the individual) and is dislocated from his prior integration into the environment, that is, "doesn't fit in the square." The rehabilitative process attempts to rectify this displacement either by restoring function in the individual (not yet possible with ALS) or by expanding access to the environment (i.e. providing ramps and assistive devices). Adapted with permission from: Brandt EN and Pope AM (eds). *Enabling America.* Institute of Medicine Report, National Academy Press, Washington D.C., 1997.

The Rehabilitation Team

Rehabilitation is a team effort. The team may consist of some or all of the following individuals: physiatrist, neurologist, physical therapist, occupational therapist, speech therapist, respiratory therapist, dietitian, psychologist, social worker, and, most important, the patient and family or caregivers.

Two groups of physicians specialize in rehabilitation: physiatrists, who practice the specialty of physical medicine and rehabilitation, and neurologists with special training in neurorehabilitation. Physical Medicine and Rehabilitation (PM&R) is a relatively young medical specialty. It developed following World War II because of the need for rehabilitation of veterans with disabling war injuries. As of 1997 there were more than 5,000 board-certified physiatrists in the United States. Physiatrists must complete at least one year of general medicine and three years of training in PM&R after medical school. They care for a broad range of patients with physical disabilities resulting from many disorders, including neuromuscular diseases, brain injury, spinal cord injury, stroke, orthopedic injuries, burns, arthritis, amputations, and sprains, strains, and other acute musculoskeletal problems. The one thing that these diverse groups of patients share is a disability that has compromised their ability to function independently and/or optimally. The physiatrist's goal is to use a combination of medicines, exercise, therapies, and environmental modifications to maximize function.

Neurologists recently have also begun to subspecialize in rehabilitation. Neurologists with expertise in neurorehabilitation receive one to two additional years of training in rehabilitation after having completed their regular neurology training. They treat patients with disabilities caused by neurologic problems such as neuromuscular diseases, brain injury, spinal cord injury, and stroke. Either the physiatrist or the neurorehabilitation neurologist is best suited to coordinate the overall rehabilitation effort and the work of other team members in the care of the person with ALS.

Physical therapists (PTs) are trained to work with ALS patients on issues related to mobility and exercise. They assess difficulties with walking and transferring (getting your body from one seat or position to another) and may recommend techniques that improve mobility, assistive devices (such as canes or walkers), foot braces (called ankle-foot orthoses or AFOs), or wheelchairs. They are trained to help patients develop safe and appropriate exercise programs and can teach family members and other caregivers how to physically assist the person with ALS without injuring themselves.

Occupational therapists (OTs) provide some of the same treatments as physical therapists when the physical problem involves the arms rather than the legs. They also often work with physical therapists in prescribing wheelchairs. Occupational therapists evaluate the patient's ability to perform activities of daily living (ADLs) such as dressing, bathing, feeding oneself, preparing meals, and more complex tasks such as those required for a specific job or hobby. They teach compensatory strategies and recommend assistive devices and equipment that will make it easier for the person with ALS to maintain his independence with ADLs. Some occupational therapists will evaluate the skills necessary for driving and make recommendations to improve driving safety or to modify the car to make it easier to operate.

A speech therapist (formally referred to as a speech and language pathologist, or SLP) is important for ALS patients with bulbar symptoms. He or she is trained to work with problems associated with speaking and swallowing. When dealing with speech difficulties, the SLP can teach the person with ALS compensatory strategies both to make him more easily understood and to minimize voice fatigue. The SLP can also help the person to evaluate and select alternative means of communication if necessary. Speech therapists evaluate swallowing function both by observing patients while they swallow and by performing radiographic (videofluoroscopy) studies of swallowing. They recommend changes in food consistencies and special swallowing techniques to help prevent aspiration (accidentally getting food into the lungs) and/or choking.

Respiratory therapists teach patients and their caregivers to operate and troubleshoot with equipment used to assist breathing. The therapist may teach patients with weak coughs how to cough more forcefully or to use devices to increase their coughing ability so that they can adequately clear their lungs of secretions. Equipment that the respiratory therapist may assist with includes a manual resuscitation bag, portable ventilators, BiPAP machines, in-exsufflator ("coughing" machine), and suction machines.

A psychologist may help both the patient and his family members adjust to the changes in physical function, family roles, and financial status that often follow the diagnosis of ALS. Many people become depressed after being diagnosed with ALS, and depression may prevent them from using rehabilitation services to maximize their function, independence, and quality of life. The psychologist's assistance may decrease the intensity or length of this period of depression. Acceptance of death and dying is another process with which many patients and families require assistance.

The social worker is a critical member of the rehabilitation team. He assists patients to navigate through the red tape involved in obtaining insurance to cover rehabilitation services and home assistance. He also provides guidance about applying for Social Security disability benefits, Medicare, Medicaid, and so forth, and may be able to provide additional information about community services for people with disabilities.

Rehabilitation Settings

Rehabilitation services can be provided in outpatient clinics, inpatient settings, or in the home. Patients who are fairly mobile usually receive therapies (physical, occupational, speech, etc.) in the outpatient departments of hospitals or in freestanding therapy practices. These settings are preferable to therapy in the home because the therapist is generally able to spend more time with the patient and has more equipment available. Because ALS is relatively rare, many therapists may not have any experience with it. Thus the ideal therapy setting is the outpatient department of a teaching hospital or a rehabilitation hospital where the therapists at least have experience working with patients with neurologic impairments. Compared with other neurologic disorders, ALS is unique because of its rapid rate of progression. The therapist must remain one step ahead of the disease so that equipment that will not be usable by the time it arrives is not ordered. Therapy in the home setting is often preferable for patients with extremely limited mobility. An advantage of therapy in the home is that the PT and/or OT can assess the home environment and recommend modifications that will improve safety and independence, such as grab bars and ramps. Assessing the patient in the home environment may also demonstrate a need for additional assistive devices, which may not be apparent in the therapy gym. Family members and caretakers can be trained to safely transfer the patient in his home setting.

Most people with ALS do not receive rehabilitation in an acute rehabilitation hospital inpatient setting. However, a short "tune-up" stay is appropriate when multiple complex rehabilitation issues need to be addressed simultaneously. To qualify for an inpatient stay (based on the rules of most insurance companies and Medicare), a patient must require intensive therapy for a total of at least four hours per day from a combination of at least two different therapy disciplines. An example of a patient suitable for a one-week "tune-up" rehabilitation admission might be someone who needs to be fitted for a wheelchair, have family members learn how to transfer him safely, learn how to use a ventilator for nighttime ventilatory assistance, and explore augmentative communication systems. All of this could be accomplished during a short intensive inpatient stay but could easily require four to six weeks (time that might not be available) on an outpatient basis.

When Is Rehabilitation Necessary?

Rehabilitation is necessary during all stages of ALS. As the disease progresses, however, rehabilitation strategies and needs change. Most therapies will be intermittent. For example, a person with early ALS may be referred to a physical therapist for help with designing an appropriate aerobic exercise and strengthening program. As increasing spasticity develops, she may return to PT for a few sessions on stretching and range of motion exercises. If a footdrop develops and a brace is prescribed, she may again return for a few sessions of gait training with the new brace. As weakness increases, additional sessions of PT may be necessary to teach the spouse to effectively transfer the patient.

Insurance carriers will often deny coverage of continuing therapy to patients with ALS because they consider it maintenance therapy since no "improvement" is expected. This is faulty reasoning about which health care providers need to educate insurers. Amyotrophic lateral sclerosis is not a static disease, and additional therapy may be required as function changes. In addition, therapy is sometimes required in order for the patient to maintain function or slow the decline in function.

Exercise and Prevention of Disability

Rehabilitation should begin early in the course of ALS to prevent or delay the onset of disability. This concept is known as "prehabilitation" because it is a preventive form of rehabilitation. One important method of prehabilitation is exercise. Three types of exercise are important for all individuals, whether they have ALS or not: flexibility or stretching exercises, strengthening exercises, and aerobic exercises.

Stretching, or range of motion exercises, is very important for people with ALS. Range of motion exercises maintain the normal movement of joints and muscles. As muscle weakness develops, joints that are not used will lose their ability to move freely. This may cause pain, which in turn will interfere with function. For example, as shoulder weakness develops, a person can no longer raise his arm overhead. If he does not make an effort to maintain range of motion in the shoulder joint, the shoulder will become "frozen." Then, if a caregiver tries to assist the person by lifting his arm over his head, he will fail because of pain and tightness of the tissues around the joint. Stretching is also important when spasticity is present. Spastic muscles tend to become permanently shortened—a condition called a contracture—when not stretched regularly. This also can limit function and produce pain and discomfort. Patients can be taught specific stretching techniques that actually decrease the severity of—or help to abort—painful muscle spasms.

Unfortunately, there have not been any good studies on the effect of strengthening exercises in patients with ALS, so their use in ALS is somewhat controversial. However, based on research done on patients with other neuromuscular diseases such as muscular dystrophy and inherited neuropathies (such as Charcot-Marie-Tooth disease), it appears that muscles that are only mildly affected by the disease process can be strengthened by a moderate resistance strengthening program (3). The stronger a muscle is when a strength training program is started, the better the muscle responds. I recommend that interested ALS patients begin a strengthening program as soon as possible after diagnosis. Its objective is to maximize the strength of unaffected or mildly affected muscles in an attempt to delay the time when function will be impaired. For example, if an elderly person must use 90 percent of the strength of his leg muscles to rise from a chair before he develops ALS, he will be unable to arise from a chair after losing only 10 percent of his muscular capacity. If another individual requires only 50 percent of his maximal leg strength to rise from a chair before developing ALS, he will remain independent much longer, even if the disease progresses at the same pace.

Many physicians have expressed concern about the development of overuse weakness as a result of strength training in patients with neuromuscular diseases. There is no good evidence that overuse weakness actually develops in people with ALS who have antigravity strength (the ability to lift a limb against gravity) in their muscles and who exercise at a moderate intensity. I recommend that any weight-training or strengthening exercise be performed with a weight that the individual can comfortably lift 20 times; this guideline will prevent overworking the muscles with excessively heavy weights. People who weight-train often use weights that they can lift only 8 to 10 times before fatigue produces failure; this intensity of weight-training is not recommended for people with ALS. Another general guideline is that an exercise regimen is too strenuous if it consistently produces muscle soreness or fatigue lasting longer than one half hour after exercise.

Aerobic exercise is exercise that raises the heart rate and is sustained continuously for a period of at least 15 to 20 minutes. Examples include rapid walking, running, cycling, or using an exercise machine such as a rowing machine, stair-stepper, and the like. Aerobic exercise helps maintain fitness of the heart and lungs, and it is recommended for patients with ALS as long as it can be performed safely without risk of falling or injury. In addition to the physical benefits, this form of exercise often has a beneficial effect on mood, psychological well-being, appetite, and sleep.

Maximizing Mobility

An important aspect of rehabilitation is helping the person with ALS maintain in-dependent mobility in the community and his environment for as long as possible. Interventions that allow people to maintain mobility include assistive devices such as canes, walkers, braces, wheelchairs, and scooters; medications to decrease spas-ticity; home equipment such as grab bars, raised toilet seats, shower benches, and lifts; home modifications (ramps, wide doorways); and automobile adaptations such as hand controls.

Both bracing and wheelchairs are best prescribed by multidisciplinary teams. Many rehabilitation centers have Brace Clinics that are staffed by a team consist-ing of an orthotist (the person who makes the brace), a physical therapist, and a physiatrist. There is a surprisingly large array of options when it comes to pre-scribing something as seemingly simple as an ankle-foot orthosis (AFO), a brace to prevent footdrop. The brace may be constructed of a number of different mate-rials, may have several different types of ankle joints, may have special features built in to help control spasticity, and may even be designed to help control knee motion. An experienced team is best equipped to prescribe the most appropriate brace for a given person.

Many rehabilitation centers use a similar team approach for wheelchair pre-scription. The Wheelchair Clinic typically is staffed by a physical therapist, an oc-cupational therapist, and a physiatrist. Numerous options are available in a wheel-chair, and, as with the AFO, a multidisciplinary team is best equipped to prescribe the most appropriate (and economic) wheelchair.

Maximizing Independence with Activities of Daily Living

The term *activities of daily living* (ADLs) describes basic tasks such as bathing, dressing, and feeding oneself. The term *instrumental ADLs* refers to more complex tasks such as shopping, meal preparation, and the performance of household chores. The occupational therapist helps people with ALS to remain independent in ADLs for as long as possible. They may be taught energy conservation tech-niques, be provided with dressing aids (buttoners, sock pullers, reachers, Velcro fasteners for clothes), and given adapted kitchen utensils and writing tools (built-up handles, universal cuffs, plate guards, dicem pads). Various hand splints constructed by an occupational therapist may improve grip, making ADLs easier to perform.

Pursuit of Vocation and Avocation

Helping the person with ALS continue to work and pursue his hobbies and interests for as long as possible is another function of the rehabilitation team. The team may be able to assess the worksite and recommend environmental modifications that will allow the person with ALS to continue to perform his job. Voice-activated software may be recommended for people who use computers and have hand weakness. Other modifications might include the installation of ramps and the use of a scooter at work or other interventions discussed previously that allow maintenance of mobility and independence with ADLs.

Communication and Swallowing

Another area typically addressed by the rehabilitation team is speech and swallowing function. In addition to the speech therapist, a physician and occupational therapist are often involved in addressing these issues.

Adequate swallowing function is needed to maintain the nutritional status of the person with ALS unless he has a feeding tube. If nutritional status is not properly maintained, patients tend to burn up muscle for energy and thus lose muscle mass and strength earlier than they otherwise would. Swallowing dysfunction can also precipitate pneumonia and/or respiratory failure when food goes into the lungs instead of into the esophagus and stomach; this is called aspiration. A speech therapist or rehabilitation physician often recognizes swallowing difficulties before the person with ALS is aware of them. People with mild swallowing difficulties can be taught compensatory techniques to prevent aspiration and choking. Food consistencies also often require modification.

The ability to effectively communicate is extremely important for psychological and physical well-being. The rehabilitation team can use a variety of tools to ensure that the person with ALS is able to effectively communicate. Interventions include speech therapy to teach techniques to increase intelligibility of speech, palatal lifts, voice amplifiers, and augmentative communication devices, which may be as simple as a letterboard or as complex as a computer with a voice synthesizer.

Pulmonary Rehabilitation

Preventing and managing respiratory failure associated with ALS is of concern to the rehabilitation team because patients must be able to breath adequately and comfortably in order to have optimal function and quality of life. As mentioned previously, an important preventive measure is trying to avoid aspiration when swallowing. Physical therapists may instruct patients and family members in methods to assist coughing that allow the lungs to be cleared of mucus and help prevent infection. The rehabilitation team may also recommend physical medicine aids to assist with breathing. These may include machines to assist with coughing, methods of providing range of motion exercises to the lungs to prevent them from becoming excessively stiff, and machines to assist with breathing. Some physiatrists have special expertise in the use of noninvasive ventilation techniques; this term refers to ventilatory support that does not require tracheostomy.

The rehabilitation team may also assist the patient in making decisions concerning whether or not to pursue long term ventilatory support. Rehabilitation experts have experience working with patients with a variety of diagnoses who require ventilatory support and have a good understanding of the type of family support required, the necessary home equipment, and the level of independence and function the patient will be able to achieve.

Caregivers' Role in Rehabilitation

The family members and/or caregivers of people with ALS are a critical part of successful rehabilitation interventions. The rehabilitation process must focus on the caregivers as well as on the patient. Caregivers require instruction from physical therapists in how to properly transfer the patient so that they do not injure themselves. They also require instruction in the maintenance and use of any home equipment provided for the patient. The rehabilitation team should be sensitive to the psychological and physical well-being of caregivers because their ability to assist the person with ALS will have a direct impact on his level of function and independence.

Assistive Technology

Some rehabilitation hospitals have assistive technology centers that specialize in using technology to help people with disabilities overcome their limitations. Assistive technology centers are staffed by a multidisciplinary team that consists of physicians, physical therapists, occupational therapists, speech therapists, rehabilitation technologists, and neuropsychologists. These centers provide expertise in augmentative communication, complex seating and wheelchair prescription (i.e., power wheelchairs), environmental control systems, and worksite modification. Assistive technology allows people to do things like wave a hand to turn on a light, use a puff of air to control a wheelchair, and use voice to activate an appliance. The assistive technology team determines what assistive equipment will best serve the patient, customizes the device to the patient's needs once it has been purchased, and trains the patient and caregiver to use the equipment. In areas without a consolidated assistive technology program, these services are provided via a variety of different therapists and clinics.

Case Study

This case study briefly outlines the various rehabilitation interventions used by one patient throughout the course of her illness and illustrates the fact that rehabilitation is an ongoing process. Mrs. A developed right leg weakness at age 50 and was subsequently diagnosed with ALS. She was in good physical condition and had no medical problems before the onset of her leg weakness. Her first rehabilitation intervention was a few sessions of physical therapy to work on gait training with a cane. She soon developed a right footdrop, and an AFO was prescribed. Following receipt of her AFO, she returned to physical therapy for a few additional sessions of gait training with the AFO.

She subsequently began to develop weakness in her left leg and both arms; to slur her speech; and to require assistance to rise from chairs, shower, and use the toilet. She was admitted to a local rehabilitation hospital for a one-week stay and received daily physical, occupational, and speech therapy. Her gait was evaluated while she used a variety of assistive devices, and she was discharged using a rolling walker. Her husband was trained to assist her with transferring in a safe manner so that he would not injure his back. A raised toilet seat and a shower chair were ordered for the home. Her therapists made a home visit and made several recommendations designed to increase her safety and function; these included removing throw rugs, rearranging the kitchen, and obtaining some adaptive kitchen utensils. Mrs. A worked with a speech therapist who evaluated her swallowing and recommended that she avoid thin liquids because she tended to aspirate them. She was taught to slow down and overarticulate her speech so that she could be more easily understood. Mrs. A was also evaluated for a power wheelchair because her disease appeared to be progressing rapidly. Arrangements were made to have a rental power chair available in her home as soon as she thought she needed it. All of these rehabilitation interventions could have been performed on an outpatient basis but probably would have taken at least four weeks instead of one. Because Mrs. A's disease was progressing rapidly, she had multiple rehabilitation needs that were most efficiently addressed with a short inpatient stay.

A few months after Mrs. A's discharge from rehabilitation, she was having such difficulty eating that she had lost 30 pounds. A feeding tube was placed. She also was sleeping poorly and was very fatigued during the day. She was evaluated by a physiatrist specializing in pulmonary rehabilitation, who found that her vital capacity was only 25 percent of predicted and recommended that she begin to use noninvasive positive pressure ventilation at night. She and her husband were instructed in the use of the new equipment by a respiratory therapist who made several follow-up visits to their home. She gradually adjusted to using the ventilator all night, and as time went on she began using it for rest periods during the day.

Mrs. A's arm and leg weakness progressed, and she was no longer able to lift her arms over her head. A physical therapist came to the home for two visits to teach Mr. A how to assist her with range of motion exercises. The therapist also instructed him in some additional transfer techniques since Mrs. A was requiring substantially more assistance with transfers. She was no longer able to walk more than a few steps, and the power wheelchair was rented.

Mrs. A's speech continued to deteriorate so that only 30 percent to 50 percent of her words could be understood by those who were not family members. She visited a speech therapist who specialized in augmentative communication, was evaluated using a number of communication devices, and decided to order a dedicated communication device with a voice synthesizer. At the time of this initial visit, she had enough hand strength for direct selection with the communication device.

Within a few months, Mrs. A's arms and hands were too weak to drive her power chair or use the keyboard on her communication device. She also was having difficulty holding her head up and needed better head support for her wheelchair. She made a final visit to the rehabilitation center, where she attended its Wheelchair Clinic and was prescribed a manual chair that caretakers would have to push. The chair had a high back, a head rest, a ventilator tray, a lap tray for her communication device, and the ability to tilt in space for pressure relief. She also was reevaluated by the speech therapist specializing in augmentative communication; her communication device was modified so that she could use a scanning mode instead of direct selection, and she tried a variety of switches until she found one she could operate.

Shortly after returning home from the rehabilitation center, Mr. A again began to have difficulty transferring his wife because she could no longer assist in any way. Their physician recommended a TransAid lift. A rental lift was obtained, and the physical therapist returned to the A's home to instruct them in using the lift.

This case demonstrates the ongoing rehabilitation needs of ALS patients. At five different times during the course of Mrs. A's ALS, she either attended physical therapy or had a physical therapist work with her in the home. Similarly, she had multiple speech therapy interventions. She also worked with occupational and respiratory therapists and attended a Wheelchair Clinic. This combination of rehabilitation interventions allowed Mrs. A to remain at home with assistance from her husband and thus significantly improved her quality of life.

References

1. DeLisa JA. *Rehabilitation medicine*. Hagerstown, Md.: Lippincott-Raven, 1993.
2. Kottke FJ, Lehman JF. *Krusen's handbook of physical medicine and rehabilitation*. Philadelphia: WB Saunders, 1990.
3. Aitkens SG, McCrory MA, et al. Moderate resistance exercise program: Its effect in slowly progressive neuromuscular disease. *Arch Phys Med Rehabil* 1993; 74(7):711–715.

Suggested Reading

1. Bach JR. *Pulmonary rehabilitation.* Philadelphia: Hanley & Belfus, 1996.

2. Bach JR, Neurorehabilitation. *Semin Neurol* 1995; 15(1).

3. Bohannon R. Results of resistance exercise on a patient with ALS: A case study. *Phys Ther* 1983; 63:965–968.

4. Kazandjian MS. *Communication and swallowing solutions for the ALS/MND community: A CINI manual.* San Diego: Singular Publishing Group, 1997.

5. *Living with ALS: Functioning when your mobility is affected.* Woodland Hills, CA: The ALS Association, 1997.

6. *Living with ALS: Adjusting to swallowing and speaking difficulties.* Woodland Hills, CA: The ALS Association, 1997.

7. *Living with ALS: Adapting to breathing changes.* Woodland Hills, CA: The ALS Association, 1997.

8. Mitsumoto H, Chad DA, Pioro EP. Physical rehabilitation. In: *Amyotrophic lateral sclerosis.* Philadelphia: FA Davis, 1998:360–381.

9. Sanjak M, Paulson D, et al. Physiologic and metabolic response to progressive and prolonged exercise in amyotrophic lateral sclerosis. *Neurology* 1987; 37:1217–1220.

10. Siegel IM, Casey P. *101 Hints to "Help-with-Ease" for Patients with Neuromuscular Disease.* Muscular Dystrophy Association, 1996.

7

Physical Therapy

Vanina Dal Bello-Haas, B.Sc.P.T., M.Ed

As a member of the multidisciplinary rehabilitation team, the physical therapist (PT) can assist the individual with amyotrophic lateral sclerosis (ALS) to maintain optimal functional independence, reduce the effects of disability, and enhance quality of life. This is accomplished through education, rehabilitation programs, psychological support, the provision of appropriate equipment, and referrals to community resources (1). This chapter describes the profession of physical therapy, outlines its role in managing typical problems encountered by people with ALS, and describes some of the most common equipment recommended for people with ALS.

WHO ARE PHYSICAL THERAPISTS? WHAT DO THEY DO?

Physical therapists are health care professionals who are educated at the college or university level and are licensed in the state or states in which they practice. In some states you must be referred to physical therapists by a physician. In other states a physician's referral is not needed to see a physical therapist. In general, physical therapists help (1) prevent and/or address the onset and progression of impairments, functional limitations, disabilities, and changes in physical function and health status resulting from injury, disease, or other causes; (2) restore, maintain, and promote overall fitness, health, and optimal quality of life; and (3) alleviate pain (2).

As clinicians, physical therapists engage in examination and evaluation processes that assist in determining the most appropriate intervention for the individual. In an initial examination or reexamination, the PT will take a history to obtain an account of past and present health status and will conduct a systems review to gain additional information about general health. After analyzing all relevant information gathered from the history and systems review, she will administer one or more specific tests and measures to identify existing and potential problems (2). Tests and measures of pain, joint range of motion (ROM), muscle strength, muscle tone, flexibility, posture, edema, skin integrity, sensation, coordination, balance, transfers, gait, locomotion, endurance, aerobic capacity, and/or safety in the home and community are commonly used by physical therapists in examining people with ALS.

Based on the data gathered and the findings of the examination, the PT will make a clinical judgment (evaluation), determine a physical therapy diagnosis and prognosis, and design a plan of care (2). All of the data gathered, the physical therapy diagnosis, prognostic predictions, and patient goals are integrated and incorporated into establishing a plan of care (2). The plan of care for the individual with ALS may include recommendations for therapeutic exercise; interventions for pain, muscle cramps, spasticity, fatigue, and respiratory dysfunction; and assistive, orthotic, supportive, and/or adaptive devices.

THERAPEUTIC EXERCISE

Therapeutic exercise includes a broad group of activities intended to (1) prevent dysfunction; and, (2) maintain or improve strength, mobility, flexibility, endurance, cardiovascular fitness, breathing, coordination, motor function, posture, skill, and balance (2,3). Therapeutic exercise is an important component of a physical therapy plan of care for a person with ALS, and various types of exercises may be recommended—strengthening, ROM, stretching, and endurance.

Strengthening exercises may be isometric, isotonic, or isokinetic. Isometric exercises involve contracting a muscle, but no joint movement, and are used to maintain muscle strength. Isotonic exercises may be concentric (muscle shortening) or eccentric (muscle lengthening) and involve muscle contraction and movement of the joint during the contraction. They may be performed with or without weights or resistance and are used to increase muscle strength and prevent muscle wasting. Isokinetic exercise involves moving the joint at a constant velocity with varying resistance and requires specialized equipment (3).

It is not known whether muscles affected by ALS can be improved through strengthening exercises. Thus strengthening exercises are usually prescribed for unaffected muscles. When designing a strengthening exercise program for an individual with ALS, the PT considers two factors: (1) prevention of overuse/overwork fatigue/damage, the permanent or temporary loss of muscle strength due to excessive exercise; and (2) disuse atrophy, the lack of use leading to a decrease in muscle mass, strength, and endurance. There is research evidence from people with other neuromuscular diseases that highly repetitive or heavy resistance exercises can cause overwork damage in weakened, denervated muscle. On the other hand, a marked decrease in activity level because of ALS can lead to cardiovascular deconditioning and disuse weakness beyond the amount caused by the disease itself. Therefore, the PT will carefully monitor the intensity of the exercise program so as not to unduly cause fatigue, while simultaneously promoting optimal use of intact muscle groups.

Range of motion exercises involve moving each joint through the normal extent of movement. Active range of motion exercises are performed independently, whereas active-assisted range of motion exercises involve using an external force (mechanical device or another person) to assist the individual to perform the movement. Passive range of motion exercises involve the use of an external force to perform the movement without any voluntary muscle contraction from the individual. Range of motion exercises may be recommended to (1) prevent the development of limited mobility due to muscle shortening and/or tightness in the joint capsule, ligaments, and tendons (contractures); and (2) to maintain joint mobility and muscle strength (3).

Stretching exercises are designed to lengthen shortened soft tissue, such as muscle, thereby increasing range of motion. Stretching exercises differ from range of motion exercises. With range of motion exercises the joint to be exercised is moved, whereas with stretching exercises a position of stretch is maintained for a period of time. Stretching exercises may include manual passive stretching, mechanical passive stretching, and flexibility exercises (self-stretching).

Endurance exercises involve sustained, rhythmic movements of large muscle groups and include walking, swimming, rowing, and stationary bicycling. They may be recommended to increase or maintain aerobic capacity and to prevent deconditioning.

Regardless of the type of exercises, they should be performed in moderation, and you should not exercise to the point of fatigue.

The literature describing and examining the efficacy of exercise programs for people with ALS is very limited. In one study by Bohannon, a 56-year-old non-ambulatory woman with ALS performed resistive exercises to her upper extremities using what is termed *proprioceptive neuromuscular facilitation* patterns over a period of 75 days. Isometric strength measurements of nine upper extremity muscle groups using a strain gauge obtained initially and at the conclusion of the study showed that 14 muscles had increased strength (7%–96%), whereas four muscles lost strength (10%–21%). Baseline manual muscle test scores for the upper extremities remained unchanged after training. Although no specific functional tests were performed in this study, the author reported that the patient noted improvement in transfers and wheelchair propulsion (4). In another study by Sanjak and coworkers, a 46-year-old man with ALS performed upper extremity and lower extremity strengthening exercises using an Air-Dyne bicycle ergometer for six weeks. The man had only upper motor neuron signs in the upper extremities and mixed upper and lower motor neuron signs in the lower extremities. Isokinetic strength and cardiopulmonary responses to exercise improved in the upper extremities following two weeks of training, but not in the lower extremities (5). Although functional benefits have yet to be determined, exercise programs may have positive physiologic and psychological effects for patients with ALS, especially when implemented before significant muscular atrophy occurs. More research needs to be done in this area.

INTERVENTIONS FOR PAIN, MUSCLE CRAMPS, SPASTICITY, AND FATIGUE

People with ALS may experience a variety of symptoms such as pain, muscle cramps, spasticity, and fatigue.

Pain may have several causes. It may be directly caused by muscle strains, joint sprains, acute injuries (such as from falls), spasticity, and preexisting conditions such as arthritis. Indirectly, weakness can produce pain because it may result in shortened muscles (contractures) or hypomobile joints that may cause pain when stretched. Compensatory movement patterns may develop due to muscle weakness; as a result, muscles and surrounding soft tissues and joints may be injured. Strong muscles may be overused, leading to pain, and joints may become unstable or sublux due to muscle weakness. In addition, poor resting positions may strain muscles or unstable joints. People with ALS most commonly develop pain in the shoulder joint. Because the muscles around the shoulder become weak, he is unable to move his arm. As a result, the soft tissues around the shoulder become tight, causing a "frozen shoulder."

Depending on the cause of the pain, the PT may recommend or perform range of motion exercises, joint mobilizations, massage, passive stretching, and education about correct positioning and joint protection. In addition, she may use physical agents and electrotherapeutic modalities to address the pain. Physical agents include thermal modalities such as superficial heat (hot packs), deep heat (ultrasound, diathermy), and cryotherapy (cold packs, ice massage). Electrotherapeutic modalities may include transcutaneous electrical nerve stimulation (TENS) and iontophoresis, the introduction of topically applied medication prescribed by a physician into the skin using electrical stimulation (2).

A muscle cramp is an abrupt, involuntary, and painful muscle shortening that is accompanied by knotting. Muscle cramps are common in the quadriceps (front thigh) muscles, the hamstring (back thigh) muscles, and the gastrocnemieus (calf) muscles, but it can also occur in the abdomen, arms, neck, and jaw (6). Muscle cramps can be alleviated and addressed by massage and stretching.

Spasticity is a state of sustained muscle tension (resistance) when the muscle is moved passively (6). Heat and cold can temporarily decrease spasticity. In addition, physical therapists can perform and show caregivers slow, prolonged stretches and passive ROM exercises to help relieve spasticity.

Fatigue is a common symptom of ALS and can be helped by a program of energy conservation. These suggestions for changing daily routines and lifestyles will minimize fatigue and avoid exhaustion. Principles of energy conservation include:

1. *Balancing rest and activity.* Resting is one of the best ways to manage symptoms of fatigue and can be accomplished in various ways: total body rest (nap), resting a specific joint or muscle group, and emotional rest (relaxing). It is important to learn your own tolerance and rest before the point of fatigue, take a "time-out" if an activity becomes too tiring, and schedule rest breaks into daily routines, such as taking a nap or resting 10 minutes out of every hour.

2. *Organizing work.* This may include by planning ahead, scheduling, setting priorities, and pacing; alternate periods of work, activity and exercise with rest periods; spread activities that are difficult or tiring throughout the day; alternate heavy jobs with light ones and change positions often

3. *Making work easier.* Is the task necessary? Is there an easier way to do it? Can some of it be done tomorrow? Can someone else do it?

4. *Working in comfort.* This can be accomplished by organizing work areas; placing articles between shoulder and waist level for easy reach; minimizing unnecessary straining, stooping, twisting and bending; siting comfortably instead of standing (25% of your energy can be saved); and using recommended assistive devices your therapist recommends.

5. *Relaxing.* Stress is fatiguing. It is important to work at a comfortable pace and schedule time to relax. Find pleasant relaxing activities and outlets.

6. *Planning work or play.* These activities should be done at times of the day when energy is the highest. In addition, plan rest periods when considering daily schedules, and save energy for the activities you most enjoy.

ASSISTIVE DEVICES—AMBULATORY (WALKING) AIDS

An assistive device is a piece of equipment that is used to provide support or stability while walking. Because of muscle weakness, balance problems, and/or spasticity, the PT may recommend a walking aid to enhance mobility and provide additional support. The PT will help determine which aid will best meet your needs, will determine the correct height for the walking aid, and will provide instruction on its proper use. The type of assistive device recommended is determined by the amount of leg and trunk weakness, mobility and strength of the arms, extent and rate of progression of the disease, acceptance of the aid, and economic constraints. In addition, she can also provide information on where to purchase the walking aid.

Three main categories of walking aids are canes, crutches, and walkers.

Canes

Canes provide minimal to moderate support. A cane is carried in the hand opposite to the affected leg and requires good upper extremity (arm) strength. Canes can be used on stairs. See Table 7-1.

Table 7-1. Types of Canes

Standard wooden	Least expensive; can be adjusted shorter, not longer; may wobble
Aluminum adjustable	Easily adjustable for various heights; handle may be slippery
Aluminum adjustable with angled handle, flattened grip	Easily adjustable for various heights; weight directed over tip in contact with floor; easier to grasp for those with hand muscle weakness
Quad cane	Greater stability than straight cane, but all tips must be in contact with the ground for stability; size of base can vary; heavier to lift

Crutches

Few people with ALS use crutches because they often find them too bulky and extremely difficult to manage (Table 7-2).

Walkers

Walkers provide greater support than canes and crutches but use up more space. Various types are available and they can be modified to suit your walking environments and needs (Table 7-3).

ORTHOTIC DEVICES

An *orthotic device* is used to correct or straighten a deformity or to provide support. Orthoses may be recommended for people with ALS to (1) improve function by offering support to weakened muscles and the joints they surround, (2) decrease the stress on compensatory muscles, (3) minimize local or general muscle fatigue, (4) prevent deformity, and (5) conserve energy.

Table 7-2. Types of Crutches

Standard axillary crutch (wooden or aluminum)	Requires good arm and trunk strength; requires good balance
Adjustable aluminum Lofstrand crutch (forearm, Canadian)	Handle can be freed for standing tasks without having to release the crutch; requires good arm and trunk strength
Adjustable aluminum platform crutch on the platform	Upper extremity weight can be placed

Ankle-foot orthoses (AFOs) are probably the most common type of orthotic devices recommended. Prefabricated AFOs may be purchased "off the shelf" or they may be custom-made. The orthoses must be lightweight to allow the user to expend the least amount of energy while using the device.

An AFO may be solid or hinged at the ankle joint; each has advantages and disadvantages. A solid AFO is usually prescribed for quadriceps (front thigh) muscle weakness in addition to ankle weakness and instability. Because the ankle is held in a fixed position, getting up from sitting, going up and down stairs, and going up inclines may be difficult. A person with mild ankle weakness and adequate knee muscle strength during walking may be prescribed a hinged AFO, which allows a certain degree of ankle motion. The degree of ankle motion can be adjusted depending on your stability and need for support.

SUPPORTIVE DEVICES

Supportive devices include therapeutic appliances that are designed to support weak or ineffective joints or muscles. People with ALS may develop cervical extensor muscle weakness (muscles at the back of the neck). Early complaints may

Table 7-3. Types of Walkers

Standard aluminum	Least expensive; very stable; adjustable; must be picked up and lowered to take steps; may be heavy to lift
Aluminum with wheels	Rolls forward easily; does not need to be lifted; may move too quickly
Folding aluminum with or without wheels with rear brakes	Rear brakes secure walker when taking steps; stores easily; portable
Specialized wheeled walker	Most expensive; large wheels good outdoors or on rough ground

include neck stiffness, heaviness, and fatigue in holding up the head. You may notice difficulties in keeping the head upright with unexpected movements. If weakness is more severe, the head may begin to fall forward (6). The PT may recommend a neck collar to help with this *cervical extensor* muscle weakness. The type of collar recommended depends on the amount of weakness and its acceptance by the user. Several different types of collars can support the head, protect weakened muscles, and prevent further deformity.

A soft, foam collar may be recommended for mild to moderate weakness. This type of collar limits neck movements to a certain degree and usually is comfortable and well-tolerated.

A semirigid collar, such as the Philadelphia™ collar or Newport collar may be recommended for moderate to severe weakness. If the user has a tracheostomy, a Miami-J® collar or a similar collar that allows for anterior neck access will be prescribed. These collars provide firm support, but they can be very warm and may make the wearer feel confined.

These devices may not be effective when severe or intractable neck droop is present, in which case you may be referred to an orthotist or biomedical engineer for a custom-made neck collar.

ADAPTIVE DEVICES

Adaptive devices are apparatuses or pieces of equipment that are designed and fabricated to improve performance of *activities of daily living.*

People with ALS who have leg weakness may find it difficult to get up from a chair. Initially, difficulty rising from a seated position to standing may be helped by placing a firm cushion, 2 to 3 inches thick, under the buttocks in the chair so that the hips are higher than the knees. Or, the chair itself may be raised by placing the legs in prefabricated blocks to make rising easier. Self-powered lifting cushions, such as the UPlift Seat Assist™ are relatively inexpensive, portable devices that provide assistance for rising to standing and gently ease the body's weight into the chair using hydropneumatics. These devices can be purchased through several catalog suppliers. Although much more expensive, powered seat lift recliner chairs are also available for rental or purchase. They enable a person to rise to a standing position or recline by activating an electric control.

A transfer board or sliding board is a device made of plastic or wood with a very smooth surface. It can be used if you are unable to stand because of leg weakness, to move from bed to chair, or to transfer in and out of a wheelchair. The transfer board may be used alone if you have adequate arm strength and good sitting balance, or you can be assisted by another person.

People who have difficulty transferring from place to place (bed to chair, chair to a commode, and so forth), even with the assistance of a caregiver, may require a mechanical lift. Lifts most frequently recommended are the Easy Pivot™, the Hoyer Lift, and the Trans-Aid Patient Lifter.

Chair glides and stairway lifts can be purchased for people who live in multi-level homes but who cannot or should not climb stairs. They are measured and custom-made for individual staircases and are quite expensive. Insurance companies usually do not reimburse for stairway lifts, but some medical supply companies offer "rent-to-own" options. In addition, local ALSA chapters and/or Muscular Dystrophy Association chapters may have lifts that have been recycled.

Other useful devices are transfer belts and swivel cushions/seats. Transfer belts vary in design, but they all allow a caregiver to grasp the belt instead of the individual during transfers. This makes transfers easier on the caregiver and prevents pulling on the arms, which may cause shoulder problems. Swivel cushions/seats are lightweight, cushioned seats that swivel in both directions and make getting in and out of a car easier.

INTERVENTIONS FOR PULMONARY DYSFUNCTION

People with ALS may have difficulty coughing and may develop shortness of breath and/or pulmonary infections. Physical therapists can perform or show caregivers techniques that optimize the cough mechanism and gas exchange and that reduce the accumulation of lung secretions and facilitate their removal.

A person with ALS may find it difficult to generate enough force to cough. This may be due to muscle weakness, the inability to close the glottis, or an inability to build up enough pressure in the chest cavity or the position. To increase the effectiveness of a cough:

1. If possible, sit in a forward-leaning position (sitting is usually best). This pushes up the diaphragm. Some people are able to cough more effectively in a side-lying position.

2. Take in the biggest breath possible.

3. If you are able to, place both hands (one on top of the other) in the center of the abdomen, just below the chest or encircle the arms around the rib cage (a caregiver can assist at this step). Apply pressure as the breath is let out and a cough is attempted. A variation is to squeeze the arms against the side of the chest.

4. "Huff" with the mouth open.

5. If this is not possible, the physical therapist can show the caregiver other techniques to assist with coughing.

Postural drainage and manual techniques such as percussion and vibration can decrease the retention of secretions and assist the person with ALS to mobilize secretions. In addition, breathing exercises can be taught that will maximize ventilation (gas exchange within the lungs).

In addition, a person with ALS who experiences shortness of breath may benefit from resting in relaxed positions.

SUMMARY

"Rehabilitaire" (the Latin root of rehabilitate) denotes "to supply again with means." Physical therapy is an integral part of the rehabilitation team and can provide education and direct intervention to address various problems seen throughout the course of ALS.

REFERENCES

1. Dal Bello-Haas V, Kloos A, Mitsumoto H. Physical therapy for the stages of amyotrophic lateral sclerosis: A case report. *Phys Ther* 1998; 78(12):1312–1324.
2. The American Physical Therapy Association. Guide to physical therapy practice. *J Am Phys Ther Assn* 1997; 77(11): PAGES.
3. Kisner C, Colby LA. *Therapeutic exercise: Foundations and techniques,* 3rd ed. Philadelphia: FA Davis, YEAR.
4. Bohannon RW. Results of resistance exercise on a patient with amyotrophic lateral sclerosis. *Phys Ther* 1983; 63(6):965–968.
5. Sanjak M, Paulson D, Sufit R, et al. Physiologic and metabolic response to progressive and prolonged exercise in amyotrophic lateral sclerosis. *Neurology* 1987; 37:1217–1220.
6. Mitsumoto H, Chad DA, Pioro EP. *Amyotrophic lateral sclerosis.* Philadelphia: FA Davis, 1998.
7. Dal Bello-Haas V, Kloos AD, Mitsumoto H. Physical therapy for a patient through six stages of amyootrophic lateral sclerosis. *Phys Ther* 1998;78:1312–1324.

8

Occupational Therapy

Patricia Casey, MS, OTR/L

Occupational therapy (OT) is a systematic therapeutic program designed to maximize a person's functional capacity. Independence is usually the goal. However, ALS presents unique challenges as progressive physical changes occur, and the purpose of occupational therapy is to maintain or improve the self-care abilities of the person with the disease. The functional abilities of the caregiver are also a major concern. Occupational therapists should focus on your immediate problems and present possible solutions for them. An experienced therapist will try to suggest fairly simple solutions without offering "too much" information or "too many" alternatives. Therapists must remember that a person changes the way he performs a task only if the change makes accomplishing the task easier, and nobody changes the way he does something unless he must.

For psychological and physical benefit the person with ALS should continue to exercise for as long as possible. Table 8-1 summarizes an appropriate exercise program.

Table 8-1. Exercises for Patients with ALS

Breathing
Breathe in a big breath through your nose, with your mouth closed. Pucker your lips as if you are going to whistle. Slowly blow out as long as you can, pulling your abdomen in as best as you can. Do this only three times at any given time. You may do this once every hour during the day (10–15 times per day).

Arm Exercises
Lie on your back on your bed. Scoot down on the bed so you have enough room to raise your arms over your head. Then raise both arms over your head with your elbows bent. Use one hand to help lift the other if needed. If your shoulders are stiff, raise them as far as they will go. Rest your hands on your chin, your forehead, or the pillow under your head. Press your elbows and shoulderblades into the pillow. Once you have them in the best position, gently make small circles at the shoulder to stretch the ligaments and tendons around the shoulder joints. You will feel stretching or pulling in your muscles, but you should not feel sharp pains. If you do experience pain, stop and gently lower your arms. Call your physician. This is a gentle exercise to maintain your range of motion and to prevent stiffening of the shoulder joint. Raise your arms in this manner once in the morning before you get out of bed and once in the evening before you go to sleep. The (10) rotations should provide enough stretching.

Leg Exercises
These exercises can be done once an hour while you are sitting in a firm chair. Raise each leg with knee straight and your toes pulled toward you as far as they will go. Rotate your foot three times each way. Lower that leg. Raise the other leg. Do the same motions. Repeat these exercises at least once per hour, alternating legs three times.

Hand Exercises
Turn both palms up. Arms should be held with elbows against your ribs. Pretend you are pulling your fingers into a ball of clay and you want to make your fingerprints in the clay. Aim your thumb toward your little finger. Don't forget to look at each finger while you are pulling. Then turn your hands over and pretend you are pushing your fingers into the clay until they are fully outstretched. Then, with fingers extended, pull your wrist back. Feel the stretch. Repeat this once an hour.

Walking
Walk every hour. Make an imaginary exercise path inside your home or office. Stand up and walk every hour. Go as far as you are comfortable, 1 minute, 5 minutes, or 10 minutes. If you cannot walk, stand by your walker, desk, or kitchen counter for balance and shift weight from one foot to the other for five minutes every hour.

The advice of an occupational therapist will be especially helpful when you must make environmental adaptations and need new information about:

- assistive devices
- practical solutions for self-care or work station activities
- upper extremity joint mobility and support
- postural support and control
- home modifications
- collaboration with physical therapy, speech therapy, nutrition, nursing and social service

Environmental adaptations for ALS include physical, mechanical, or procedural changes needed to accomplish activities of daily living (ADLs). Adaptation may require assistive devices or medical equipment, proper placement of furniture, utensils, or tools, or a change in the method of operation (i.e., pushing or sliding an object instead of lifting or carrying it).

Several factors affect the ability to make adaptations to the physical changes that occur with progression of the disease. People with ALS and their caregivers may have different perceptions of immediate and long-term needs and the degree to which increasing physical limitations will affect their lives. They may be in different stages of the grieving process, with denial and depression making any change more difficult. They may have different learning and problem-solving capacities that limit resolution. Finally, families have different lifestyles and varying social and financial resources. All these factors need to be considered when a therapist assesses environmental adaptations for short-term and long-term needs.

Progressive physical limitations require the use of a variety of assistive devices (Table 8-2). The use of these appliances may mean modifying time, space, and the location of activities. It will eventually become necessary for a caregiver to perform activities such as feeding, washing, and dressing. Occupational therapy in your home as well as in the clinic permits periodic reevaluation to assess your changing family priorities, the need for additional information, and your readiness to adapt the environment to maintain or improve function.

Recommendations for environmental adaptations are based on physical limitation rather than on stage of the disease because a patient may present with more or less disability at any stage. Along with the physical needs of the person with ALS, the therapist must consider the abilities of caregivers and the availability of insurance (Medicare, public assistance, managed care policies) to purchase assistive equipment and environmental adaptations.

Table 8-2. Recommended Assistive Equipment and Devices

Lightweight manual wheelchairs
    Companion model: Everest and Jennings (E&J)
    Other models with or without quick release wheels: E&J, Invacare, Quickie

---

Power or manual wheelchair
    with Tilt-in-Space frame
    with or without Reclining back
    with attendant control, ventilator add-ons, environmental control: E&J, Invacare, Quickie

---

Adult Stroller: Pogon

Motorized carts (POV) with adjustable tillers, hydraulic seat options, seating options

---

Cushions and seating systems: air, gel, gel/foam, contour, pressure-relief
    Gel or T-foam cushions: Jay, Roho, Varilite, Ultimate
    High-back seating (make sure a headrest bracket can be attached),
        With lateral supports or contoured low-back with lateral supports
        With headrest supports, ventilator trays, electronics to accommodate joystick or head control, environmental control switches, remote control

---

Wheelchair ramps: prefabricated, custom-made

Power seat lift recliner chair: purchase or rent

Padded shower commode on casters with U-shaped cushion, push handles, footrests:
    Activeaid models JTG 605, 462-5, 463-5, 496; Invacare, Lumex

---

Bath tub seat and bench, bathtub lift, bathtub attachment with separating sling or bath sling:
    Hoyer, Transaid, Invacare, Lumex

Patient lift with separating sling: Hoyer, Transaid, Invacare; Easy Pivot

---

Hand devices: Enrichments catalog for self-care, work, leisure activities

---

Hand splints, wrist supports, mobile arm supports: OT evaluation

---

Infant monitor: Fisher Price

WALKING WITH ASSISTANCE

Frequent falls occur when ankle weakness results in "drop foot" and weakness in the quadriceps causes the knees to "give out." Lightweight, plastic ankle-foot orthoses (AFOs) with 5–10 degrees of plantar flexion can usually stabilize walking. People who wear braces and live in apartments or homes with stairs are a problem because standard orthoses usually decrease the ability to climb stairs. Articulating ankle joints may be considered when prescribing braces, but these preclude the floor reaction effect of the brace that is necessary for knee stability. Careful assessment is required by a physical therapist and an orthotist, a specialist in fitting supportive devices of various types.

If upper extremity weakness is severe, a rolling walker may be helpful because it need not be lifted for smooth ambulation. A gait belt is often useful when assisted ambulation is necessary.

Trilevel, bilevel, and two-story homes with turning stairways are the most difficult to maneuver. Solutions depend on family resources. Stair lifts are a solution for families who are unable or unwilling to move. It is possible to rent stair lifts, which help in short-term and long-term planning. The most feasible solution may be to move the patient to the most accessible level of the home, with some changes made for toileting and bathing needs. Finally, porch lifts can be installed inside homes to gain access to two levels with easy access to front and back doors, garages, and bathrooms.

WALKING WHEN ENDURANCE IS LIMITED

Once walking is affected by weakness, decreased endurance, or fatigability, assistive equipment will be required for continued functioning at work, in the home or community, and for leisure. Careful selection of manual and power wheelchairs with seating systems should be determined by the person with ALS, the therapist, and a seating specialist, and depends on the rate of disease progression. Most patients with lower extremity weakness require a lightweight manual wheelchair that can be placed easily in the back seat or trunk of a car. The caregiver's ability to lift and transport a wheelchair must be considered when prescribing such equipment. A suitable lightweight gel or dense foam cushion is always needed for adequate trunk and pelvic support. An adult stroller may be more supportive than a wheelchair for patients who have neck and shoulder weakness because it has a high back and a slightly reclined seat/back angle and offers the advantage of easy portability. A reclining back wheelchair is bulky and difficult to transport in a car, although it sometimes is useful for people with neck and trunk weakness who remain at home or use a van with a lift. The tilt-in-space style frame offers more relief for seat, low-back, shoulder, and neck pressure areas than the recliner back. The wheelchair prescription should be determined in consultation with an occupational therapist or physical therapist and a seating specialist.

Some people with ALS, especially those who are working or are socially active, are interested in using motorized scooters. The rental or loan of such equipment is appropriate if the rate of progression of the disease is slow to moderate. Sitting posture, shoulder and hand function, and hip strength must be assessed to ensure proper seating support. An adjustable tiller control or a hydraulic seat may be necessary.

Depending on the family's needs and resources, information may be provided about wheelchair racks and lifts, as well as lifts for motorized scooters and power wheelchairs for cars and vans.

When fatigability results in poor walking endurance, respiratory function may be at risk (see Chapter 12). Some thought may have already been given to the possibility of needing ventilator assistance, and guidance is needed in selecting a power recliner or manual wheelchair with a ventilator tray.

Once the decision is made that a wheelchair is needed, easy entrance and exit from the house, car, and office must be considered. Portable wheelchair ramps provide the simplest means of negotiating one or two steps. Two motorcycle ramps are usually less expensive than a single wheelchair ramp. Wooden or metal ramps come in all shapes and sizes, depending on the configuration of front doors, walkways, shrubbery, and the location of your house in relation to the sidewalk. Walkways along the side of the house allow space for a long ramp. A Z-shaped ramp is necessary when a short frontyard or backyard does not provide adequate length for a safe, long incline. A platform level at the door before the ramp inclines is needed to rest the wheelchair safely while opening and closing the door. Ramp inclines 1:12 (1-inch incline for every foot of distance) but not more than 1.5:12 are safe and easy to climb. Hydraulic porch lifts or elevators may be the most economical or even the only architectural choice for some homes. Local building ordinances must be taken into account.

TRUNK AND HIP WEAKNESS

Initially, difficulty rising from a seated position to a standing position may simply require adding a firm 2" or 3" cushion to the sitting surface. Sometimes it is necessary to sit on a firm chair with supportive back and arms. More often the purchase or rental of a power seat lift recliner chair will be needed to provide independent change of position either to a standing, seated, or reclined position. In the bathroom, using a plastic molded raised toilet seat is a simple solution for initial weakness. A padded shower commode with a U-shaped cushion on casters incorporates features required for problems of progressive weakness. It can be used over the toilet by the patient and easily removed by other family members. It provides a high seat and back support, removable armrests, and a large opening for hygiene purposes. It can be placed at the bedside to avoid the hazards of walking to the bathroom at night.

Various bathtub seats, benches, lifts, and accessories are available to enhance both independent bathing and assisted bathing. Their selection depends on the design of the bathroom and willingness to make minor changes if expensive renovation is not feasible. A tiled floor with a recessed drain allows access to a remodeled shower area using a rolling shower commode. A standard shower stall with a 3"–4" rim can be modified with a simple wood deck and removable ramp for access with a shower commode. Bathroom doors can widened with inexpensive offset hinges. Commode chairs on casters usually clear doors because they measure only 20–21 inches in width.

Early use of a full electric bed (one that raises from the floor electrically) to facilitate safe standing and sitting can save energy and maintain independence. If space is adequate, a hospital bed frame (80") without a headboard can be clamped to an extra-long twin bed frame (80") to form a king-size bed, allowing spouses to continue sleeping together while providing power-operated assistance for positioning support. Some insurance companies underwrite a queen- or king-size electric bed, but these beds usually do not raise to assist standing; other companies cover only hospital beds.

When standing is no longer possible, a hydraulic or mechanical lift can be used for lifting in and out of bed, wheelchair, commode, seat lift recliner chair, or car. A full-size separating sling is easily placed under the patient and removed without lifting him. The extra-long model provides head and neck support. New pivot lifts facilitate transfers and toileting.

Electric ceiling lifts are commercially available but are expensive. Less expensive adaptations have been devised by some families to provide consistent, safe, and easy lifting. One innovative person devised a ceiling lift using a garage door opener track and motor with an attached swivel bar (from a standard lift) and sling. Another family living in a bilevel home installed an I-beam and quarter-ton hoist on the ceiling. An attached swivel bar and sling allowed transport of the patient over the stairwell from top to ground level. The set of lower steps were placed on rollers. When they were rolled out of the way, the wheelchair could be positioned directly below the hoist. This inexpensive renovation (under $2,000) allowed the family safe and easy access to both levels of their home. It was considerably less expensive than installing an elevator or double stair lift. It also precluded the need to move to a one-level home.

NECK AND SHOULDER WEAKNESS

Self-care, work, and leisure activities are difficult to perform when the neck and shoulder muscles are weak. Assistive devices will be needed to promote proper positioning and support, to relieve strained muscles, and to allow continued performance of desired activities. Patients with mild to moderate weakness of the neck and shoulders may request a soft cervical collar or a clavicle splint to provide support. A plastazote Philadelphia collar offers additional support without restricting neck muscles, but patients cannot eat, speak, or drive a car while wearing this appliance. It also may not provide adequate head support while walking. The Headmaster lightweight tubular frame collar gives unrestricted neck support with adequate head support. The Oxford wire spring support collar allows some head motion for eating and speaking and gives lightweight support while walking. It also offers unrestricted neck support for suctioning or mechanical ventilation to patients who have a tracheostomy. A sterno-occipital-mandibular immobilizer (SOMI) assures adequate head and neck control while walking or sitting. A simple sling should provide maximum support for frail upper extremities and minimize pressure on weak shoulder and neck muscles. Arm support while sitting can be provided by an adjustable overbed table and properly positioned pillows.

UPPER EXTREMITY WEAKNESS

Weakness and atrophy in the shoulders and upper arms may prevent placing the hand in a functional position. Weakness in the elbow, forearm, wrist, and hand limit using the hand to manipulate tools and utensils for self-care, work, or leisure activities. Intrinsic muscle weakness and atrophy affect grasp and prehension. Because many assistive devices are available for these conditions, careful selection is required to promote function for as long as possible and reduce frustration for both patient and caregiver.

Mobile arm supports (MAS) allow both horizontal and vertical motion. Additional features can provide wrist support and allow for limited supination. Self-feeding and some grooming and personal care can be accomplished with the MAS once materials have been set up. It is possible to operate computer keyboards and communication devices using the MAS system.

Ergonomic computer keyboard forearm supports to prevent carpal tunnel syndrome are now available. They resemble the MAS but do not have the same horizontal range for shoulder motions or vertical range for reaching the face and mouth. However, wrist supports could be riveted to the forearm trough. These are useful at home or work for computer enthusiasts.

Other useful devices for eating include lightweight wrist splints, utensil holders, foam or cork tubes for utensils, plastic or long-handled utensils, extra-long straws, lightweight large-handled cups, plate guards, and suction holders or non-skid pads. Key holders, doorknob extenders, light switch extension levers, lightweight reachers, self-opening scissors, and cardholders assist with some usual daily activities. Button and zipper hooks, long-handled sponges, lightweight electric shavers, an adapted floss holder, a rechargeable electric toothbrush with rotary brush, and velcro fasteners facilitate hygiene, grooming, and dressing.

Communication aids include use of a rubber thumb, pencil grips, writing splints, Magic Slate or MagnaDoodle® (erasable writing boards), book holders, tilt-top overbed table, lap-style AbleTable®, portable phone, speaker phone, use of telecommunication devices for the deaf (TDD) assistance through the phone company, infant monitor system, or small bell. Various augmentative electronic speech devices are used by those who have adequate hand function to operate a keyboard, and single switch computer systems are available for those who do not.

COMFORT IN BED

When muscle atrophy affects the shoulder and pelvic areas, artificial padding will be needed for sleeping comfort. Also, comfort must be ensured for patients who spend more time in bed. Gel and foam mattresses with sheepskin padding are used by some people with ALS. Contour neck pillows, foam boots, elbow and heel pads, and blanket supports are sometimes helpful. An adequate communication system should be in place by this time whether it is activated by eyeblinks, facial expressions, or a computer with a speech synthesizer.

SUMMARY

ALS initially forces a person to adapt to his environment. He changes the way he performs tasks in order to function as independently as possible. As weakness increases, however, the environment must be adapted to fit the patient's and caregiver's needs, to make function possible, if not easier. Each patient and family has its priorities, and each has its own style, format, and unique sense of timing. The occupational therapist intervenes in this dynamic process to help both patient and caregiver function as well as is possible for as long as is feasible.

SUGGESTED READING

1. *ALS: Maintaining Mobility.* New York: Muscular Dystrophy Association, 1987.

2. Caroscio J (ed). *Amyotrophic lateral sclerosis: A guide for patient care.* New York: Thieme Medical Publishers, 1986.

3. Foyder JE. *Family caregiver's guide.* Cincinnati: Futuro Company, 1985.

4. Hamilton L. *Why didn't somebody tell me about these things?* Shawnee Mission, KS: Intercollegiate Press, 1984.

5. *Living with ALS.* A series of manuals. Woodland Hills, CA: ALS Association, 1997.

9

Wheelchair Selection

Catherine Balsdon Richer, OTR/L

The prospect of obtaining a wheelchair can be daunting. Gone are the days when you go to your neighborhood drugstore and pick out your wheelchair from a shelf filled with "one size fits all" models. With the recent advances in technology and the savvy of today's health care consumers, wheelchairs can now be custom-prescribed and custom-built for the individual user. This means choices for you as a consumer—and plenty of them! This chapter takes you through the process of selecting a wheelchair system and answers some questions most commonly asked by consumers.

When Is It "Time" to Get a Wheelchair?

When is the "right time" to get a wheelchair? Good question—and a difficult one at that. Should you wait until your doctor tells you it is time? Should you wait until you are at risk for falling when you walk? Probably not. Reflect back on your lifestyle over recent weeks, or months, or over the past year. Have you given up activities that are enjoyable or meaningful to you because you have difficulty walking? Is most of your strength and energy being used up for locomotion? If your answer to either of these questions is yes, consider this—if using a wheelchair allowed you to conserve precious energy or to resume activities that you value, would it be worth it? This is a very individual decision and one that only you can make based on your personal values and beliefs. Consult your loved ones—they often have useful insight.

For some people, the need to use a wheelchair seems to be a marker of how far the disease has progressed and from that moment on "things can only get worse." This certainly is not the case. Your decision to use a wheelchair need not be a self-imposed, life-long sentence of sitting. Early on in the disease process, a wheelchair may be used intermittently for traversing long distances such as the local mall or park or when traveling—a wise way to conserve energy. It may be premature for you to purchase a permanent wheelchair system at this time; you currently do not need it for "regular" use, and your needs probably are going to change over time as your symptoms change. In this instance, obtaining a wheelchair on a temporary basis (short-term rental or loan from your local ALSA chapter, church, friends, or family) makes sense. This way your resources (personal or medical insurances) remain intact for your future needs. Also, if you are undecided about whether you "need" a wheelchair, the temporary use of one is a great way to test the waters and see if it makes a difference in the quality of your life. When you find yourself using the wheelchair regularly to perform activities throughout the day or week, it might then be the "right" time to consider purchasing a permanent wheelchair that is customized to your individual needs.

Can't I Just Go to the Store and Pick Out a Wheelchair?

Yes, you can. The greatest risk that you take in selecting and purchasing a wheelchair directly from a salesperson is that you purchase a piece of equipment that is not the most appropriate choice for you, particularly as your symptoms change. Some, although certainly not all, people who sell durable medical equipment such as wheelchairs have the medical background to fully appreciate the disease process. Model "XYZ" may be impressive from a showroom floor, but it may not meet your future needs. If you use your insurance benefits to purchase a wheelchair system that is not a good choice, your insurance source may deny covering a second wheelchair (because they expect that the first one they paid for should be meeting your needs). The expectation is that you will get it right the first time—this can be an expensive lesson to learn.

It may require a bit more time and effort on your part, but by seeking the input of a skilled professional you can be better assured you will receive a wheelchair system that is tailor-made to meet your individual needs both now and in the future. Look for a Wheelchair/Seating Clinic in your area; you may find one at many inpatient and outpatient rehabilitation centers. If no such clinic exists in your area, inquire at local hospitals that have an outpatient therapy department. The Rehabilitation Engineering Society of North America (RESNA) is an interdisciplinary association that is devoted to the advancement of assistive technology. RESNA publishes a list of their membership that can help you locate a specialist in wheelchair evaluations in your area.

Clinic-based wheelchair evaluations are most commonly done by an occupational therapist (OT) and/or a physical therapist (PT). He or she may work alone or in conjunction with a treatment team, which can consist of a physician, a rehabilitation engineer (who specializes in the design of the equipment), and/or an rehabilitation technology supplier (who will sell you the equipment). Even if there is no specialist in your geographic area, seeking the professional input of an OT or a PT is invaluable to the selection process. Your therapist may not know everything there is to know about wheelchair pieces and parts, but he or she is trained to evaluate your physical and functional status; a salesperson (dealer) can fill in the blanks about what equipment will best fulfill these needs.

It is essential that you obtain a physician's prescription for the therapy evaluation *before scheduling;* you will be required to produce this documentation for your evaluator. Also, most medical insurance companies require a physician's prescription or referral to consider funding the cost of the therapy visit(s) required to complete the full evaluation of your wheelchair system needs.

What Does a Wheelchair Evaluation Involve?

A thorough wheelchair evaluation can take a minimum of one lengthy visit to a clinic. Depending on the complexity of your needs and the complexity of the device, it may take a series of visits. Your initial contact with the evaluator will involve information gathering and should include:

- A thorough review of your medical history and ALS symptoms (including your pattern of muscle weakness, breathing and swallowing problems, skin problems—particularly on weight-bearing surfaces— weight loss, pain, and so forth), your vision, and any orthopaedic issues

- An evaluation of your ability to complete activities of daily living that are part of your everyday routine such as eating, dressing, bathing, toileting, transferring between seat surfaces, home management and work-based tasks, and leisure activities

- A discussion of the physical environments (indoor and outdoor) in which you will be using the device—home, workplace, church, local neighborhood, special events, and so forth. General physical layouts, specific door frame measurements, table and desk heights, vehicle information (for transport), and descriptions of any transitions (ramps, thresholds) are all valuable.

- A review of any mobility device(s) that you are currently using. How and where do you use it? How long have you had it? How was it purchased and from whom?

- Your goals—WHAT DO YOU WANT TO BE ABLE TO DO?

The more information you can provide the better. Don't forget to take your medical insurance information to the evaluation; in fact, it is a good idea to contact your insurance carrier *before* the evaluation to verify your coverage for durable medical equipment such as a wheelchair. Having a general idea of any potential out-of-pocket expense can certainly influence your decision making.

The evaluator will then complete a hands-on physical evaluation, during which he or she will assess your:

- sitting balance
- sitting posture and spinal alignment
- range of motion at all major joints (including ankles, knees, hips, back, shoulders, elbows, wrists, hands, and neck)
- arm and leg strength and muscle tone
- neck strength and head positioning
- hand function
- body measurements (to ensure a good fit of the wheelchair)

The information gleaned from the interview and physical evaluation is critical and heavily influences the recommendations your evaluator will make with regard to options in wheelchair styles and postural supports appropriate for you. The evaluation process is also meant to be collaborative. There should be open and honest dialogue between you and your therapist so that the best decisions possible will be made.

What Kind of Wheelchair System Is Right for Me?

A wheelchair system consists of the wheelchair itself—or "base"—and the postural supports or "seating" on or into which you sit.

Wheelchair Base Types

Manual Wheelchairs

Manual wheelchair frames consist of two small front wheels, called *casters* that swivel and are used to steer the wheelchair, and two larger rear wheels. They can be propelled using the arms and hands, the legs and feet, or both. The back and seat surfaces are fabric (nylon or vinyl) unless otherwise specified. There commonly are rear push handles that allow someone else to push you in the wheelchair if necessary. Arm and foot supports come with the wheelchair for your comfort and convenience.

Manual wheelchairs are categorized as follows:

1. *Standard weight.* Standard wheelchairs are heavy-duty wheelchairs that typically weigh between 40 and 50 pounds—the ones that you most often find offered as courtesy wheelchairs at the local shopping mall, hotel, or hospital. These frames tend to be very durable (almost indestructible) and are made from low-grade steel. The weight of the

frame, however, can make these wheelchairs difficult to push and to lift and load into your vehicle for transporting. They are the least expensive option in manual wheelchair frames.

2. *Lightweight.* Lightweight wheelchairs typically weigh between 30 and 40 pounds. The frames are made from strong lighter metals such as aluminum. The lighter weight makes them attractive for ease of propulsion (energy conservation) and transporting. There typically are more options available on lightweight frames (compared with standard frames) to allow customization of the wheelchair for your needs.

3. *Ultra-lightweight.* Ultra-lightweight wheelchairs are "sportier," have the most frame adjustments to customize for fit, and are most often prescribed for very active users (including wheelchair athletes) or for those whose limited energy reserves severely restrict their activity. The frames are constructed from extremely light, more expensive materials such as titanium or carbon fiber, which keeps the weight well under 30 pounds.

Power Wheelchairs

A power wheelchair base consists of two direct drive motors (one to power each drive wheel of the wheelchair), two deep-cycle rechargeable batteries, and the electronics or the "brains" of the wheelchair. Belt-driven power wheelchairs are still available, although they have fallen out of favor because of the greater power of the direct drive motor. A power wheelchair is operated using a drive control, most commonly a joystick (similar to video game joysticks).

Power wheelchairs are categorized according to the placement of the drive wheels that power the wheelchair:

1. *Rear Wheel Drive (RWD).* On an RWD power wheelchair, the drive wheels are positioned to the rear of the base, behind you. Rear wheel drive power wheelchairs tend to be quite stable because your weight and the weight of the wheelchair usually are well distributed across the total length of the wheelchair. As such, they are able to smoothly handle changes in gradient, such as ramps and curb cuts. Rear wheel drive power wheelchairs, however, require more space to maneuver in terms of turning radius (compared with a mid or front wheel drive power wheelchair) and therefore may not offer the accessibility needed to navigate within small or cluttered environments or to make tight turns from narrow hallways.

2. *Mid Wheel Drive (MWD).* The drive wheels on MWD wheelchairs are positioned directly under you. This effectively allows the wheelchair to spin on its base much like a "lazy Susan." MWD power wheelchairs offer the smallest full (360°) turning radius and therefore provide optimal access in tight spaces such as galley-style kitchens or bath-

rooms. Because the center of gravity of the wheelchair is shifted forward under the seat, this style of power base has a tendency for some forward instability, which feels like a slight forward rocking of the wheelchair with abrupt stops or when traveling down a ramp or hill. Although all MWD wheelchairs are equipped with front antitip devices to prevent forward tipping of the wheelchair, you may find this slight rocking motion unsettling. At higher speeds, MWD power wheelchairs tend to "fish-tail" a bit, which requires corrective steering on your part. In addition, they inherently have some difficulty negotiating steeper inclines—the antitip devices that protrude from the front of the wheelchair can lift the drive wheels off the ground in some situations.

3. *Front Wheel Drive (FWD).* The drive wheels on a front wheel drive power wheelchair are located in the most forward position of any other power wheelchair base. This style of wheelchair base offers optimal stability (compared with RWD and MWD bases), so no antitip devices are needed. FWD power wheelchairs navigate environmental obstacles such as curbs better than MWD or RWD wheelchairs and offer maneuverability and accessibility comparable to that of a MWD wheelchair.

There have been tremendous technological and design advances in the power wheelchair industry over recent years. The technology exists to allow you to operate a power wheelchair with almost any part of your body that you are able to move reliably, including your head, chin, arm, finger, foot, tongue, or even your breath. Although hand-operated joysticks are "standard," careful consideration must be given to what type of drive control will work best for you, based on your abilities and disease symptoms.

The electronics that run the drive control are mini, on-board computers. The wheelchair is programmed to operate in accordance with your abilities, needs, preferences, and environmental demands. There are varying levels of sophistication in the electronics packages that are used on power wheelchair bases. With more basic electronics packages, you may be able to adjust only the maximum speed. On the other hand, high-end electronics can offer you complete freedom in programming all parameters of how your wheelchair system will perform, including maximum speed, acceleration and deceleration, turning speeds, torque, and so forth. This allows the operation of the wheelchair to be fully customized to match your changing physical abilities. Some of the high-end electronics packages will also interface with other assistive technologies. Interfaces can permit your wheelchair control device to also run your computer, television, and lights.

Which Is Better for Me—
A Manual Wheelchair or a Power Wheelchair?

There are many factors to consider when deciding between a manual wheelchair and a power wheelchair. If you choose to purchase a manual wheelchair, there undoubtedly will be a point at which you are no longer able to propel yourself in it and will have to rely on someone else's assistance to move from one place to another. This is acceptable to some individuals. Other people choose power mobility because they want to be able to maintain independent mobility for as long as possible. This is a *very important and personal* decision—one that only you and your family can make. Power wheelchairs certainly cost more than manual wheelchairs, and the more sophisticated your power wheelchair system, the more the cost will increase. If you are required to make an out-of-pocket contribution toward the purchase price, the cost of a power wheelchair system may be prohibitive. Consideration must be given to how you will transport the device. How will you lift and load the device into your vehicle? Which vehicle do you travel in most? How large is the trunk or cargo area? Certainly, in the area of transportation, manual wheelchairs are more portable than power devices. A number of power bases are marketed as "portable," but they generally require some assembly and disassembly; taking apart and putting together a power wheelchair system may be a major inconvenience in inclement weather. In addition, despite the "portability" of a power base, someone still needs to be capable of lifting the motors and wheelchair frame (which together may range in weight from 30 pounds to over 60 pounds) in and out of your vehicle. One alternative would be to purchase a power hoist for your vehicle. Another choice would be to purchase a lift-equipped van that is designed for wheelchair transportation. Either of these options can involve a significant out-of-pocket expense because many insurance sources do not consider vehicle modification to be a medical necessity. Another option would be to purchase (or borrow) a second wheelchair (a manual one) for community outings.

Power-Operated Vehicles

The term *power-operated vehicles* refers to a category of devices more commonly known as "scooters." Power scooters typically have three wheels (although four-wheeled models are available), a platform base, a tiller style drive control that typically has handle bars (similar to those of a bicycle), a motor(s), and one or two deep-cycle rechargeable batteries. The throttle is usually either a thumb throttle or a squeeze throttle—either, however, requires relatively good hand control and muscle endurance to safely operate the device. By design, scooters are intended to be driven by users who have relatively good use of both arms and both hands and who have good control of their back muscles to maintain an erect sitting posture. It becomes infinitely more difficult to steer and maneuver this type of device when arm, hand, and/or back weakness worsens. Although this type of device may be well suited to you in the early stages of ALS, perhaps when long-distance walking is difficult, the use of a scooter may be limited in later months or years as your muscle weakness progresses. This may cause problems with funding of a new device if your medical insurance(s) was involved in the previous purchase of a scooter; most insurance companies consider a scooter to be a power mobility device and therefore may not fund a second power wheelchair device.

Customizing the Wheelchair Features for You

Prescription wheelchairs are built at the factory to meet your individual specifications. Once you have decided on a type of wheelchair base, manual or power, you and your evaluator will begin customizing the features and options to meet your personal needs.

Wheelchair Dimensions

The size of the wheelchair is heavily influenced by your height, weight, and body dimensions. However, accessibility is also a consideration. For example, your hip width may measure 18 inches, but a wheelchair with an 18-inch wide seat may be too wide overall to fit through your doorways. A 16-inch wide seat may be a bit skimpy but may keep the wheelchair narrow enough to allow free movement around your home.

Wheels

1. *Mag or molded.* The term mag refers to magnesium, which was originally used to create a wheel in the molded style. Mag wheels are now made of a solid or composite material, usually nylon, plastic, or aluminum. Mag wheels are standard on all power wheelchairs but are an option on manual wheelchairs. They are virtually maintenance-free and require only periodic cleaning. There is no risk of corrosion in damp conditions because they are made of synthetic materials. However, they are slightly heavier and have more limited shock-absorption qualities than a spoked wheel.

2. *Spoked.* Spoked wheels resemble bicycle tires and are available only on manual wheelchairs. They are lighter than mag wheels but require more maintenance, including periodic adjustment of the spokes (to maintain proper tension) and replacement of broken or bent spokes. Additionally, spoked wheels are more difficult to maintain in damp climates because of the risk of corrosion.

Removable or "quick release" rear wheels and/or casters are an option on some manual wheelchair frames. This feature can be useful in making the frame lighter for lifting, or smaller for transporting in vehicles with smaller cargo areas.

Tires

1. *Polyurethane.* Polyurethane or solid rubber tires do not require air and therefore are considered maintenance-free. They roll easily on smooth surfaces but offer little shock absorption on rough or uneven terrain and less traction on wet surfaces. They also are heavier than an air-filled

tire. Manual wheelchairs may be ordered with polyurethane tires front and back, but they are offered only as a caster option for power wheelchairs.

2. *Pneumatic.* Pneumatic tires are air-filled inner tubes with a tread. They offer the best shock absorption and optimal maneuverability and traction on rough or uneven terrains. However, just like the tires on your car or bicycle, they require regular maintenance to maintain air pressure, and there is a risk of getting a flat.

3. *Flat-Free.* In a flat-free tire, a solid insert replaces the inner air tube. With this, you have a no-maintenance tire with the benefit of tread for traction. Flat-free tires are somewhat heavier than air-filled tires and offer slightly reduced shock absorption, but for many users the benefits (no flat tires and no maintenance of tire pressure) outweigh these drawbacks.

Wheel Size

"Standard" rear wheels used on adult manual wheelchairs are 24 inches in diameter, but 22-inch and 26-inch tires are also available. The choice of wheel size is in part determined by your body size (how well you are able to reach the wheel), but ease of propulsion and overall seat height (the larger the wheel, the higher the seat height) are also considerations. Large rear wheels (at least 20" in diameter) are paramount if your family or friends will be "bumping" you in the manual wheelchair up and down stairs (consider places where you travel where there are no ramps)—smaller wheels are unable to climb the gradient between most steps.

"Standard" rear wheels on direct drive power wheelchairs are usually 12 inches or 14 inches in diameter. Either size is capable of handling outdoor terrains with no difficulty.

Wheel Locks

Wheel locks are used to prevent rolling of the wheelchair at rest. WHEEL LOCKS ARE NOT BRAKES! They are not designed to slow down or stop a moving wheelchair—in fact, you may incur injury if wheel locks are used in this manner. The wheel locks on a manual wheelchair are most commonly located in front of the rear wheels, just below the level of the seat. They may be "push to lock" or "pull to lock" operated. Pull to lock wheel locks generally move the wheel lock lever out of way for side-to-side transfers in and out of the wheelchair. Extension handles for wheel locks are helpful if your hands are weak because they reduce the amount of power needed to engage the wheel locks.

Power mobility devices (wheelchair and scooters) are equipped with an automatic braking systems that allows them to stop and remain stationary on flat surfaces as well as inclined and declined surfaces.

Caster Size

Casters also come in different sizes, and size must be specified on the prescription.

1. *Larger casters (8").* Eight-inch casters are better able to overcome environmental obstacles, such as cracks in the sidewalk or the gap in the elevator, but they require more space to maneuver. They are well-suited to outdoor use.

2. *Smaller casters (6", 5", 3", etc.).* Smaller casters increase the turning maneuverability of the wheelchair, but greater personal strength is needed to get across door thresholds or to overcome other environmental obstacles.

Back Height

The height of the back support provided by the wheelchair is dictated by the length of your upper body and the strength of your trunk. On some wheelchair styles, the rear back posts are height-adjustable, which offers you the option to later raise the height of the back support (a few inches maximum) if necessary. Typically, back support that is lower requires good trunk strength and balance.

Seat Height

Seat height is measured from the floor to the level of the seat surface and is determined in part by your lower leg length as well as by whether you want your feet to contact the ground (for foot propulsion of a manual wheelchair frame or for transfers). Seat height is an important consideration for environmental access, including knee clearance under tables and vehicle access. Don't forget to factor in the thickness of your seat cushion when calculating the overall seat height of your wheelchair system.

Armrests

When well fitted, armrest supports should support the forearm without raising or lowering the shoulders and should increase your stability and balance when sitting. They also provide a surface to push against to relieve sitting pressures (push ups) and to transfer out of the wheelchair. When deciding on an armrest style, consider whether you will want the armrest support to swing out of the way/flip back and/or remove from the wheelchair frame altogether (relative to your transfer method, need for tabletop access, etc.).

1. *Swing-away.* Swing-away armrest supports typically are tubular with a layer of thin foam padding. They are the lightest style of armrest support, but they also tend to be the least durable over time.

2. *Full-length.* As the name implies, full-length armrests run the full length of the seat. Full-length armrest supports provide a greater surface area on which to rest your arms, which may affect your comfort.

The longer pads may assist you in using your arm strength to rise to standing or to control a descent into the wheelchair. Additionally, this style of armrest is more conducive to using a lap tray support. However, the length of the pad may prevent you from gaining close access to tabletop surfaces for eating meals, using a computer, and so forth, unless the armrests are moved out of the way.

3. *Desk-length.* Desk-length armrests are shorter and allow you tabletop access with the armrests in place. The shorter length of the armrest may make independent or assisted transfers in and our of the wheelchair more difficult because you must reach farther behind your body to access the support surfaces.

Both full-length and desk-length armrests may be ordered with either fixed height or a height-adjustable feature. Because fixed-height armrests are non–height adjustable, they are slightly lighter in weight than height-adjustable armrests. The height of the fixed armrest should allow you to use the support without reaching. Adjustable height armrests are needed if fixed-height armrests are too low for you.

Foot Supports

Foot supports or "footrests" are used to support the legs and protect the feet from dragging on the ground or getting caught in the front casters. When the footrests are adjusted appropriately, your hips and knees are level; the weight of your thighs should then be evenly distributed on the seat surface, which will add to your comfort. If the footrests are adjusted too short, you may experience excessive pressure on your buttocks, your feet may slip off the footplates when traversing bumpy surfaces or during quick changes in direction, or your legs may roll outward (frog's legs) or inward (knock-knees). Conversely, if they are adjusted too long, you will experience excessive pressure behind the knees and possibly low back pain. It is ideal to have at least 2 inches of clearance of the footplate from the ground to clear uneven surfaces.

Most footrests can swing out of the way and/or remove altogether, which provides for less interference during transfers in and out of the wheelchair. The angle at which the footrests protrude forward may be specified for 60°, 70°, or 90° on some models, depending on how flexible your knees are, which position is most comfortable, and your accessibility needs—the farther they stick out, the more overall space is needed to turn and maneuver the wheelchair. Tapered footrests are available on some models; these position your feet closer together and may improve your accessibility (by requiring less space for turning). The footplates on tapered footrests tends to be smaller than those on nontapered front rigging and may not provide a large enough surface to adequately support your feet.

Footrests with an elevating feature are called "legrests." They allow the lower leg to be elevated slightly if swelling, knee pain, or knee range of motion is a problem. Legrests do add weight and greater length to your wheelchair system, which may affect accessibility.

Seat Cushions

Wheelchair seat cushions are used to keep you comfortable when sitting for long periods in the wheelchair. They also serve to position your pelvis and legs and to better distribute the pressures incurred on your buttocks and thighs when sitting. Wheelchair seat cushions are made from a variety of materials. People who spend greater time sitting in a wheelchair usually require greater pressure relief than those who use a wheelchair only occasionally. The most common seat cushions are made from foam (polyurethane, latex, or viscoelastic). The foam compresses to conform to the contours of your body when you sit. Foam cushions tend to be lightweight, low-maintenance, and the least expensive. Foam does "break down" over time, losing its ability to "spring back" and provide support. Foam cushions that are used daily need to be replaced at yearly intervals. Other seat cushion mediums include gel, viscous fluid, water, and air. These cushions are designed to "float" bony areas, such as your tailbone or sitting bones, and to prevent them from butting up against a firm surface, which can obstruct the circulation of blood to the skin. Although these cushions are designed to allow you to sit more comfortably for longer periods, they certainly do not replace the need for you to move between seat surfaces periodically throughout the day to avoid the development of pressure ulcers. These types of cushions are more expensive than foam cushions, and some makes and models require routine maintenance. However, with appropriate care they may not need replacing for years.

Some considerations when selecting wheelchair seat cushions (and covers) are:

- the weight of the cushion (particularly if you are self-propelling in a manual wheelchair)
- the ability of the cushion to repel fluids, bodily (perspiration, urine, etc.) or otherwise
- the air exchange properties of the cushion (remembering what it is like to sit on vinyl car seats on a hot day!)
- how the cushion is cleaned—many may be wiped clean with a cloth using a gentle cleanser such as dishwashing liquid, and others can be thrown right into your washing machine!

The surface of a wheelchair seat cushion may be flat (planar) or may have some shape (contoured). Your evaluator will offer valuable input as to which style of seat cushion he or she would recommend for you based on the results of the physical evaluation (i.e., depending on how much support and positioning you require to maintain good sitting posture). You also will want to consider ease of movement in sitting—seat cushions with contours can restrict your lower body movement.

Back Supports

The purpose of a wheelchair back support is to maintain the natural curves of your spine. Wheelchair systems, particularly manual ones, often have an upholstered or fabric back support. This may be adequate for the occasional or light user. An upholstered back support is light and allows a collapsible frame to be easily folded. However, the fabric does stretch or hammock with use and requires replacing at routine intervals, depending on how much the wheelchair is used.

An upholstered back support may not provide enough support for many people who experience weakness and/or fatigue of the muscles of the back. A wide variety of backrest inserts can be used in addition to the upholstery or can replace it altogether. An insert that is used in conjunction with the upholstery has the added benefit of being transferable to any wheelchair or chair (at home, in your car, etc.). An insert that replaces the upholstery consists of a firm padded shell; it must be removed before a collapsible wheelchair frame can fold. This may sound inconvenient, but, in fact, assembly and disassembly are relatively quick and easy. For those of you who use more than one wheelchair system, this also allows the back support to be transferable between wheelchairs (using extra hardware packages). These inserts generally offer the greatest amount of support. Like seat cushions, back supports may be flat or contoured, depending on your needs, and may be padded with different mediums such as foam, fluid, or air. Again, your evaluator will likely offer his or her recommendation based on the results of the physical evaluation (i.e., depending on how much support and positioning you require to maintain good sitting posture).

Head Supports

Head supports or headrests can be added to most wheelchair systems and are used to prevent the head from falling backward into hyperextension (unlike a cervical collar, which prevents the head from falling forward onto your chest). Detachable or flip-down hardware is most convenient because it allows the head support to be moved out of the way, particularly for assisted transfers in and out of the wheelchair. Headrests also may be flat or contoured. Many of the contoured supports are adjustable if the prefabricated shape does not match what you need. The headrest should support your head well both at the base of the skull and at the back of your head.

Pelvic Positioning Strap

A pelvic positioning strap, or lap belt, is used to help keep your hips positioned to the rear of the seat if sliding forward is a problem. It is not intended to be used as a restraint device like the seatbelts in your car.

Trays

A lap tray or tray table is a portable tabletop surface that attaches to your armrest supports via velcro strapping or "quick release" clamping hardware. A lap tray is useful for arm and hand positioning if standard armrest supports are inadequate. It also allows for easy transport of a communication device, a laptop computer, and so forth.

If you plan to use a machine to assist with your breathing (e.g., BiPAP, ventilator), make certain that your wheelchair system can be equipped with a means of carrying the device.

Antitippers

Antitip devices are standard on power wheelchairs (except FWD) but are an option on most manual wheelchairs. These devices are a safety feature designed to decrease your risk of tipping directly backward or forward. They may be mounted on the front (MWD) or the rear of the wheelchair frame (manual, RWD). For MWD power wheelchairs, these front-mounted antitip devices can pose problems in some situations—they can get in your way during transfers in and out of the wheelchair, they can limit the angle of incline that can be traversed (such as ramps), and they can prohibit you from traversing obstacles (usually more than 3"–5" high) (refer to "Power Wheelchairs—MWD" for more details). Front-mounted antitip devices can be adjusted upward and can be equipped with suspension systems, but this will increase the forward rocking of your MWD power wheelchair.

Tilt and Recline Features

Postural adjustments in a wheelchair system may be made by changing your body position relative to gravitational pull. When you sit fully upright, the force of gravity pulls directly downward through your head, neck, and trunk. If your muscles are weak or easily fatigued, this can result in poor sitting posture—slouching forward or listing to the side. By adjusting your body position relative to the force of gravity, you may actually succeed in maintaining a better, more erect sitting posture. There are generally two ways to achieve this:

1. *Recline.* When you recline, you open up the angle between the seat and back surfaces. Essentially your buttocks and thighs stay where they are, while your head, neck, and trunk lean back.

2. *Tilt-in-space.* When you are tilted, your seated position remains constant, and the entire system is "tipped" or angled backward. Your seated posture is the same when vertical as when tilted.

Tilt-in-space and recline features may be used alone or in combination with one another. They may be fixed (i.e., nonadjustable) or adjustable. Some of the benefits of using postural adjustments (tilt or recline) include:

- Pressure relief—when you recline back, you increase the surface area of your body used for weight bearing. With tilt, you displace the pressures from your buttocks and thighs to your back.

- Gravity-assisted positioned—with either tilt or recline, gravitational pull can be manipulated to pull you into the seat, back and head supports (versus pulling you forward and out when you are sitting fully upright).

This is a particularly good tool for positioning the head and neck. Tilt and/or recline may assist to reduce or eliminate the need for a chest harness (which can interfere with ease of breathing) to prevent forward instability of your trunk if your muscles are very weak.

- Sitting tolerance—tilt or recline can increase the overall length of time you are able to remain sitting. Because your position can be adjusted for comfort and in accordance with your level of fatigue, you can conceivably increase your sitting tolerance and reduce time spent lying down.

Your evaluator will consider a number of other medical issues when recommending tilt, recline, or both, including your transfer method, hip range of motion limitations, muscle spasticity, and so forth.

Tilt and recline features can be manually operated (i.e., you need someone's assistance) or power-operated (i.e., you can adjust your posture independently) and should always be used in conjunction with the appropriate head support.

Seat Elevators

Power-operated seat elevators or seat lifts are available on some power bases. A power-operated seat lift allows you to raise the height of the seat surface approximately 6 to 8 inches from its lowest position. This feature may be used to assist you to safely transfer in and out of the wheelchair if leg weakness is a problem. It also allows you access to tabletops, countertops, and cupboards from a seated position if it is no longer safe for you to stand.

Batteries and Battery Chargers

Batteries are used to power the drive motors of power wheelchair bases and to operate power options on your wheelchair system such as tilt, recline, or a seat lift feature. The batteries used on wheelchair systems are deep-cycle, rechargeable batteries and are designed to be regularly discharged slowly over time and then recharged. They differ from the batteries that you use in your car, which are designed for quick bursts of power (to start the car) followed by recharging by an alternator. Marine batteries often are not deep-cycle batteries.

Deep-cycle batteries can be wet lead acid or sealed lead acid, typically called "gel cell." Wet lead acid batteries are generally less expensive than sealed lead acid or gel cell batteries, and they also offer longer running time. However, wet batteries require higher maintenance than sealed lead acid and gel cell batteries and are a potential safety risk because of the risk of contact with battery acid. Only gel cell batteries are approved for airline travel at this time. Batteries will usually last for approximately one year before they need replacing, although this may vary depending on how much you use your wheelchair and on inherent features of the batteries themselves—some simply last longer than others! You typically can get a full day's use from a single charge; if not, it may be time to replace them.

Battery chargers can be on-board or off-board. On-board chargers are convenient in that you can plug in your wheelchair for charging almost anywhere there is an available electrical socket. On-board chargers may be preferable if you travel a lot.

> ** *All new wheelchair systems come with an owner's maintenance manual that provides invaluable information regarding the features you have selected for your wheelchair system and their care and maintenance. Review this manual with care.* **

Which Manufacturer Should I Choose?

When deciding on a particular manufacturer for your wheelchair, it is important to consider not only cost but also the warranty, local servicing, and availability of parts. You will want repairs done expeditiously, and waiting for parts from halfway around the world can put a crimp in your plans!

Will My Insurance Pay for My Wheelchair System?

Most medical insurance sources will consider funding wheelchair equipment, provided the equipment is considered "medically necessary"—in other words, the expense is justified by your medical condition. This is where the knowledge and skill of your evaluator becomes integral. He or she often will assume the responsibility for preparing the justification strategy or documentation that systematically outlines the medical need for all the pieces and parts of your system. The more thorough the medical documentation, the less likely your need(s) will be questioned, and the more likely your insurance coverage for the purchase will be optimized. Most (if not all) insurance sources require a medical prescription for the wheelchair system, so talk to your physician in advance.

Carefully consider your options. If you are at all interested in power mobility, preserve your medical insurance coverage for the purchase of a power wheelchair. Choose a system that is modular, where changes can readily be made relative to your changing abilities—it is far easier to justify the medical need for modifications to an existing wheelchair system than it is to justify the need to replace the system altogether.

Medicare

As your primary insurer, Medicare generally will pay for 80 percent of a preestablished fee for your wheelchair. You or your coinsurance(s) (if you have any) will be responsible for the remaining 20 percent of the cost.

With manual wheelchair frames, Medicare operates under a "capped rental program." This means Medicare pays your dealer (the company from whom you purchase your wheelchair) a monthly fee, which is intended over time to cover the purchase cost of the frame as well as the cost of routine maintenance and repairs; these payments continue for 15 months. However, before the full 15 months have expired, you should written receive notification from your equipment dealer asking whether you wish to continue renting the wheelchair or if you wish to purchase it. In the event that you opt to purchase the wheelchair, the payments that Medicare has made thus far are converted toward the purchase, and the wheelchair becomes part of your estate. Medicare generally will continue to cover the cost of maintenance and repairs that are considered "reasonable." If you choose to continue renting the wheelchair, Medicare will continue to pay for routine servicing of the wheelchair, but it will have to be returned to your dealer when you no longer need it.

Medicare usually purchases power mobility bases (wheelchairs or scooters) outright and usually will cover the cost of routine servicing and repairs. Seating items such as seat cushions and customized back supports, whether used on a manual or on a power mobility base, are considered purchase items because of the intimacy of contact associated with their use.

Medicaid

As your primary insurer, Medicaid usually will pay for most or all of the cost of a wheelchair system that is considered medically necessary, although every state has its own policies and procedures. Detailed medical justification and preauthorization are common in most states, so the process of obtaining coverage for purchase of a wheelchair can be quite lengthy (months).

Private Medical Insurance Policies

Private insurance coverage for durable medical equipment such as wheelchairs varies greatly—from no coverage at all to 100 percent coverage. Verify the specifics of your policy either by reviewing your contract at home or by contacting your insurance provider directly.

Coinsurance

If you are fortunate enough to have more than one medical insurance source, the secondary and tertiary coverage sources often will consider paying for the portion of the cost of your wheelchair system that is not covered by your primary provider. Coinsurance sources typically will not pay for a wheelchair system if the claim has been denied by your primary insurance provider.

How Long Will It Take for Me to Get My Wheelchair?

The medical review process begins once the necessary documentation is provided to your insurance source. During the review, your primary insurance source reviews the claim and determines your eligibility to receive this insurance benefit. This internal review process by your insurance carrier can take from one month to several months to be completed. The ordering, shipping, and fitting of your system can add another few weeks to the process, so be proactive relative to obtaining your wheelchair. Anticipate your future needs as best as you can, and do not wait until you are in crisis before you initiate getting a wheelchair.

What If My Insurance Denies My Claim?

In many cases when insurance sources deny requests for funding of wheelchair systems, it is because they need additional information (i.e., the medical necessity on the original claim was not clear enough). You may request that your claim be re-reviewed by your primary insurer, at which time additional relevant information should be submitted relative to your medical need for the equipment. Self-purchase remains an option in the event that insurance funding is denied. Alternative funding sources include the Department of Veterans Affairs (for some veterans), charitable funding from local social service agencies, and donations from family, coworkers, and/or friends.

Where Should I Buy My Wheelchair?

Some insurance sources allow you to use the dealer of your choice, whereas others, particularly health maintenance organizations (HMOs), have "preferred providers" for durable medical equipment. For you as the consumer, this means your coverage (percentage of the total cost of the wheelchair system paid by your insurance) is better if you use one of the equipment dealers specified in their list of preferred providers. If you choose to use a dealer outside this provider network, you likely will incur a penalty (which often amounts to greater out-of-pocket expense). Your medical insurance source can provide you with a list of preferred providers in your area.

Certain industry standards can be used in researching a reputable wheelchair dealer in your area. Find out if the company you are considering is approved by The Joint Commission for Accreditation of Healthcare Organizations (JCAHO). JCAHO is an independent, not-for-profit organization whose mandate is to establish minimum professional standards for the industry and to regularly evaluate the compliance of the company against these standards. JCAHO accreditation is recognized throughout the health care industry as representative of quality service. You also may wish to inquire whether the dealer has employees who are members of the National Registry of Rehabilitation Technology Suppliers (NRRTS). NRRTS was established to credential individuals who provide rehabilitation technology equipment such as wheelchairs. It has standards of practice and ethics to which each member must adhere in order to maintain membership. In addition, seek the frank opinions of other consumers who use wheelchairs. If you do not know anyone personally, check with your local ALS Society. Go on the Internet. Ask your evaluator who he or she recommends in your area. Inquire about each company's reputation regarding customer service, reliability, and both routine and emergency maintenance issues. Will they offer you a "test drive" of the wheelchair equipment you are considering? Although the trial equipment may not have the exact features and proportions for you, a "test drive" will provide invaluable information about the equipment that you cannot possibly learn from a brochure—how the equipment drives, its maneuverability, how well it fits into your home or car, and so forth.

Summary

Consumers need to be proactive with regard to their personal well-being. Selecting a wheelchair system can be challenging, but, like anything else, the more information you have, the more educated your decisions will be. A carefully selected wheelchair system will allow you to continue at your maximal level of independence and comfort—certainly for much longer than an inappropriate wheelchair.

SUGGESTED READING

1. Bhasin C. Seating and wheelchair prescription for the non-specialized therapist. Presented at the Ohio Occupational Therapy Association Conference, Cleveland, Ohio, October 1994.

2. Brubaker, CE. Ergonomic considerations. *J Rehab R&D* 1990; (Suppl 2):37–48.

3. Christie S. Designing supplemental wheelchair seating systems. *ADVANCE for Directors in Rehabilitation* 1996; 5(10):11–13.

4. Fields CD. Groundwork: Wheels of fortune. *TeamRehab Report* 1992; 28–31.

5. Health Care Financing Administration (1998). Region B DMERC supplier bulletin. Indianapolis, IN: AdminaStar Federal.

6. Invacare Corporation. Rehab group catalogue [brochure], 1998.

7. Joint Commission on Accreditation of Healthcare Organizations (1999). Facts About the Joint Commission on Accreditation of Healthcare Organizations [on-line]. Available: www.jcaho.org.

8. Kreutz D. Power tilt, recline or both. *TeamRehab Report* 1997; 8(3):29–32.

9. MED Group. Product information for customers: power wheelchairs and scooters, 2nd ed. [brochure], 1997.

10. MK Battery. The HME battery guide [brochure], 1998.

11. National Registry of Rehabilitation Technology Suppliers (1999). NRRTS [on-line] Available: www.teamrehab.com/nrrts/intro.html.

12. Perr A. Elements of seating and wheeled mobility intervention. *OT Practice* 1998; 3(9):16–24.

13. Ragnarsson KT. Prescription considerations and a comparison of conventional and lightweight wheelchairs. *J Rehab Res Dev* 1990; (Suppl 2):8–16.

14. Reed S. When was the last time you made a housing adjustment? *Quickie News* 1996; 85:4.

15. Reed S. Front frame angles and front rigging angles. *Quickie News* 1995; 76:4.

16. Reed S. Wheels—the first step to a comfortable pair of shoes *Quickie News* 1995; 68:5.

17. Reed S. Wheels, casters and tires: Is it time for a new pair of shoes? *Quickie News* 1994; 67:6.

18. Rehabilitation Engineering and Assistive Technology Society of North America, (1999). RESNA [On-line]. Available: www.resna.org.

19. Shepherd, M. Tuning your lightweight wheelchair. *Action Digest* July–August 1992.

20. United States Department of Transportation, (1999). New horizons: Information for the air traveler with a disability [on-line]. Available: www.dot.gov/airconsumer/ horizons.htm.

10

Managing Communication and Swallowing Difficulties

Lisa Adams, M.A. CCC-SLP, and Marta Kazandjian, M.A.CCC-SLP

The role of the speech language pathologist (SLP) in ALS extends beyond the traditional boundaries of "speech" or "language" treatment. The SLP is part of the interdisciplinary team that will help you to manage the disease. This requires an awareness of how important communication is in the life of every individual. The person with ALS who remains cognitively intact despite severe limitations in physical mobility must have options for communication even when speech fails.

Speech may be disrupted due to the weakness of muscles involved in speaking and/or to tracheostomy and ventilator dependence. Many options are available that allow vocal and/ or nonvocal communication. If you are experiencing respiratory difficulty, communication management may involve working closely with the respiratory therapist and physician to allow airflow through the upper airway or voice box in order to both speak and safely swallow. The therapist must use techniques such as tracheostomy tube cuff deflation and one-way speaking valves to achieve these goals.

Swallowing function may decline as the muscles involved in speech and swallowing become increasingly weak. The degree and nature of the swallowing impairment can be tested. As the disease progresses, dietary changes can be used to avoid choking and aspiration or the entrance of food or liquid into the lungs. Techniques to supplement or augment communication can also be used to assist the person with ALS to communicate messages when speech becomes increasingly difficult to understand. It is the role of the SLP who specializes in diseases such as ALS to continually reevaluate your communication and swallowing needs as they change. This proactive approach will enable you to work with the SLP to anticipate problems before they occur. In a proactive approach there is always a plan to maintain or compensate for the loss of function. This chapter discusses the various management techniques used to facilitate communication and swallowing throughout the disease process, as well as discussing the other team members who assist in meeting these goals.

Early Communication Management

A person with ALS who begins to experience changes in speech clarity or intelligibility may be diagnosed as having *dysarthria*. This speech impairment results from a weakness of the articulation and breathing muscles. You and the speech pathologist may begin to hear imprecise articulation or slurred speech sounds, nasal-sounding speech quality, decreased loudness, and short rushes of speech that sound as if you are running out of breath. People often report better communication with familiar people as well as better message exchanges in quiet, one-to-one interactions during the early hours of the day.

Some people with ALS have good articulation but reduced loudness or breathlessness as a result of excessive air loss through the nose. If this is the case, a device designed to lift up the soft palate or *velum* to reduce loss of airflow from the nose may be appropriate. This device is called a *palatal lift* and is custom-produced by a prosthodontist. Palatal lifts are expensive and often require multiple fittings before they are completed to ensure that airflow is stopped and comfort is maintained. Some people report restoration of louder and more understandable speech. The palatal lift may decrease the feeling of "breathlessness" caused by loss of air out the nose. Unfortunately, speech muscle deterioration can occur quickly in some people, and a palatal lift may be a short-lived therapeutic option.

Speech that is reduced in loudness may be improved through amplification. Vocal amplifiers range in size and are an option even when it is difficult to hold the microphone. Headsets or lapel microphones can be purchased to eliminate this problem. Many people have difficulty abandoning the practice of speaking to each other from distant rooms. This communication pattern creates frustration for both parties. A powerful amplifier or intercom in the home may be helpful in this case. A strategy of *breath grouping* is also highly effective for people who "run out of air" during speech. This usually occurs because a lengthy sentence is produced on one short breath. As a result, the beginning of the sentence is understandable, but the end is not. The breath-grouping strategy limits the number of words produced per breath to only about three or four. A new breath must be taken for each group of words. With this technique, overall speech rate is reduced and intelligibility and volume are improved by the added airflow and breath support.

Speech clarity may be further complicated by difficulty articulating words.

The SLP can introduce compensatory strategies that will improve the intelligibility of speech so that there can be a more successful exchange of messages between the person with ALS and a variety of communication partners. One compensatory technique is referred to as "speech supplementation," in which an alphabet board is used as an adjunct to speech. The person points to the first letter of each word as the word is produced. If the word is not understood after two or three attempts, it is spelled out on the board. Many people who have adequate use of their hands will write to supplement messages that are not easily understood. Magic Slates or easily erasable boards are helpful. An occupational therapist might assist in recommending methods of maintaining writing through assistive devices or splinting.

Middle-Stage Communication Management

As speech musculature weakens and verbal communication becomes more difficult to understand, reliance on supplemental or *augmentative methods of communication* increases. Augmentative communication refers to the use of nonverbal and/or nonvocal communication strategies that are combined with speech. These strategies may include alphabet spelling on a board or a list of frequently used messages that are needed throughout the day. In middle-stage communication management, these techniques are often coupled with the use of speech for messages easily understood by familiar communication partners such as family members. The SLP who specializes in augmentative communication will work closely with the patient to meet his communication needs as physical motor function changes. An *augmentative communication evaluation* is often recommended during this stage of the disease.

The augmentative communication evaluation can be conducted in a clinic, a hospital, or the home. You should be optimally seated and positioned in the place you spend most of your time (i.e., easy chair, wheelchair, bed). The SLP, often with the assistance of an occupational therapist or a physical therapist, will assess your current motor movements to determine one that is most *functional*. A functional motor movement may be any small movement of a muscle or body part that you can readily control consistently and reliably. This single motor movement can then be used as a signal to control the communication system. The physical motor movement or technique that you use to communicate is called an *access method*. This method of access may change as the disease progresses and motor movement becomes less reliable.

Direct selection is often the access method of choice during this stage of communication function. It is considered the quickest method of access because a body part, such as a finger for pointing or typing, selects the desired letter or key. It is sometimes necessary to provide adaptive equipment to make the arm or hand functional. For example, if the shoulder or wrist is weak, assistive devices to support the arm may make the hand and fingers more reliable for typing and using as a direct selection method. Assistive devices are prescribed and implemented by the occupational therapist or physical therapist. They will work closely with the SLP as physical motor function changes in an effort to maintain and compensate for decreased muscle strength.

Low-Technology Options

Communication options have a range of sophistication and complexity. Your specific communication needs often will determine which ones are chosen. Options include a variety of communication partners, a variety of environments in which message exchanges take place, vocational needs, literacy, and so forth. *Low-technology* options involve handmade or prefabricated alphabet-phrase boards or picture boards. These boards may be small enough to fit in a pocket and can be used in combination with speech or as an alternative to speech with unfamiliar listeners. Eye gaze is an extremely useful method of selection for patients who want to communicate rapidly but cannot point with a finger. The Eye Link™ (Figure 10-1) is an example of a low-technology option that uses eye gaze as a direct selection method. This device, which is commercially available or can be created at home, has letters of the alphabet organized on a piece of clear plastic. The listener holds the clear plastic with the letters facing the person with ALS. He or she looks directly at each letter of his message. The listener or communication partner follows the patient's eyes and "links" eye gaze as each letter is deciphered. The process continues for each letter until the message is completed.

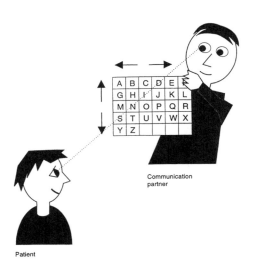

Figure 10-1. Instructions for using an Eye-Link. (From *Communication and Swallowing Management of Tracheostomized and Ventilator Dependent Adults* by K.J. Dikeman and M.S. Kazandjian, 1995, p. 211. San Diego, CA: Singular Publishing Group, Inc.. Copyright 1995. Reprinted with permission.)

High-Technology Options

There has also been research and development into electronic eye gaze systems in which a person can select letters by looking at them. Eye movements are electronically tracked, and a selection is made when the patient sustains eye gaze at an item for a predetermined amount of time. This high-level technology allows very disabled users to use a rapid direct selection technique for communication.

During middle-stage communication management, the person with ALS may begin to have significant difficulty with speech, especially with unfamiliar listeners or in noisy environments. However, he or she may still be physically active, either walking or moving about in a wheelchair. The following section reviews options that allow for maintaining communication in social settings through speech, over the phone, and through writing.

Many people with ALS seek assistance in maintaining phone use even when speech becomes too difficult to understand when not face to face. If he or she has finger use for typing, a Telecommunications Device for the Deaf (TDD) may be considered. Although this device is designed for people who are deaf, it may help maintain phone use for those who are speech impaired. The user types in the message instead of speaking over the telephone. The message is sent to another TDD and can be read on a display. If the communication partner does not have a TDD available, a third party or a relay operator reads the message aloud. The communication partner replies verbally to the patient. The telephone company offers this service through their "Services for People with Disability."

Many patients use desktop personal computers for work or pleasure, primarily to produce written text, to send electronic mail, or to use on-line services. People with a moderate degree of physical motor deterioration and who still have hand function can use a personal computer with ongoing modifications. People who have difficulty controlling the movement of a mouse or manipulating the click button on the mouse can explore alternatives to the standard mouse. One alternative is a trackball, which can be rolled in a variety of directions using very small finger movements. Many programs are now equipped with a *dwell* feature in which an icon is automatically "clicked" when the mouse cursor is left in one area for a specified amount of time. Many alternative mouse products can be purchased in standard computer stores.

When alternatives to the standard mouse are used, they are commonly coupled with *onscreen keyboards* to allow ongoing direct selection. Communication software programs are available that bypass the standard keyboard and allow a person with limited physical motor control of his hands and/or fingers to select each desired letter shown on the computer screen. Those who do not have good hand function but who maintain good head movement may be able to operate a computer through the use of a *head mouse*. The user wears a small sensor strapped to the forehead. When interfaced with the computer, it directs a beam of light to the computer screen. The mouse is controlled by small movements of the head. The mouse click can be accomplished via the dwell feature. Specialized software is also available that provides *keystroke saving options.* These options enhance the speed with which a person can type by providing *word prediction* and *abbreviation-expansion.* Word prediction is a typing or rate enhancement tool in which the software attempts to "guess" what the user is trying to say. As he or she types, a prediction box appears on the screen. The user checks to see if the correct word or phrase is being predicted from the few letters that have been typed. If the word is available in the box, the user need only choose a single number. This saves time and energy for the typist. Abbreviation-expansion is a method of abbreviating frequently used word, phrases, and sentences. Lengthy items can be retrieved by simply typing in two or three letters. For example, TM = "Hi, this is Tom Murray. I am using a computer to help me communication with you." This type of software is designed to work well with other standard computer software programs. An additional benefit to using specialized communication software is that *environmental control* options are often built into the software. Environmental control is a function that allows the computer user to manipulate appliances in the environment through the computer. This may include lights, television, or an electric bed. Each appliance is fit with a small module that permits it to be controlled by a computer. This may be highly beneficial for individuals who continue to work and require increased independence in manipulating the environment.

Although the personal computer is an excellent tool for in-home use, it does not address the communication needs of the person with ALS who needs to communicate in other settings. When speech becomes too difficult to use with less familiar people or in groups, a portable communication device is recommended. This may be a *notebook or laptop computer.* It can also be a *dedicated communication system.* "Dedicated" means the system was developed solely for use by people who are communicatively impaired. The degree of portability needed will vary from person to person. For some, "portable" means a device that is small and lightweight enough to be carried around freely by hand. Some devices are small enough to be carried in a handbag. Other devices cannot be carried but can be *mounted* or fixed on a wheelchair. A laptop computer is often considered too heavy for most disabled users to carry but can be easily mounted.

The features offered within a dedicated system may be more desirable for the person with ALS who can walk but cannot speak. Ambulatory individuals need truly portable systems. A dedicated communication system will run for 8 to 10 hours on a single battery charge, making it easy to use in all communication settings. Most dedicated systems include high-quality synthetic speech output that substitutes for the user's actual voice. Many highly portable devices also offer *digitized speech* as an alternative to synthetic speech. Digitized speech is recorded and therefore has a more authentic voice quality than synthetic speech. However, devices using digitized speech are usually limited to a finite number of minutes of speech output and often speak only a preset group of messages. This differs from synthetic speech, which offers a *text to speech* option in which any message the person types is spoken aloud. There is no limit to the number of messages that can be spoken. Users can explore devices that offer both digitized speech and synthetic speech as options. The dedicated device may also offer printed output, which is known as *hard copy*. Sometimes a printer is "built in" to the device, although it often will have "strip" style printers in place of full-sized paper. Some devices do not print on their own and must be coupled with a full-sized printer to produce written output. Some dedicated devices offer an enhanced two-way screen so that a message can be read when facing the person, as shown in Figure 10-2. This unique feature allows normal face-to-face communication to take place instead of side-by-side message transfer.

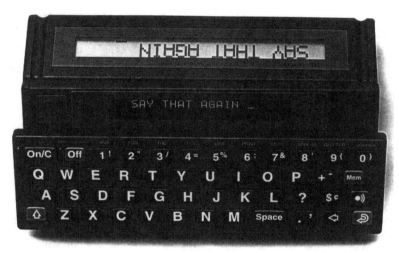

Figure 10-2. An example of a portable communication device with a two-way message display. (Photo courtesy of Zygo Industries, Inc. Manufactured by Toby Churchill Ltd., U.K. Distributed in North America by Zygo Industries, Inc.)

Although dedicated computer systems meet the communication needs of many people with ALS, there also are disadvantages in choosing a dedicated communication system. Some systems are better designed for individuals who have hand and finger function. The device may or may not continue to be usable when these movements deteriorate. Because the device is designed to be small and highly portable, it is not equipped with all the features of a less portable system, such as a large screen. It also does not have the option to run a variety of software programs or provide E-mail and Internet access. E-mail and Internet access allow even the most physically disabled patient to communicate with an unlimited number of people around the world without ever leaving the home. The Internet or "information superhighway" provides vast resources for people to obtain information on an unlimited number of subjects.

To obtain the advantages of a personal computer, you need to sacrifice portability and select a laptop or notebook computer. This type of communication system provides all the advantages of a desktop computer in a more portable form. This includes a screen that is easier to read, printed output, and access to a wide variety of software, including Internet access. However, a laptop system is far less compact than a dedicated system. Each component, such as the printer, is an additional component that is added to the computer communication system. A laptop will only run for 4 to 5 hours on a single battery charge. An AC adapter or portable battery pack can be used, but this increases the weight of the system.

Late-Stage Communication Management

In the late stages of ALS, speech as a reliable mode of communication is often lost. Significant physical motor weakness throughout the body may prevent the person with ALS from using his hands or fingers as a method of directly accessing a communication device. However, residual or minute motor movements throughout the body may be used to control communication, such as a slight bend of a finger, a head turn, a jaw clench, an eyebrow raise, or any movement of the eyes. At this point many patients are fit with a *switch*. Each time he or she acts on the switch, an activation signal is sent to the device. The switch can be fit anywhere on the body where there is a consistent, reliable motor movement, including areas of the face and eyes. Switches work in various ways. Some must be activated by pressure, whereas others react to minute movements and will sense a head turn, finger bend, or deep muscle movement. An *infrared switch* is an example of a switch that can be triggered by small movements. This type of switch casts out a beam of light. The user must execute a small motor movement such as an eye blink or a downward movement of the eye to break the beam of light. Figure 10-3 shows an infrared switch mounted on a headband. Once fitted with a switch, the person can control an electronic communication system using only a single, small motor movement. Fitting the person with a switch requires experience and is best done by a speech-language pathologist, occupational therapist, or rehabilitation engineer who has a good working knowledge of switches and switch interfaces. Accurate positioning of the switch is crucial and may require input from several members of the treatment team.

Coded Systems

Switch access is provided when direct selection techniques are no longer functional and alternate access methods are required. A switch is a piece of equipment that allows a person to bypass the keyboard. One technique that may be beneficial to a person who can activate one or two switches is *coding*. In a coded system, the person uses a code that is deciphered by the listener. The code is a combination of smaller units that stand for larger units, such as letters of the alphabet or phrases on a board. Using a brief code to represent longer messages saves time. Coding is very useful for people who want to access a large amount of language rapidly but do not have the physical ability to accomplish it. The most commonly used code

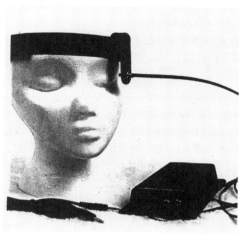

Figure 10-3. A fiberoptic infrared switch mounted for use with an eyeblink. (Photo courtesy of Empowering Resources, Inc.)

is *Morse code.* The individual using Morse code may be able to activate a buzzer system. When the buzzes are combined, they stand for letters of the alphabet. Coding can be used in a low-technology, nonelectronic system, such as an *E-Tran,* as shown in Figure 10-4. It also can be used as a way of accessing an electronic or computerized communication system. When using Morse code, the series of buzzes are automatically converted by the computer into letters of the alphabet.

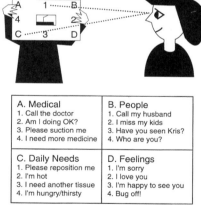

A. Medical	B. People
1. Call the doctor	1. Call my husband
2. Am I doing OK?	2. I miss my kids
3. Please suction me	3. Have you seen Kris?
4. I need more medicine	4. Who are you?

C. Daily Needs	D. Feelings
1. Please reposition me	1. I'm sorry
2. I'm hot	2. I love you
3. I need another tissue	3. I'm happy to see you
4. I'm hungry/thirsty	4. Bug off!

Figure 10-4. An example of encoding through the user of an E-Tran. (From *Communication and Swallowing Management of Tracheostomized and Ventilator Dependent Adults* by K.J. Dikeman and M.S. Kazandjian, 1995, p. 215. San Diego, CA: Singular Publishing Group, Inc.. Copyright 1995. Reprinted with permission.)

Scanning

Scanning is another access method used by people who have a functional residual motor movement but cannot rely on direct selection options because of severe physical motor weakness. Scanning with an alphabet board is a widely used method of communication for nonspeaking patients. During scanning the alphabet is accessed in groups. When row-column scanning is used, as illustrated in Figure 10-5, each row of letters is scanned through until the desired row is presented. The user then executes a predetermined motor movement, such as upward eye gaze, to select that row. Each letter within the row is scanned until the desired letter is presented. The patient then executes the motor movement to select the letter. The process is repeated until each letter of the word is selected. Lengthy messages can also be spelled.

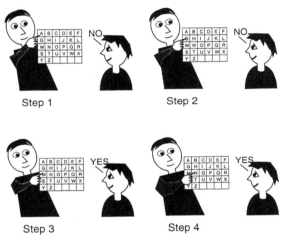

Figure 10-5. An example of row-column scanning. (Adapted from *Electronic Communication Aids, Selection and Use* by I. Fishman, 1987, p. 71. San Diego, CA: College-Hill Press. Copyright by I. Fishman.)

Scanning can also be accomplished electronically with a computer-based communication system. Many dedicated systems offer scanning as a method of input, but this should be investigated before purchase. Specialized computer software for desktop or laptop computers generally offer scanning as a method of input. To use an electronic communication system via scanning, the user's functional motor movement must be paired with a switch. The switch controls a moving cursor on the screen. Each time the switch is activated, the cursor movement is stopped and a selection of a letter, word, or number can be made.

Many people with ALS use multiple communication systems, including low- and high-technology devices, to meet specific communication needs in specific communication environments. For example, a low-technology row-column scanning alphabet board may be used for easy message transmission from bed, a portable electronic communication system when out at a social gathering, and a desktop computer with modifications to complete work-related tasks. The SLP who specializes in augmentative and alternative communication should assist the patient in the selection of a variety of appropriate methods of communication at each stage of the disease so that the patient's individual communication needs are always being met.

Funding Communication Systems

Once the SLP and the patient have determined the specific type or types of communication systems needed to best meet his or her needs, the SLP will formulate a prescription for the communication device. This prescription is often in the form of an evaluation, detailing the patient's physical motor status and current method of communication, and naming the desired device, software package, and switch access if one is needed. The managing physician then approves this prescription. Once this is accomplished, the SLP can seek an appropriate funding source to assist in payment for the communication equipment. The funding process varies widely from state to state. Some people with ALS are entitled to communication equipment through their state Medicaid or Medicare program. If the patient is privately insured, his or her insurance company should be approached to determine whether communication equipment could be funded. Policies on granting communication equipment vary widely from one insurance company to another.

Other funding sources may also be explored, including local churches or temples and organizations that perform charitable works such as fund-raising. Patients and caregivers may receive important information through their local ALS Association chapter and Muscular Dystrophy Association (MDA). Some chapters may provide equipment loan banks for communication devices and other daily care items. Some people with ALS purchase second-hand equipment from an individual who no longer can use it. The SLP who frequently works in the area of ALS acts as the patient's primary advocate in the area of funding. She may also use the services of a public interest attorney in appealing to state and private organizations.

Tracheostomy

At times, speech articulation remains intact but the presence of a *tracheostomy tube* creates an interruption in speech production. A *tracheotomy,* or the surgical creation of a hole in the neck, is performed to provide assistance in breathing and for removal of secretions. A tracheostomy tube is placed through the hole, below the level of the *vocal cords,* as shown in Figure 10-6. Air must go through the vocal cords for voice or sound to be produced. Some tracheostomy tubes contain a *cuff.* This is a balloon on the end of the tube that, when inflated, prevents air that is coming out of the lungs from escaping up through the vocal cords, mouth, and nose. This results in a condition known as *aphonia,* or the absence of voice. Figure 10-7 illustrates airflow that is passing around the tracheostomy tube cuff

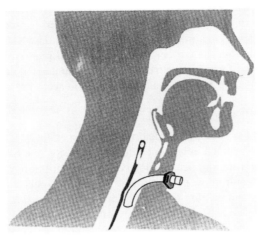

Figure 10-6. A tracheostomy tube in place. Note its position below the level of the vocal cords. (From *Communication and Swallowing Management of Tracheostomized and Ventilator Dependent Adults* by K.J. Dikeman and M.S. Kazandjian, 1995, p. 54. San Diego, CA: Singular Publishing Group, Inc.. Copyright 1995. Reprinted with permission.)

during *de*flation and air that is stopped from reaching the vocal cords during cuff *in*flation. When the tracheostomy tube cuff is deflated fully or even partially, air can potentially be directed upward around the sides of the tracheostomy tube, through the vocal folds, mouth, and nose. Speech can be produced when the tracheostomy tube is occluded by a finger or other device that stops the air from moving out the tracheostomy tube. Tracheostomy tube cuffs are designed for two purposes: to stop large amounts of oral secretions from being *aspirated* or entering the lungs and to allow a patient to receive the correct amount of air that a mechanical ventilator or respirator is set to provide. Cuffs are not designed to stop large amounts of food or liquid from entering the lungs. Speech and safe swallowing can be facilitated by deflation of tracheostomy tube cuffs. When even a small amount of air is removed from the cuff, the cuff can move more easily within the neck. This allows the person to return to a more normal pattern of swallowing and to potentially produce voice. The SLP works closely with the respiratory therapist and physician to allow air to travel up through the vocal cords or voice box while ensuring that the patient on a ventilator maintains breathing.

When a patient is able to tolerate full cuff deflation, a one-way speaking valve can be considered to assist in verbal communication production. One-way valves stop air from escaping out the tracheostomy tube by redirecting the air that is breathed in, or *inspired,* and allowing it to travel up to the vocal cords. Figure 10-8 illustrates the airflow that is used for speech production when a one-way valve is placed on the tracheostomy tube. One-way valves can be used for patients who are on or off

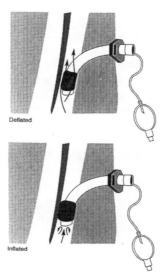

Figure 10-7. A cuffed tracheostomy tube in place. Arrows indicate upward airflow. (From *Communication and Swallowing Management of Tracheostomized and Ventilator Dependent Adults* by K.J. Dikeman and M.S. Kazandjian, 1995, p. 72. San Diego, CA: Singular Publishing Group, Inc.. Copyright 1995. Reprinted with permission.)

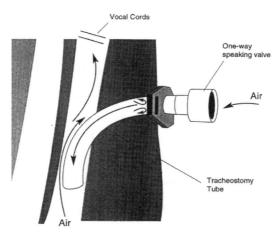

Figure 10-8. The redirection of airflow when a one-way valve is in place on the tracheostomy tube. (From *Communication and Swallowing Management of Tracheostomized and Ventilator Dependent Adults* by K.J. Dikeman and M.S. Kazandjian, 1995, p. 165. San Diego, CA: Singular Publishing Group, Inc., Copyright 1995. Reprinted with permission.)

ventilators. A patient is considered a candidate only if full cuff deflation is accomplished and there is sufficient oral motor strength to mouth understandable words.

Swallowing Disorders

The loss of motor movement that results in the progressive deterioration of speech also typically results in the progressive deterioration of swallowing. The normal swallowing process is interrupted by changes in the strength and range of movement of the lips, tongue, jaw, soft palate, and vocal cords, as illustrated in Figure 10-9. An impairment in swallowing function is known as *dysphagia*. The swallowing ability of a person with ALS changes gradually. The progressive weakening of each of the oral motor structures yields its own set of problems. The loss of lip strength may make it difficult to hold food, especially liquids, in the mouth. The loss of tongue strength alters the normal movements of the tongue that are required to safely swallow foods. This includes the side-to-side movement the tongue makes that enables food to be swept onto the molars for chewing. If this movement is not accomplished, food will remain unchewed. It also includes the upward movement of the tongue that enables food to be pushed toward the back of the mouth. People with ALS often have to manage this backward food propulsion by using many swallows. When viewed by the SLP, the patient appears to be "pumping" the tongue to get it to do its work. If the tongue is weak, food may not be gathered into a *cohesive bolus,* or mass. This may result in small food particles being deposited into the crevices around the lips or adhering to the hard palate.

As food leaves the mouth, the soft palate closes to keep food from entering the nasal cavity and being pushed out the nose. The food or liquid enters the throat or

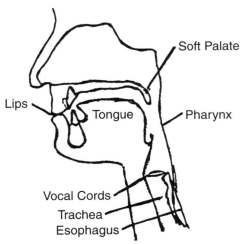

Figure 10-9. A schematic of selected structures involved in the swallowing process.

pharynx, and the next stage of swallowing begins. It is at this point that the actual swallow occurs. The back of the tongue has moved backward, and the muscles of the pharynx begin to contract to push the food downward. At the same time, the entrance to the windpipe or larynx closes tightly as the *larynx* moves upward. The *vocal cords* are contained within the larynx and must close to ensure that the food or liquid, which passes directly over the larynx, does not spill into the lungs. If these precisely timed events do not occur in the appropriate order, the patient will no longer produce a safe swallow. ALS results in many changes in the strength and speed of the structures that contribute to an unsafe swallowing pattern during this stage of the swallowing process. As the muscles of the pharynx weaken, food may not be effectively pushed downward into the *esophagus* and finally into the stomach. The result may be a feeling of food sticking in the throat. Liquids may need to be taken to assist in moving the food through the throat and esophagus. However, if the finely timed event of vocal cord closure does not occur, choking or coughing may result as food or liquid enters the larynx instead of moving normally through the pharynx and into the esophagus and stomach. The entry of food or liquid into the larynx and lungs is referred to as *aspiration.* The entrance of any substance other than air has the potential of causing an infection. Some patients may develop an *aspiration pneumonia* if this occurs only once; others may be at high risk after several episodes of large-scale aspiration. It is difficult to judge how much is too much aspiration before a particular patient experiences a pneumonia. Repeated episodes of coughing when eating or drinking may indicate a risk of food or liquid entering the lungs.

Evaluation of Swallowing Disorders

The philosophy of managing swallowing problems in ALS is to teach the patient about the potential problems before they occur and to circumvent them by using compensatory strategies for as long as possible. In the early stages of swallowing impairment, the problems may be highly visible and easy to diagnose and manage. As the disease progresses, it may become more difficult to diagnose the exact nature of a problem because the structures for swallowing are not readily visible. To fully understand what aspect of the swallowing process is being disrupted, the SLP has to view the structures for swallowing. This is most easily accomplished by performing an examination known as *videofluoroscopy* or *modified barium swallow.* During this examination, the patient is asked to chew and swallow a variety of food textures ranging from liquid to smooth to coarse. The foods are impregnated with *barium,* a substance that can be tracked on an x-ray. An x-ray examination is then taken of the patient chewing and swallowing foods. This examination allows the SLP and the radiologist to determine those aspects of the swallow that are most difficult for the patient and whether aspiration of foods is occurring. The videofluoroscopy is a very beneficial tool to use when the goal is safe preservation of the swallow for as long as possible. It allows the SLP to determine whether some type of a compensatory swallowing strategy can circumvent a problem and to actually experiment with that strategy during the examination to assess its benefit.

The SLP must often justify the need for this examination to the managing physician, who views the loss of swallowing and the placement of a feeding tube as an inevitable part of ALS. Although the progressive loss of swallowing is accepted by the SLP as a possibility, the larger goal is to maintain swallowing as a means of improving the overall quality of life with ALS. The videofluoroscopy may allow the patient to continue eating safely even if full nutrition and hydration cannot be maintained by mouth. The patient may choose favorite items and eat small quantities for pleasure, while also using the strategies that have been determined as effective during the evaluation.

In many clinical settings, videofluoroscopy may not be available or recommended when the clinical signs of aspiration are already evident. Examples would include episodes of pneumonia or upper respiratory tract infections, frequent coughing, and significant weight loss. When these signs are present, the SLP may be able to determine the appropriate management techniques for safer swallowing. If the SLP is unable to use the videofluoroscopy as an assessment tool, another possible tool is a *fiberoptic endoscopic swallow study*. During this examination, a flexible fiberoptic scope is passed through the nose and suspended above the larynx, as shown in Figure 10-10. Vegetable dye is added to food and liquid. This tool allows the SLP to view the dyed food and liquid moving through the pharynx while observing the effectiveness of vocal cord closure and protection of the *trachea* (windpipe) and lungs.

The SLP may also view the structures after the patient has swallowed foods impregnated with dye. Residue of the dye will be visible in "high-risk" areas

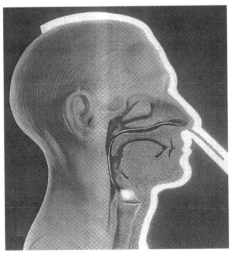

Figure 10-10. The flexible fiberoptic scope in place for viewing the pharynx. (Photo courtesy of Pentax Precision Instruments)

around the vocal cords if the patient is not swallowing safely. If the patient has a tracheostomy tube in place, secretions suctioned from the tube may be tinged with dye if the food has penetrated the trachea. These tools allow the SLP to obtain further information about the nature and extent of the swallowing impairment and to determine which treatment strategy will allow safe swallowing to continue.

Management of Swallowing Disorders

The gradual loss of swallowing, like the gradual loss of speech, presents a challenge to the SLP in attempting to stay one step ahead of the disease. Swallowing problems should be anticipated, and a consistent update about the swallowing ability of the person with ALS should be provided so that changes can be recognized. Dietary management can prevent problems and prolong safe swallowing. The SLP should consult a *registered dietitian* to assist with the diet so that the patient has adequate caloric intake and his or her nutritional needs are met. People with ALS often eliminate difficult food consistencies from their diet as swallowing deteriorates. If solid food becomes difficult to chew, prechopped or mashed foods can eliminate the need for extensive chewing. Foods that do not contain small pieces and are well moistened will move toward the back of the mouth easier. When foods are held together by a cohesive food substance, such as mashed potatoes, it is less likely that the patient will "breathe in" the food. Thin liquid consistencies present a particular challenge. Thin liquids are difficult to keep in the mouth, and they are difficult to control when swallowing, thereby resulting in coughing or choking. People with ALS often benefit from thickening liquids to a honey-like consistency. Several thickening substances are available that do not greatly alter the taste of liquid and allow the patient to achieve the safest consistency. The person with ALS may also want to eat several small meals throughout the day to reduce the fatigue that accompanies eating. Many people with ALS complain that their saliva is copious and thick. There has been varying success in controlling thick saliva with various medications. The patient's physician will attempt to determine an appropriate medication given his medical history. Strategies such as ensuring adequate hydration and avoiding dairy products and chocolates can be helpful. The use of papain (found in meat tenderizers) and over-the-counter cough medicines (Robitussin™) that contain guaifenesin have also assisted some people in managing thick saliva.

The person with ALS may also attempt to manage swallowing problems by using *compensatory swallowing techniques*. These techniques have been evaluated for their effectiveness via objective assessment, including videofluoroscopy and the endoscopic swallow examination. One technique involves placing food toward the rear of the mouth to reduce the use of tongue pumping. Another technique involves teaching the patient to "hold" his or her breath and "bear down" during the swallowing process, which may forcibly close the vocal folds for better protection. Another technique teaches the patient to swallow many times to clear residue from the throat. Yet another involves teaching the patient to "cough" after the swallow to clear any residue that may have fallen around the vocal folds. Through the use of careful testing, dietary management, and compensatory swallowing techniques, the patient may continue to swallow safely until a significant amount of motor deterioration has occurred. At that time, an alternative method of swallowing such as a gastrostomy tube may be recommended. The placement of a gastrostomy tube may be recommended when the patient cannot manage to take a sufficient amount of food by mouth to maintain adequate nutrition and hydration. However, small amounts of oral intake can be continued in the presence of a gastrostomy tube. This will provide another source of pleasure and improve the quality of life for the individual with ALS.

Conclusion

Amyotrophic lateral sclerosis challenges the therapist's training in the area of rehabilitation. A philosophy of maintenance and compensation must be used if the person with ALS is going to be managed by the SLP. Technology is constantly opening new doors to provide improved quality of life through communication for the person with ALS and has made communication a reality for everyone with ALS. The provision of high-quality synthetic and digitized speech, written output, and access to on-line services can restore a high degree of independence. The philosophy of maintenance and compensation can be applied to the changes in swallowing that occur in ALS so that another aspect of the patient's functioning can be preserved for as long as possible. By working with a team of highly trained professionals, the person with ALS can manage the disease from a position of knowledge and strength. Through ongoing education and research, the highest quality of life can be maintained for this population of individuals.

SUGGESTED READING

1. Adams L, Connolly MA. Nonvocal treatments for short term and long term ventilator patients. In: M. Mason (ed.). Speech pathology for the tracheostomized and ventilator dependent patient. Newport Beach, CA: Voicing!, 1993:288–335.
2. Beukelman DR, Yorkston KM, Dowden PA. Communication augmentation: A casebook of clinical management. San Diego, CA: College-Hill Press, 1985.
3. Dikeman K, Kazandjian M. Communication and swallowing management of tracheostomized and ventilator dependent adults. San Diego, CA: Singular Publishing Group, 1995.
4. Esposito SJ, Mitsumoto H, Shanks M. Use of palatal lift and palatal augmentation prostheses to improve dysarthria in patients with amyotrophic lateral sclerosis: A cases series. *J Prosthet Dent* 2000; 83: 90–98.
5. Fishman I. Electronic communication aids and techniques. Boston: College-Hill Press, 1987.
6. Kazandjian M (ed.). Communication and swallowing solutions for the ALS/MND community. New York: Communication Independence for the Neurologically Impaired, 1997.
7. Yorkston KM (ed.). Augmentative communication in the medical setting. Tucson, AZ: Communication Skill Builders, 1992.

11

Maintaining Optimum Nutrition

**Carmen Blakely-Adams, R.D., L.D.,
and Eileen M. Carr-Davis, R.D., L.D., M.B.A.**

Chewing and swallowing may become more difficult as amyotrophic lateral sclerosis (ALS) progresses and the muscles around the face and throat weaken and the tongue and lips lose their strength. It also may take more time and energy to finish a meal. Taken together, these conditions lead to an inability of the body to meet its nutrient needs, resulting in uncontrolled loss of body weight and malnutrition. It is therefore important to address nutritional problems in the early stages of the disease.

Registered dietitians provide nutritional counseling through diet management to promote good nutrition while preventing malnutrition. They are available to:

- Assess your nutritional needs based on the progression of the disease

- Identify malnutrition

- Recommend changes in your diet to assist in the treatment of the disease

- Develop an individualized care plan to promote good nutritional status

- Adapt the consistency of foods and liquids when swallowing becomes difficult

- Provide suggestions to maximize calorie and nutrient consumption

- Recommend alternate forms of nutrition, such as tube feeding, if you are unable to obtain adequate nutrition by mouth

- Provide education on care and administration of tube feedings

Working with speech pathologists, registered dietitians can identify swallowing weaknesses that can interfere with safe food and/or fluid intake. Speech pathologists may perform examinations to identify the source of chewing and swallowing problems and help the registered dietitian recommend modifications in the daily diet, depending on your individual needs. This may mean that the consistency of certain foods will be changed and the nutritional value maximized.

Identifying Nutritional Problems

Assessing Weight Changes

The initial assessment is very important because it gives an overview of your nutritional status and a point for comparison over time. At this time it is important to assess weight changes because muscle-wasting is part of ALS and can contribute to weight loss if caloric intake is insufficient. An increase in weight may be due to improvement in food consumption or tolerance of oral supplementation or tube feedings. It may also be related to fluid retention if weight gain is greater than two pounds per week, in which case the doctor should be notified.

Height is another factor in a nutritional assessment. A dietitian can help you determine how close you are to your ideal body weight. A weight 125 percent above "ideal weight" is considered overweight for height; 90 percent to 125 percent is a desirable range for weight, and anything less than 80 percent of ideal weight indicates severe loss and possibly poor nutritional stores, and may be of concern. A registered dietitian can determine whether you are well nourished or malnourished, depending on a variety of factors, including percent of ideal body weight.

Effects of Muscle Weakness

People in the early course of ALS generally lose lean body mass and have an increase in body fat because of decreased physical activity. Once problems with chewing, swallowing, and weight loss become more significant, both lean body mass and body fat become depleted. Chewing and swallowing problems are assessed by asking questions such as: How long does it take you to eat a meal? Are you having difficulty chewing, swallowing, or moving food around in your mouth? Do you choke on thin liquids such as water or on dry, crumbly foods such as crackers or popcorn?

Significant increases in the time that it takes to eat meals may be due to weakness in the arms and hands, causing difficulty using spoons, knives, and forks. Difficulty with chewing and swallowing also increases the time it takes to complete meals. People who take longer than 20 to 30 minutes to complete a meal may be showing evidence of difficulty in chewing and/or swallowing. A speech pathologist can examine and evaluate swallowing to determine any chewing or swallowing problems and recommend diet changes in liquids and solid foods.

Assessing Hydration Status

Adequate fluid is important to replace normal body losses, ensure good digestion and intestinal function, and prevent dehydration. It is generally recommended that everyone drink at least six to eight cups of fluid per day. If a person is having difficulty swallowing, however, this can become more difficult and even dangerous. In this case, the consistency of the fluids taken must be changed to help avoid aspiration of liquids.

Changes In Bowel Function

It is important to discuss any signs of constipation or diarrhea with the dietitian during the nutritional assessment. Constipation may occur because the muscles that assist defecation can become weak, especially if physical activity lessens. Also, the fiber content of the diet may drop if softer foods are eaten, making it difficult to maintain regular bowel movements. Diarrhea can occur because of a particular food item, viral illness, or a tube feeding formula. Problems in these areas should be discussed with your dietitian so that modifications to the diet or tube feeding can be considered to alleviate any discomfort if there are no medical issues.

The Effects of Past Medical History

Past medical problems can be an obstacle to adequate nutrition and diet. People with ALS may not have other significant medical problems, but any history of heart disease, diabetes, cancer, renal disease, stroke, or other conditions should be discussed with the dietitian. The dietitian will help assess whether past dietary restrictions should be continued, liberalized, or discontinued based on current nutritional status. It may be appropriate to adjust some existing diet restrictions if you experience poor food and/or liquid consumption, chewing and/or swallowing problems, and weight loss. This should be done only after consultation with a registered dietitian.

Follow-Up and Reassessment

Follow-up with the dietitian is important because it can help address any new issues that have occurred since the last assessment. Your weight should be checked at every visit, and chewing and swallowing should be reevaluated. Reassessment may result in changes to your diet prescription, oral supplementation, recommendations for enteral tube feedings, providing high-calorie recipes, or simply a continuation of the current diet regimen. Each follow-up visit will address issues needed to continue your optimal nutritional status.

Recommendations to Improve Nutrition and Fluid Intake

Adapting Food and/or Fluid Consistencies

If chewing and swallowing become difficult, it is important to change the consistency of foods to make them easier and safer to swallow. The diet usually will change to mechanically softened with chopped meats, casseroles, well-cooked vegetables, and soft fruits, or a pureed diet, which provides a blenderized consistency for all food items. All foods should be well moistened with gravy, butter, and/or sauces to make them easier to swallow. Dry and crumbly foods such as crackers, potato chips, pretzels, and muffins may cause problems and therefore should be avoided (Tables 11-1 and 11-2).

Maximizing Calories and Nutrients

When any weight loss is noted, oral supplementation with commercial or home-prepared products is encouraged to increase calorie and protein content and to prevent continued weight loss or minimize any loss of lean body mass. Oral supplements should be consumed at least two to four times per day, depending on your nutritional needs and the amount of solid food eaten. Some people with ALS complain of excess phlegm with consumption of dairy products. Most oral supplements either are made with milk or have a milky consistency, and they may need to be discontinued to alleviate the excess phlegm. Alternative supplements made with fruit ice, juices, and egg whites or nonfat dry milk to add protein can substitute for the thicker products.

Other ways to increase calories include adding gravy, cream sauces, sugar, honey, and butter to foods (Table 11-3). Calories and protein can be added to the diet with items such as nonfat dry milk or egg whites mixed with other foods. Although adequate dietary protein is important, insufficient calorie intake is the primary problem that most people experience and should be the focus of nutritional supplementation.

Some people with ALS complain of becoming full early while consuming a meal. Eating six small meals per day may alleviate this problem. Drinking fluids while eating may contribute to a feeling of fullness, and drinking fluids between meals and after meals may increase the amount of food tolerated, unless drinking while eating helps the swallowing process.

Maintaining Adequate Hydration

It is important to drink at least six to eight cups of fluid per day to maintain good hydration. You may have difficulty with thin liquids, making this goal for fluid intake very difficult to achieve. Commercial thickeners added to thin liquids or the use of naturally thick liquids may be helpful. Commercial thickeners can be purchased without a doctor's prescription. Naturally thick liquids may also be used, such as milkshakes, ice cream, cream soups, puddings, tomato juice, nectars, and gelatin (see Table 11-2).

Table 11-1

Selecting Easy To Swallow Foods
FLUIDS: 6 to 8 8-ounce cups per day

Select	Select, only if thin liquids are tolerated
Sherbet and sherbet shakes Ice Cream Milk shakes Gelatin Pudding Fruit ice Orange juice with gelatin added Pureed fruits	Water Coffee Tea Soft drinks Thin juices Hot chocolate Thin soup Chunky-style soup

PROTEINS: 2 to 3 servings per day

Select	Avoid
Moist, ground or pureed meat and poultry Tender fish without bones Eggs	Tough, dry meats Dry poultry or dry fish Peanut butter

DAIRY: 2 to 3 servings per day

Select	Avoid
Creamy cottage cheese Yogurt Ice cream without nuts, raisins, or candy Milk, buttermilk (if thin liquids are tolerated), and milkshakes	Dry cottage cheese Ice cream with nuts, raisins, or candy

STARCHES: 6 TO 11 SERVINGS PER DAY

Select	Avoid
Bread or toast buttered or dunked in liquid Cold cereal soaked in milk or cream Cooked cereal Pancakes Pasta Casseroles Rice with gravy or sauce Moist cookies or quick breads without coconut, raisins or nuts Baked, mashed or boiled potatoes with gravy, cream, or margarine	Crumbly bread Hard rolls Bread with nuts, seeds, coconut, or fruit Bread with cracked wheat particles Sweet rolls Waffles Doughnuts Coffee cake English muffins Dry cereal flakes Dry toast, crackers, Melba toast, dry rice, or dry cookies

Table 11-1 *(cont.)*

FRUITS: 2 to 4 servings per day

Select	Avoid
Soft, fresh or canned fruits with seeds, pits, and skin removed Chilled applesauce or pureed fruit Poached fruit in gelatin Ripe bananas	Raw fruits with skins Stringy pineapple Dried fruit

VEGETABLES: 3 to 5 servings per day

Select	Avoid
Soft, canned vegetables or well cooked fresh or frozen vegetables Scalloped tomatoes	Raw vegetables Firm cooked vegetables, stringy vegetables with hulls (such as corn, spinach, or firm peas)

SOUPS

Select	Select only if thin liquids are tolerated
Thick soups such as cream soups or thickened broth-based soups (any vegetables should be well-cooked)	Broth and thin soups

DESSERTS

Select	Avoid
Fruit whip Gelatin Cobblers Apple or peach crisps Moist cookies without nuts or raisins Custards Puddings Hard frozen sherbet or ice cream	Dry, crumbly cakes and cookies Desserts with raisins, nuts, seeds, or coconut

FATS, SNACKS, AND OTHER FOODS

Select	Avoid
Butter or margarine Gravy Sour cream Melted cheese Honey Jelly Plain chocolate without nuts Chocolate mint patties	Popcorn Potato chips Corn chips Pickles Seeds Whole spices Nuts

Table 11-2

CREATING THE BEST TEXTURE

To thicken foods and liquids, try . . .

- Adding mashed potatoes, potato flakes, sauces, or gravies to pureed vegetables, casseroles or soups
- Adding plain gelatin, cooked cereal, or flaked rice cereal to pureed fruits
- Cooking canned fruit with tapioca or corn starch to create a thick pie-filling texture

---

To thin foods or make dry foods moist, try . . .

- Adding broth, gravies, sauces, milk, cream, butter, or margarine to hot foods
- Adding fruit juices, pureed fruit, cold milk, cream, yogurt, or liquid plain gelatin to cold foods

---

To make your foods softer, try . . .

- Using your favorite foods in casserole recipes when suitable
- Grinding meats with vegetables in a blender or food processor
- Mashing fruit or vegetables
- Cooking meat in broth or soup to keep it moist
- Poaching fish in milk to keep it soft

Table 11-3

BOOSTING CALORIES

Instead of . . .	Try . . .
Hot cereal	Hot cereal with butter or margarine, cream and honey, or sugar
Plain eggs	Scrambled eggs with butter or margarine, melted cheese, and cream
Plain pancakes	Pancakes topped with plenty of syrup, whipped cream, butter, or margarine
Baked potato	Potatoes mashed with cream and butter or margarine, or topped with sour cream, Parmesan, Romano or other cheeses, and butter or margarine
Fresh apple	A peeled, cored apple baked with brown sugar and butter, topped with cream
Regular pudding	Pudding made with cream and topped with whipped cream
Plain ice cream	Premium ice cream topped with your favorite flavored syrup and marshmallow cream
Milk (if thin liquids are tolerated)	Make thick milkshakes by adding ice cream, your favorite syrup, and an instant breakfast mix

Adequate fluid intake will help to relieve constipation as well as maintain hydration. Soft, fiber-containing foods may also be recommended, and bulking agents can be tried. If diarrhea occurs as the result of consumption of a particular food, such as milk, that food item should be omitted from the diet. Medical treatment may be needed if the diarrhea is caused by diseases rather than diet. Increasing fluid intake is also appropriate to help replace fluid losses from diarrhea. Patients on tube feeding may have diarrhea because of a concentrated formula (more than 1 calorie per milliliter), the rate at which the tube feeding is being administered, or too high a volume. You should contact a dietitian for recommendations to change the tube feeding formula, rate, and/or volume to maintain appropriate fluid, calories, and protein to meet your nutritional needs.

If you begin to have difficulty with chewing or swallowing, increased time to consume meals, and weight loss, meeting nutritional needs by mouth may no longer be possible. When these signs begin to appear, it is important to begin to discuss the option of having a feeding tube placed. It is important to understand that tube feedings may be safer and easier than trying to meet all your nutrient needs by eating and drinking by mouth. If increased time to consume a meal is primarily a result of inability to handle and manipulate spoons, knives, and forks, rather than difficulty chewing and/or swallowing, an occupational therapist may be able to recommend utensils that can help with eating. If the weakness also involves difficulty chewing and/or swallowing, tube feedings will be the most effective option.

Tube Feeding

Tube feedings are an alternative form of meeting nutritional needs if eating by mouth has become difficult, dangerous, or insufficient. The option of having a feeding tube placed should be discussed when it becomes apparent that eating is affected by weakness. Subjective signs, such as taking longer to finish meals, coughing or choking with foods or beverages, difficulty moving food around in the mouth, or difficulty chewing, are signs that eating is becoming more difficult and that maintaining intake by mouth alone may not be feasible. It is very important to realize that receiving a feeding tube early in the disease provides a better outcome.

Weight loss, a more objective sign that adequate caloric intake is not being achieved, also indicates that tube feeding may be necessary. It has been suggested that a weight loss of 5 percent of usual body weight along with signs of chewing and swallowing difficulty should be a starting point for discussions of receiving a feeding tube. Weight loss of more than 10 percent of one's usual weight over a short span of time (2 to 3 months or less) or of more than 20 percent overall, is considered severe. Tube feeding options should be discussed by the time weight loss has reached these levels. Although there is no definitive point at which feeding tube placement is considered "ideal," tube feeding placement is often better tolerated by a well-nourished person who has a well-maintained breathing capacity (vital capacity greater than 50% of normal). Also, the presence of a feeding tube does not need to interfere with food intake by mouth but can supplement regular oral intake. Tube feeding allows people to achieve all of their food and fluid requirements.

There are a variety of feeding tubes, and selection will depend on your medical condition and the expected length of time that the tube will be required. Tube types and their advantages and disadvantages are summarized in Table 11-4. Tubes that extend from the nose into the stomach are often used for short-term feedings, that is, a few weeks or less. They may cause irritation to the throat and nasal passages over longer periods and are somewhat obtrusive to the user, and therefore are not the typical tube used for long-term feeding as is necessary with ALS.

Instead, *gastrostomy tubes* are most commonly used by people with ALS. They are placed directly into the stomach through an incision in the outside of the abdominal wall. They can easily be kept out of sight when not in use and generally do not cause physical discomfort or irritation after the original incision has healed. The most common gastrostomy tube is called a *percutaneous endoscopic gastrostomy* (PEG) tube. This tube is placed by a gastroenterologist or surgeon and requires only local anesthetic for placement. Patients are usually discharged from the hospital the day after tube placement. Feedings usually are administered in 4 to 5 feed-

Table 11-4

TUBE TYPE	USUAL FEEDING SCHEDULE	BENEFITS	LIMITATIONS
Nasogastric (NG)	Feedings can be given in bolus form (large doses in a relatively short time) several times each day.	Least traumatic to the body for placement	Irritating to the nasal cavity over time (so usually only used for a few weeks duration). May be considered obtrusive as it dangles from the nose.
Percutaneous Endoscopic Gastrostomy (PEG)	Usually bolus feedings, several times each day.	Minimal trauma, requires overnight hospitalization, uses local anesthesia and muscle relaxants.	Requires some sedation therefore pulmonary function is a concern. Otherwise, generally well tolerated
Jejunostomy (J tubes)	Feedings must be run slowly over several hours, usually at least 12 hours per day, continuously.	Placement of the tube lower in the gastrointestinal tract may or may not reduce risk of aspirating feedings.	If surgically placed, will require general anesthesia. If placed endoscopically, the anesthesia is minimized. Feeding scheduling options most limited.

ings-per-day schedules (depending on food intake) each taking about 10 to 20 minutes to infuse via a syringe and 20 to 30 minutes dripping from a tube feeding bag.
PEG tubes are available in a variety of tube or button forms (Figure 11-1). Jejunostomy tubes, which are inserted directly into the jejunum, are also available. These
tubes require slower infusion rates than gastrostomy tubes. The physician placing
the feeding tube should discuss the appropriate tube options for your situation.

Once a feeding tube (usually a PEG tube) has been placed, you will be taught
the proper use and care of the feeding tube. Formula types and volumes should be
chosen, extra water requirements should be calculated, and all steps of the feeding
procedure should be carefully taught. For proper care of a PEG tube, you will need
to flush the tube carefully with water each time the tube is used (whether for feeding or for medication administration). You also should be instructed as to the
proper steps for dealing with the potential trouble areas, such as a clogged feeding

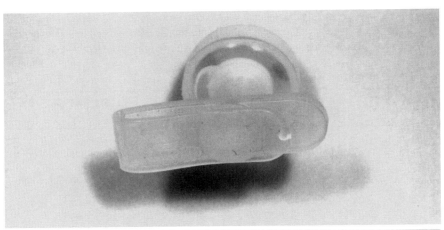

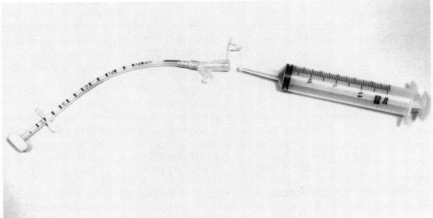

Figure 11-1. Percutaneous endoscopic gastrostomy (PEG) tubes.

tube or difficulty tolerating feedings because of diarrhea, constipation, abdominal discomfort, or nausea. You should call your physician immediately if you experience any vomiting, aspiration, irritation or redness at the PEG site, accidental removal of the PEG tube, or if any other problems continue to interfere with achieving the goal of the tube feeding plan. Tube feedings will be easiest to manage if all steps of the feeding process and any potential problems are discussed before discharge. Tube feeding schedules and formula types can also be adjusted as needed with the help of the dietitian or doctor as the tube is being used at home.

Why Should You Consider a PEG Tube Feeding?

Because it is a simple, practical, highly effective, and efficient way to provide necessary nutrition and water for anyone who has difficulty eating from the mouth. Having a PEG tube inserted is a simple, minimally invasive procedure. There is little risk associated with the procedure, and the benefits of good nutrition will assist in maintaining your strength.

Percutaneous indicates a tube that is placed from the skin surface of the abdomen; *endoscopic* means that the procedure is performed under the stomach scope; *gastrostomy* means that a direct connection is placed to the stomach.

All necessary foods fulfilling daily calorie requirement and water will be given through a feeding tube, but this does not mean that you cannot eat by mouth. In fact, patients frequently are allowed to take their foods by mouth as long as they feel comfortable. Patients need not struggle to eat to maintain their calorie and water requirements but can enjoy foods for pleasure just like anyone else. A majority of patients are reluctant to consider such a procedure; some patients do not wish to even discuss it or want to defer the decision because an artificial route to take food is not appealing. It is not uncommon for some patients to defer the decision until they become unable to eat by mouth. When this occurs, a simple procedure may become a risky one because breathing capacity may be reduced and malnourishment may have weakened the overall body defense.

The American Academy of Neurology recommends that PEG should be placed before vital capacity is below 50% of normal. This recommendation is based on previous studies showing that patients with ALS who had low vital capacity at the time of PEG procedure did poorly afterward. It does not mean that the procedure cannot be done in those who have poor breathing capacity, but the risk is not negligible. It is ideal to have the procedure done by a gastroenterologist or a general surgeon who has extensive experience with people with ALS. It is essential to have close follow-up by the doctor who performed the procedure and by a dietitian.

PEG Procedure

Before your PEG

Before having a PEG placed, a gastroenterologist will review your medical history with you and give you instructions regarding medication that you may be taking and answer any questions. The physician will schedule the procedure and give you preprocedure instructions.

What to Expect When Getting a PEG Tube

On the morning of the procedure, you will report to a procedure area at the hospital. You may not eat or drink anything for 8 hours before the procedure. You will be asked to change into a hospital gown, remove your eyeglasses and dentures, and have your vital signs taken. A nurse or a doctor will review your current medication with you and take a brief medical history. An intravenous catheter will be placed in a vein in your arm.

When the physician is ready, you will be taken into a procedure room that has all the equipment necessary for the PEG placement. The nurse will put a blood pressure cuff on your arm and a pulse oximeter on your fingertip, which will measure the amount of oxygen in your blood. Your blood pressure, heart rate, and blood oxygenation will be measured every 5 to 10 minutes during the procedure to ensure that your vital signs remain stable.

The physician will spray a numbing medication into the back of your throat and will give medication intravenously to make you sleepy and comfortable during the PEG placement. A plastic mouthpiece will be inserted into your mouth to provide an opening through which they will pass the endoscope down to your stomach. This endoscope will in no way interfere with your breathing.

After the endoscope reaches your stomach, the physician will find the correct position for the insertion of the tube, inject a small amount of medication to numb the area, and make a small incision through which to pass the tube. The flexible tube is then passed through the endoscope into your stomach and then out of the incision, so that the end of the tube is on the outside of your stomach. Bumpers are placed on both the outside and the inside of the stomach to ensure that the tube does not become dislodged. The tube can then be capped off or connected to nutritional feedings. The entire procedure takes approximately 15 minutes.

If you have difficulty breathing, the procedure may be carried out while you are on a bilevel positive pressure machine. This is a respiratory device that can assist you with breathing. A device similar to an oxygen mask can be placed over your nose to assist in moving air into your lungs. This can help make the procedure more comfortable and lessen the risk of respiratory complication both during and after the procedure.

The insertion site will be covered with an antibiotic ointment and a gauze placed over the incision. You will be transferred to a recovery area, where your vital signs will be monitored from 1-4 hours to ensure that you are feeling well and to allow the medication sufficient time to wear off. If you have any pain, there will be medication available to make you more comfortable. You may or may not be transferred to a unit in the hospital for an overnight stay.

The day after your PEG placement, sterile water will be placed through your new tube to ensure that the tube is functioning properly. If it is and your stomach tolerates the water without problems, a tube feeding, the nutritional supplement that you will be taking as nourishment, will be given to you by a nurse or dietitian. A nutritionist will teach you and your caregiver how to administer the feeding and what type and amount of nutritional supplement to use. The nutritionist will advise you as to the calories and amount of water that will meet your daily nutritional requirements. A nurse will show you how to care for the tube and the insertion site. Care of the tube and site is simple and usually requires washing it with soap and water.

You probably will be discharged the day after your procedure. A home visit with a nurse will be set up to ensure that you are comfortable with the feeding procedure and that your PEG site is healing well.

If there are changes in your bowel habits or any difficulties with your bowels, you should speak with your dietitian to ensure that your water and nutritional requirements are being met. You should also speak to your physician to determine if you need a stool softener. It is important to follow up with the physician who placed your PEG and with your dietitian.

12

Pulmonary Management

Robert Schilz, D.O., Ph.D., and Scott Marlow, R.R.T.

Progressive weakness of the muscles of eating, swallowing, and breathing can be among the more serious complications of amyotrophic lateral sclerosis (ALS). Management of these problems may require significant changes in the daily activities and care plan of a person with ALS, including options that may involve surgery and/or advanced life support techniques. These interventions and decisions are among the most significant that you will face in dealing with the disease.

The initial portion of this chapter discusses the physiology of breathing and the changes in the respiratory system that occur in ALS. Subsequent sections explore the complications that result from respiratory muscle weakness, treatment options, and decision making, using a series of questions often asked by people with ALS and their families.

Anatomy of the Muscles of Breathing

This section reviews the anatomy of the respiratory system, with special emphasis on the muscle groups responsible for inhalation, exhalation, chewing, and swallowing. The *inspiratory muscles* are depicted in Figure 12-1. The *diaphragm* is the major muscle of inspiration. It is made up of two halves, the right and left hemidiaphragms. Each hemidiaphragm is under the control of a nerve—a phrenic nerve, which carries electrical impulses originating in the brain and directs the contraction of its accompanying muscle. Contraction of this muscle leads to the

163

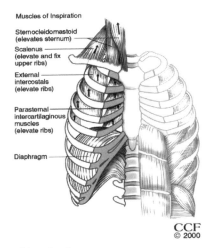

Muscles of Inspiration

Sternocleidomastoid
(elevates sternum)

Scalenus
(elevate and fix
upper ribs)

External
intercostals
(elevate ribs)

Parasternal
intercartilaginous
muscles
(elevate ribs)

Diaphragm

CCF
© 2000

Figure 12-1. Muscles of inspiration.

descent of the floor of the chest cavity, increasing the volume of the chest and creating a negative pressure or vacuum within the body. Air flows into the lung in response to this vacuum. Muscles in the shoulders, upper ribs, and chest can assist the diaphragm in the inspiratory effort and can often be seen to contract in people who have significant weakness of the diaphragm. These accessory muscles can be useful, but they are not as efficient as the diaphragm in breathing.

Weakness of the diaphragm leads to inability to create a sufficient vacuum within the chest, which in turn leads to a smaller than normal breath. Patients with significant weakness of the diaphragm often breathe rapidly and shallowly. This weakness results in breathlessness or even an accumulation of carbon dioxide in the blood if the degree of muscle weakness is advanced.

Figure 12-2 shows the muscles involved in the production of a forceful exhalation. Some muscles, particularly those of the abdomen, function to increase the pressure within the chest while the throat is closed. This "built-up" pressure exits forcefully upon opening of the throat, bringing up mucus from large airways in the lungs. Weakness of these *expiratory muscles* makes it difficult or impossible to clear secretions. These secretions can pool within the lung and increase the chance of developing pneumonia.

The Effects of ALS on the Respiratory System

Neuromuscular weakness associated with ALS leads to three major classes of respiratory disorders:

• Hypoventilation syndromes, or the inability to breathe adequately

• Obstructive sleep apnea syndrome

• Pneumonia syndromes

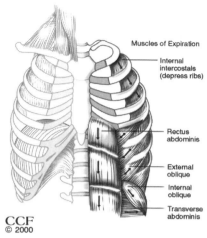

Muscles of Expiration

Internal intercostals (depress ribs)

Rectus abdominis

External oblique

Internal oblique

Transverse abdominis

CCF
© 2000

Figure 12-2. Muscles of expiration.

Each of these syndromes is discussed separately. Each section explains the symptoms that suggest the presence of any of these problems, a summary of what we know about how they occur, their impact on people with ALS, and a discussion of management of how they are managed.

Hypoventilation Syndromes

Muscle weakness that affects the muscles of respiration is one of the most serious problems in ALS, and complications of respiratory muscle weakness remains the leading cause of death. Progressive weakness of the muscles that support breathing leads to a sensation of breathlessness, an inability to cough and clear secretions, and decreased voice volume. The following section explores what may be among the most difficult questions typically asked by people with ALS.

Will my breathing muscles become weak?

Yes, even if the predominant early effect of ALS is *bulbar*—affecting the muscles of the face, tongue, and mouth. Almost everyone with the disease will ultimately face declining respiratory function. The decline of muscle strength differs in different people, but it tends to progress at a linear rate in any given person (Figure 12-3). Although isolated weakness of the respiratory muscles can occur, weakness often parallels that seen in other muscles groups such as the tongue, mouth, arms, and legs.

What are the signs and symptoms of weakness of the breathing muscles?

The earliest sign of breathing weakness is *dyspnea,* or shortness of breath during exertion. This can be noticeable in activities as simple as walking up stairs. Many people may not be aware of this limitation, especially if ALS has affected muscles

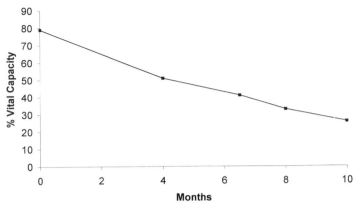

Figure 12-3. The decline of muscle strength in a patient with ALS as demonstrated by a decreased vital capacity over time.

of the legs and thus severely limited the ability to walk. In these circumstances, you may not notice a progressive decline in breathing power because you are unable to perform significant exercise. If this is the case, weakness in the breathing muscles may be noticed mainly as a decrease power of the voice, a decreased ability to cough, or breathlessness when lying down. These are all later stages of weakness characterized by a marked impairment of the muscle function. Observation of the breathing effort of people with weak respiratory muscles will often reveal a para-doxical rise of the stomach and inward motion of the chest when breathing in.

Why do I feel short of breath when I lie down but feel comfortable breathing when I sit up?

Orthopnea, or the sensation of shortness of breath when lying down, is a later stage of muscle weakness than exertional *dyspnea.* This sensation is perfectly understandable considering the anatomy of the abdominal contents and the diaphragm. When a person lies on his back, the contents of the abdomen shift to-ward the head. Inspiration requires descent of the diaphragm, which in the supine person also needs to push the abdominal contents back toward the waist. A weak-ened diaphragm may be less able to do this, and the additional work is perceived as dyspnea. Assuming an upright position allows gravity to pull the abdominal contents toward the waist, effectively unloading the inspiratory muscle and relieving the sensation of breathlessness.

How is respiratory muscle weakness diagnosed?

These symptoms in the absence of other lung or heart disorders are a clue to respiratory muscle weakness. That weakness is usually confirmed by pulmonary function testing. A person with decreased strength, in the absence of other lung or chest wall disorders, typically will show a decrease in the amount of air that can be inhaled, which is termed the *vital capacity*. This loss is paralleled by a decrease in the amount of air that can be forcibly exhaled. Maximal pressures developing during inspiration (MIP) or expiration (MEP) may also be abnormal early in the course of ALS, even when the vital capacity is normal. Maximal voluntary ventilation (MVV) is a measure of the fatigability of the respiratory muscles. The difference between pulmonary testing obtained in the seated and the supine (lying flat on the back) position may also reveal significant diaphragm dysfunction due to the physiology discussed previously. People with other lung diseases such as emphysema or fibrosis may have abnormalities of pulmonary testing that do not reflect weakness, and this complicates the interpretation of testing.

Performing the above tests requires that you be able to blow into a pulmonary testing machine with a good seal of the lips around a mouthpiece. This may be difficult if you have poor bulbar muscle function and can lead to a falsely low measurement.

Measurement of arterial blood gases is another useful test. A sample of blood taken from an artery (typically in the wrist) can be immediately analyzed for the presence of oxygen and carbon dioxide. Ineffective breathing often decreases the amount of oxygen in the blood and increases the amount of carbon dioxide—the normal waste product of oxygen use by the body. Such abnormalities if seen may signal the need to consider advanced support techniques or to test for sleep apnea.

Can the time until respiratory failure be predicted?

As stated previously, the decline of respiratory muscle strength tends to continue to progress. Many people with ALS will experience respiratory muscle paralysis or failure within 5 years of the onset of decline (Figure 12-4), but many progress over a period of months. A patient generally cannot maintain adequate gas exchange when measures of pulmonary function fall below a basic level.

However, before this point is reached, people with ALS can be at risk for rapid deterioration from aspiration due to mucus plugging or pneumonia and the increased work of breathing that these conditions can produce. Many people who ultimately remain on mechanical ventilation find themselves placed on a ventilator in the setting of an acute infection (usually pneumonia) in an intensive care unit (ICU). Medical management can often clear the infection, but the patient may remain dependent on the ventilator. This deterioration can occur over a period of hours or days even in patients who were previously stable although at a low level of muscle function. For this reason, plans regarding options for support in the setting of respiratory insufficiency should be formed at the beginning of respiratory decline and certainly when the vital capacity declines below 50 percent.

What can be done about weakening inspiratory muscles?

General measures such as optimal nutrition and rest are always important to

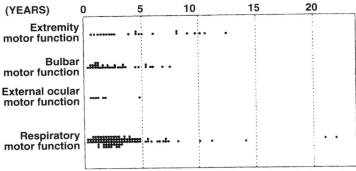

Figure 12-4. Time between diagnosis of ALS and complete paralysis of motor function in 87 patients.

optimize health and function, regardless of infirmity. Difficulties with feeding can predispose you to poor nutrition, which can decrease respiratory muscle function over and above the neuromuscular damage caused by the disease.

As with the other affected muscle groups in ALS, no medication has been shown to reverse the weakness in respiratory muscles. Newer medications such as Rilutek extend the overall lifespan, but the relationship between administration of this drug and respiratory function has not been convincingly shown. Faced with weakening respiratory muscle function, there are few options in the face of continued respiratory muscle decline. Available options are listed below. They must be considered within the context of quality of life questions and the realistic goals of treatment.

1. No mechanical support. This is best combined with symptom relief with medications and emotional support, realizing that failing or ineffective respiration will be fatal (1).

2. Consideration of ventilatory support by noninvasive means of ventilatory assist. Although devices such as pneumatic belts, negative pressure suits, rocking beds, and iron lung ventilators have been described for ventilatory assist in ALS, a face mask device, oral appliances, or nasal pillar connected to a small ventilator is more commonly used (Figure 12-5). These machines are also sometimes called BiPAP® (bilevel positive airway pressure) machines or just BiPAP®. They are usually used intermittently, often at night, and are very beneficial for respiratory symptom relief but may not be adequate to provide complete ventilation in a patient with very poor muscle strength or with diminished control of oral muscles.

3. Tracheostomy and direct mechanical ventilation (Figure 12-6).

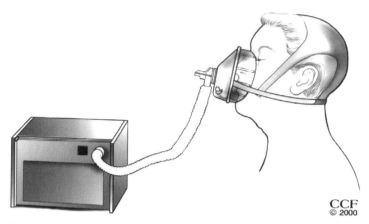

CCF
© 2000

Figure 12-5. Typical face mask in bilevel (BiPAP®) device set up.

Which option is best for me?

The ultimate choice of potentially life-sustaining treatment is a uniquely personal experience for each person with ALS. The "right" thing to do is not what any person or group of people may dictate. Rather, it is an informed choice that should be made by the person with ALS based on careful education, counseling, and, in many cases, discussion with other people with ALS and their families who are willing to share their experiences. Many patients, families, and physicians find it difficult to discuss respiratory failure, decisions regarding life support, and other advance directives difficult, and they may defer them rather than face a difficult situation. These decisions about advanced care and respiratory support should not

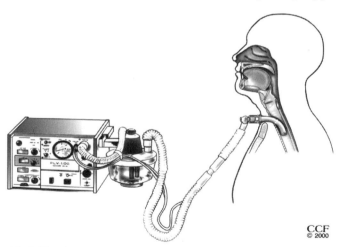

CCF
© 2000

Figure 12-6. Tracheostomy to portable mechanical ventilation.

be deferred. *Failure to initiate an open dialogue and honest appraisal of the disease course and expectations has the potential to place you and your family in situations that you did not intend, anticipate, or plan for.*

The following considerations may be helpful in the decision process, realizing that limited data exist to directly compare approaches to manage the failing muscles of respiration.

1. Patient choices and situations dictating ventilation and satisfaction.

Most (90–95%) people with ALS prefer not to undergo invasive mechanical ventilation with a tracheostomy (2). Reasons typically listed include: unwillingness to prolong what is for many an unacceptable lifestyle limitation, denial of the disease process, unwillingness to burden family members or caregivers, or the lack of resources to support mechanical ventilation. An estimated 5 percent to 8 percent of people with ALS ultimately are supported on mechanical ventilation, and most say they would make the same choice again (2).

Studies show that the initial choice for mechanical ventilation most often was made after an urgent respiratory event that placed the patient in an ICU (2). Many patients in this setting continue mechanical ventilation. However, this kind of decision making is very stressful. Rarely can a truly informed decision be made in such a setting. The resultant situation may be an adaptation to events rather than a conscious choice. Nonetheless, mechanically ventilated ALS patients typically believe that they have a quality of life that is acceptable to them in spite of profound limitation in activity (3).

2. Personal or psychological characteristics of people who accept mechanical ventilation.

As opposed to the many patients who suddenly deteriorate, a minority of patients carefully examine the benefits and burdens of invasive mechanical ventilation with tracheostomy. They consciously plan for and move to full ventilatory support as their respiratory muscle strength declines, often starting with either noninvasive face mask ventilation or 8 to 12 hours of invasive ventilation during sleep. It has been suggested—and I concur—that people who elect mechanical ventilation at home are more likely to have the following characteristics (4):

- They are highly motivated and engaged in living.
- Their ALS is progressing slowly.
- They are able to communicate and do some ADLs.
- Both patient and family understand the options.
- The family is able and wants to participate in home mechanical ventilation.
- Resources for equipment and caregivers are available.
- Experienced multidisciplinary teams are available to support the process.

Some studies have tried to determine if there is a psychological difference between people with ALS who accept mechanical ventilation and those who do not. In general, no differences in sociodemographic makeup, depression, hopelessness, overall quality of life, or psychological well-being were noted (5). However patients who chose ventilatory support had a more internal health locus of control. Caregivers supporting a patient on home ventilation described themselves as heavily burdened, with a maximal curtailing of outside activities (3).

3. Physical factors limiting choice of ventilatory assistance.

Not all options of mechanical ventilatory support are either tolerated or effective for everyone. Probably the best example is that of face mask ventilation (BiPAP®, noninvasive ventilation). Patients with poor oropharyngeal control or severe weakness of the bulbar muscles are more likely to fail in trying to use this method of ventilation (6). The absence of teeth or the particular formation of the jaw or nose may prevent effective mask fit, limiting the usefulness of this technique. Excessive secretions or mucus formation may also limit the effectiveness of a number of noninvasive techniques of ventilatory assistance.

What are the benefits of mechanical ventilation?

Mechanical ventilation, whether by mask or by tracheostomy, provides respiratory support when respiratory strength is failing. It relieves symptoms of breathlessness and prolongs life in patients who otherwise could not breath adequately by themselves. Patients undergoing ventilatory assist with face mask ventilation (6) or invasive ventilation with a tracheostomy tube (3) typically report an improved quality of life compared with previous levels without the intervention.

What are the burdens of mechanical ventilation?

1. An increase in the complexity of health care delivery.

A person who is dependent on mechanical ventilatory assistance for comfort or for provision of life-saving ventilation will require attendance by people who have been instructed in techniques of ventilator management. The amount of this additional attention will depend on how dependent he is on the ventilator. A person who uses using a face mask ventilator (BiPAP®) predominantly at night to facilitate supine sleeping but retains the ability to place the mask by himself may require only minimal supervision. However, it is more common for people requiring ventilatory support to be unable to administer the therapy on their own. People in this situation need close support and management during the period of ventilation so that adjustments and troubleshooting can occur in a timely fashion.

The delivery of invasive mechanical ventilation through a tracheostomy tube requires additional skill to manage the tracheostomy, suction the airway, and provide backup support for inadvertent machine disconnection or malfunction. Family members can be trained to do this, but providing 24-hour supervision and care is difficult at best and is often not possible without outside nursing assistance.

2. An increase in the cost of patient care.

Caring for people who require invasive mechanical ventilation is expensive. The yearly care of a ventilated ALS patient has been estimated to exceed $140,000 (2,4). This cost is beyond the means of most people, and the difference must be made up by insurance plans or other means.

3. Limitation of patient mobility.

People who require ventilatory support are typically confined to an area roughly 6 feet from the machine providing the ventilation. Portable units that use a battery or adapters, allowing operation from motor vehicles, are available but require substantial planning and technical support to provide any degree of mobility. As noted before, many people with ALS who are dependent on a ventilator are unable to participate in relocating it to facilitate mobility. Since profound weakness of other muscle groups often accompanies respiratory muscle weakness, most people who require ventilator assistance are also wheelchair bound.

4. A decrease in the quality of life of family members participating in home ventilatory care.

The intensity, duration, and effort required to support a person on mechanical ventilation is significant for caregivers. Caregivers who support a person with ALS who is on home ventilation feel maximally burdened, with a severe curtailing of outside activities.

5. The institution of mechanical ventilation may require placing patients in facilities that have skilled care to deliver mechanical ventilation.

As noted previously, the technical and caregiver support of patients who require mechanical ventilation can be extensive. Many families may not be able to provide the amount and intensity of care required. Considerations of skilled nursing facilities able to care for ventilated patients must be arranged, in addition to the other aspects of their care.

6. Discomfort of the ventilatory technique.

Although advances in ventilators continue to focus on patient comfort and better design, mechanical ventilators do not provide respiration that mimics normal breathing. Skillful pulmonary support can maximize the level of comfort, but these devices typically have some of the following shortfalls.

- An inability to deliver the duration or depth of breath required in all situations
- Asynchrony with coughing leading to inappropriate triggering of the machine
- Discomfort of the patient interface—mask or tracheostomy or other appliance

The necessity for suctioning secretions through a tracheostomy also will provoke a cough reflex. Most people using mechanical ventilation must in one way or another adapt to these limitations (7).

7. Prolongation of a chronically progressing and debilitating disease process.

Although prolongation of life is a potential benefit of mechanical ventilation, it is important to remember that not all patients see this as beneficial. Patients who are unable to effectively communicate or participate in their daily activities, yet who are able to feel discomfort and the limitation of their condition, are said to be "locked in" to their bodies by the disease process. Many people do not view this condition as providing a meaningful quality of life.

What is the optimal timing of ventilatory support if it is accepted?

Most specialists agree that mechanical ventilation should be considered in a person with ALS when

- Significant positional symptoms or dyspnea at rest is present.
- An elevated carbon dioxide level of 45–50 mmHg is present.
- There is significant hypoventilation at night.
- Vital capacity testing is less than 50 percent of normal .

None of these criteria are absolute. Conscious planning and institution of support in a controlled and intermittent fashion is preferable to urgent administration during acute events or deterioration.

What is involved in the use of mechanical ventilation?

This question comprises such a wide variety of topics that it has been subdivided into the following sections.

What is noninvasive ventilation (NIV)?

Noninvasive mask ventilation as mentioned earlier requires the use of either a volume-limited mechanical ventilator or bi-level positive pressure airway device (BiPAP®) as seen in Figure 12-5. These devices are used with a nasal appliance, oral nasal system, or a full face mask. Early noninvasive ventilation was accomplished with a home mechanical ventilator. These mechanical ventilators were used in conjunction with a nasal mask, mouth piece (8) or with a full face mask. Although this method was demonstrated to improve survival in patients with ALS (6) there are a number of practical limitations.

1. Mask interface leaks cause lower delivered support since these ventilators typically cannot deliver higher flow rates to compensate.

2. Troublesome low pressure alarms can occur requiring a caregiver to reset the alarm.

Noninvasive ventilation via pressure support or BiPAP® devices provide a way to assist ventilation which more closely follows a patient's innate respiratory pattern. Pressure support machines can sense small changes in patient breathing and increase pressure automatically to assist inspiration. The BiPAP® device then will rapidly decrease this pressure allowing exhalation when it senses the patient is stopping a breath. This action of varying inspiratory and expiratory pressure has been demonstrated to improve patient tolerance when compared to volume limited ventilation (6).

Characteristics useful for the home noninvasive ventilation should include back up respiratory rate that will automatically increase pressure even if the machine does not sense that a patient is initiating a breath. A second consideration is if the unit will require a disconnect alarm or power failure alarm. Some units have this as a feature, whereas others can connect an external alarm as needed. A third consideration includes the availability of a battery back up.

What factors influence the ability to tolerate nasal or oral noninvasive ventilation?

There are multiple factors involved with the patient's ability to tolerate noninvasive ventilation (NIV). The factors affecting the patient's ability to tolerate NIV include, but may not be limited to:

1. Difficulties with mask or system interface

2. Feeling of claustrophobia

3. Difficulties related to bulbar symptoms

4. Increased or decreased secretion problems

5. Nasal irritation

6. Pressure requirement for support

Many of these problems can be minimized with careful attention to the ventilator interface. The interface between the patient and machine can be accomplished with a nasal mask, a full-face mask, a custom mouth seal, or with a custom mouth and nose seal. Proper mask fit is essential for patient comfort and will greatly improve the patients ability to tolerate NIV. A variety of nasal mask and appliances are available. An improperly fit mask or headgear can lead to air leaks, abrasions on the bridge of the nose or under the nose, eye irritation, and ear irritation.

Careful initial fitting of masks, gradual introduction to the sensation of ventilatory support and subsequent adjustment based on patient feedback are important keys to long term comfort and effectiveness of NIV.

Mask fit and effective ventilation may be difficult or unachievable in patients with severe bulbar dysfunction. Patients demonstrating moderate to severe bulbar symptoms are twice as likely to be those noted to be intolerant of NIV, but it should be noted that those who are intolerant could have a 2.7 fold higher risk for death within the study period than those who are tolerant (6). Another factor influenced by the extent of bulbar symptoms can include abdominal distension, increasing risk of discomfort and potentially aspiration.

How is the machine adjusted?

The machine is initially adjusted to patient comfort in conjunction with a thorough description of the device's use and limitations. When the patient is initially started it is best to start both the inspiratory and expiratory pressures very low and gradually increase the pressures per patient comfort. In general the pressure levels that give relief of symptoms are typically close to the "best" levels which may subsequently be assessed by arterial blood gas analysis, end tidal CO_2 measurement, or even during a nocturnal polysomnogram (sleep study).

What are the limitations of NIV?

It is important to note that noninvasive ventilators were initially never designed as "life support" devices. A number of the factors, which make them useful for partial support, actually can hinder their use in some patients who require a ventilator to support the majority of their breathing.

1. They are not designed to deliver high pressures or predetermined volumes, which may be required for patients with profoundly weak respiratory muscles.
2. Many do not have alarms to signal potentially fatal disconnects.
3. Many simple NIV ventilators may not be able to deliver a breath unless it senses that the patient is breathing. (Although many machines now have a "backup" respiratory rate which will occur even in the absence of sufficient patient effort.)
4. NIV does not have an interface that facilitates the clearing of secretions.

What should I do if my nose bleeds or my throat becomes very dry?

With the use of the anticholinergic drugs and the increased flow created from the NIV unit, patients may complain of dryness or thicker secretions. The various modes of treatment to improve these symptoms include but may not be limited to:

1. Increasing the fluid intake
2. Adding an external heated humidifier to the NIV
3. Including lemon ice frozen dessert to the diet
4. Meat tenderizer with papase; place a few grains on the tongue and swallow
5. Adding a room or house humidifier
6. Normal saline nasal sprays

How is invasive ventilation (via tracheostomy) different from NIV?

Noninvasive ventilation augments ventilatory support via nasal and/or oral appliance, as described earlier. This is not considered a life support device and keeps intact the patient's natural humidification and body defense mechanisms of the upper oral pharyngeal cavities.

A patient undergoing mechanical ventilation via tracheostomy tube placed in the main airway (trachea) is shown in Figure 12-6. A tracheostomy tube consists of a curved round tube with an outer cannula, an inner cannula, and a flange. A small balloon device surrounds the end of the tracheostomy tube, which resides in the airway to form a seal that permits ventilation. A tract or stoma must be made in the neck and into the airway to allow placement of the tracheostomy tube. A surgeon typically performs this procedure in an operating room. Once placed, the tracheostomy tube has the following consequences:

1. It allows high pressure ventilation to occur, which can completely support the breathing needs of the patient. It does not rely on patient effort for triggering or meeting ventilatory need.

2. The tracheostomy provides a direct pathway into the lungs. This will allow caregivers to suction secretions that may not be able to be cleared by the patient but will also provide an increased chance of pulmonary infections since the upper airway defense mechanisms are bypassed. The process of suctioning induces cough with an element of discomfort in patients.

3. There are no issues with fit or intolerance of a mask.

4. The tracheostomy bypasses the "voice box" or larynx. Patients on a ventilator with a tracheostomy generally will not be able to talk unless the tracheostomy tube is temporarily plugged. This may be possible in the patient with some residual respiratory strength, who can be off a ventilator for short periods of time, but is unlikely.

What care is involved with a tracheostomy?

The aspects of care regarding a tracheostomy include:

1. Care of the tracheostomy tube and stoma

2. Suctioning of retained secretions

3. Tracheostomy tube replacement and humidification.

Once a patient is home, the family or caregivers typically adapt a clean technique for tracheostomy cleaning. Tracheostomy care involves removal, cleaning, and reinsertion of the tracheostomy tube inner cannula. Also involved with tracheostomy cleaning is the removal and replacement of the tracheostomy ties and dressings surrounding the stoma site. The stoma site is cleaned with cotton swabs saturated with a 50:50 ratio of peroxide and water. The supplies required for tracheostomy care include gloves, brush cleaner, pipe cleaners, cotton swabs , hydrogen peroxide, saline or distilled water, split gauze, tracheostomy tube holder, and a temporary inner cannula (if patient is continuously ventilated). Most of the supplies, except the solutions, are typically packaged in a sterile tracheostomy care kit.

Suctioning will be required because of the patient's progressive muscle weakness and the inability to generate sufficient cough flows. Suctioning the tracheostomy tube involves introducing a thin flexible plastic catheter through the tracheostomy tube and into the lungs. The actual technique includes preoxygenating the patient, if instructed to do so by your physician and education team, and advancing a suction catheter until a resistance is met, typically at the branch of the right and left main airways. The catheter is withdrawn approximately 2 centimeters and a vacuum is applied as the catheter is withdrawn. Suctioning should not exceed 10 to 15 seconds. Patients are often reattached to the ventilator between attempts with repeat suctioning as needed.

Remember that with any cleaning or suctioning procedure you run the risk of introducing infectious organisms. When suctioning or cleaning the tracheostomy tube care should be taken to keep the catheter or tube as clean as possible to prevent potential serious infections.

How can my family or caregivers learn how to take care of a ventilator?

Although the above procedures may seem very complicated, our experience indicates that most families can master the skills necessary to support home ventilation. Training and home preparation will typically require approximately two weeks after a tracheostomy tube has been placed. This time frame allows a caregiver conference for initial discussion and planning of home ventilation. Typically this conference will include the patient, family, hospital social worker, physician, nurse (hospital and homecare), home equipment representative, respiratory therapist, and any pastoral or supportive care. The initial conference should identify all potential caregivers and ensure that the patient and family understand that home care for the mechanically dependent individual is a twenty-four hour, seven day a week job. Practical experience has demonstrated that an insufficient *number of caregivers* can be a significant problem.

Financial support should also be evaluated at this time. The potential cost of home mechanical ventilation was previously discussed in this chapter but it should also be noted that many insurance have a lifetime capitation on spending. A few years of home ventilatory care with nursing care can easily reach this limit. If the option is available for ample home nursing assistance the issue will involve training the various nurses who assist with care in regard to the home mechanical ventilator and suctioning. While it may seem common knowledge, in a practical sense this is not always the case.

Scheduling the training sessions for caregivers and home nursing will require a large commitment from either the home care company or hospital and the caregivers. These sessions can take place in the hospital or in the home. The caregivers will be required to adequately give return demonstrations on all aspect of patient care. This care includes but is not limited to tracheostomy care, suctioning, mechanical ventilator checks, mechanical ventilator troubleshooting, maintenance, care and cleaning of all equipment, and other patient care issues, which include patient turning, skin care, cleaning, and feeding.

The *home environment* will require a hospital bed, a home suction machine, a stand for the home ventilator, a humidifier for the ventilator, adequate storage for supplies, sufficient area for cleaning of equipment, doorways adequate for wheelchair or emergency access, adequate room size for all equipment and supplies, and stairways or accessibility for wheelchair. Home care companies will typically require that the home outlets be grounded and will probably require additional electrical outlets placed in the primary living area. The wheelchair will require special adaptations to accommodate the ventilator and suction equipment. If the home has external or internal stairs, the home will require the installation of wheelchair ramps or lifts to accommodate this apparatus.

Transportation needs include the adaptation of a vehicle for wheelchair and power access for the mechanical ventilator. While these needs are not immediate they require addressing initially for patient understanding. If a patient cannot be transported in the family or caregiver's vehicle, then the option of ambulance transports needs to be considered. Most ambulettes will not transport ventilator-dependent individuals, so ambulances will be necessary.

A *portable battery powered suction machine* will be required. While there are other ways to tracheal or oral pharyngeal suction a patient, a portable suction machine with a battery back up is beneficial in power failures and during transportation.

The home care company will assist in *notifying* the local rescue personnel and emergency room. The company will also assist in notifying the local power and telephone companies. These are necessary for potential prolonged power or phone failures. It is advisable for the caregivers to spend the last day or two in the hospital performing all of the care necessary for the patient to ensure there are minimal problems when discharged.

All of these items are mentioned not to discourage the choice from noninvasive to invasive home ventilation, but rather to make the patient and caregiver aware of the multiple factors involved with home mechanical ventilation.

Can I stop mechanical ventilation if I want to?

Yes, decisions with regard to medical therapy are never "written in stone." Patients with clear goals of therapy and limitations of that therapy may discontinue ventilation when the perceived benefit of the treatment does not outweigh the burden imposed by continuing it. An inability to communicate, interact, or participate in valued activities are all reasons some patients discontinue support. As long as the intervention provides significant benefit that outweighs its potential burden, continuing the treatment should be considered. Mechanical ventilation should be withdrawn when it no longer provides acceptable benefit. The number of people who ultimately discontinue the use of mechanical ventilation is not known.

Sleep Apnea Syndromes

Although generally thought to be an uncommon problem, sleep apnea can occur in people with ALS. The term *sleep apnea* refers to a temporary cessation or decrease in the flow of air in and out of the lungs during sleep. The occurrence of this disorder in the general adult population may be as high as 5 percent. Sleep apnea occurs principally because of dysfunction of the upper airway. Normal breathing involves proper muscle function and coordination of the tongue, palate, and pharynx to maintain an open passage through the upper airway into the lung. When our brain sends signals to the muscles of breathing in the chest, it also sends continuous signals to the muscles of the throat, which helps provide an open passage for the air to travel into the lungs. For reasons not completely understood, this message is abnormal in some people during sleep. A partial obstruction of the airway can occur when muscles are weak, the tongue is large, or extra tissue is present in the throat, neck, or jaw (Figure 12-7). The resultant temporary narrowing in the respiratory pathway can lead to snoring or snorting during sleep, followed by periods of quiet when the breathing seems to stop. These periods are terminated by partial arousal, only to repeat themselves throughout the night.

What are the symptoms of obstructive sleep apnea?

People who that have obstructive sleep apnea may complain of morning headaches, poor sleep, subtle changes in personality or mood, and, in particular, daytime somnolence or excess sleepiness. During sleep, they can be observed to snore or snort with periodic pauses in the breathing with or without arousal.

What are the consequences of sleep apnea?

Although sleep apnea in itself is not fatal, it can have a number of serious side effects and should be treated when significant. In addition to daytime somnolence, it can disrupt everyday life. Transient decreases in airflow during the periods of

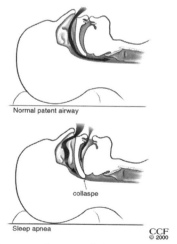

Normal patent airway

collaspe

Sleep apnea

CCF
© 2000

Figure 12-7. Normal versus obstructed airway anatomy in obstructive sleep apnea.

apnea or hypopnic episodes can lead to increased strain on the heart and lungs, increased blood pressure, and increased incidents of heart rhythm problems.

How is sleep apnea diagnosed?

Sleep apnea is confirmed by a test called *polysomnography,* which is available in most hospitals or institutions. It involves careful monitoring of heart rate, breathing, chest and stomach muscle activity, throat muscle activity, brain wave activity, and the amounts of oxygen and carbon dioxide present in the blood during sleep. After processing this information, a score of the number of times when breathing stops or decreases significantly during each hour will be calculated; this is called the *apnea hypopnea index* (AHI). It is normal for most people to have a small number of events per hour, which may range anywhere from 5 to 20, depending on age. A significantly greater number of events, especially those associated with low oxygen levels, arousal, and significant symptoms suggestive of obstructive sleep apnea, would all be reasons to consider treatment.

How is sleep apnea treated?

Treatment strategies are designed to relieve the obstruction or narrowing in the upper airway. This may be as simple as weight loss in people who have significantly increased weight as a factor causing their sleep apnea, or a change in positioning during sleeping (typically having the person lie on his side rather than supine or "flat on his back").

In ALS, sleep apnea is usually not relieved by any of these maneuvers but must be treated using a pressure mask that fits over the nose or face. The mask and pressure machines that deliver this kind of therapy together are known as CPAP or BiPAP®. These acronyms stand for *continuous positive airway pressure* and *bilevel positive airway pressure,* respectively. These systems provide air pressure in the mouth and throat that prevents the collapse of soft tissues, tongue, or muscles in the upper airway and provides an open channel for breathing during sleep. CPAP and BiPAP® masks are very effective in treating sleep apnea, and they are well tolerated by 80 percent to 90 percent of people with sleep apnea who require them at night. There are a number of masks, delivery systems, and head gear designed to improve tolerance and comfort in the treatment of their sleep apnea.

An infrequently used approach to treat mild or moderate sleep apnea can be the use of various devices designed to fit into the jaw, mouth, throat, or tongue that resemble in some respects the mouthpieces worn by professional athletes to protect their teeth. These molded orthodontic appliances maintain jaw, tongue, and soft palate position to occasionally relieve the obstruction in people who either do not tolerate CPAP or for one reason or another would prefer other options to manage their sleep apnea. They are generally not indicated in people who have severe sleep apnea that requires sophisticated management, and their applicability is limited to people who may have an obstruction in the back of the mouth or upper part of the throat that can be improved. Finally, the presence of a bulky appliance in the mouth may be uncomfortable and not well tolerated.

Surgical options to manage sleep apnea include one of two basic approaches:

1. *Resection* or cutting out areas of the tonsils, soft palate, and upper throat that may intermittently obstruct the upper airway during sleep. This surgical procedure is called *uvulopalatopharyngoplasty* or UPPP, as it is abbreviated for obvious reasons. This method has limited utility for people with ALS. Surgical removal of soft tissue in the posterior mouth and throat probably will not substantially reverse sleep apnea caused by muscular weakness.

2. The other surgical approach to the management of obstructive sleep apnea is *tracheotomy* (Figure 12-6). It involves making a small opening in the neck directly into the trachea or windpipe, which allows passage of a tube to bypass the upper airway and any obstruction in it that causes sleep apnea. This therapy is essentially 100 percent effective in eliminating sleep apnea. However, it clearly involves significant surgery and insertion of an indwelling tracheotomy tube, as well as the need to care for the appliance and the risks of infection and aspiration.

Anyone who has significant symptoms should undergo testing, although routine testing as a matter of course in the treatment of ALS is not indicated. Sleep apnea may occur alone or in conjunction with other respiratory complications related to poor pharyngeal control of feeding and secretions. Weakened respiratory muscles can cause low nocturnal oxygen levels without sleep apnea. The presence of low oxygen levels in people with ALS is typically due to hypoventilation rather that sleep apnea. If identified, treatment must be considered in the context of all potential respiratory complications.

Pneumonia Syndromes

The term *pneumonia* is synonymous with an infection in the lung, although irritations of the lung caused by food particles, dietary liquids, or stomach contents can cause the same symptoms of fever, sputum production, and breathlessness that often characterize pneumonia.

How does pneumonia occur in ALS?

Although anyone can contract pneumonia, people with ALS can be at significantly increased risk. The following mechanisms may predispose them to develop pneumonia.

1. Weakness of the expiratory muscles can lead to the decreased ability to clear secretions, mucus, or infection by coughing.

2. Significant weakness or dysfunction of pharyngeal muscles can lead to aspiration of mucus, saliva, or even food particles, thus setting the stage for pneumonia.

3. The chemical irritation of swallowed food or stomach contents can in and of itself result in a chemical pneumonia.

How is pneumonia diagnosed?

Pneumonia is typically suspected when a person develops new symptoms such as cough, fever, sputum production, chest pain, or shortness of breath. Confirmation of pneumonia is often by a chest X-ray. Laboratory culture of a coughed up specimen may or may not reveal bacteria that can cause this infection.

What are the consequences of pneumonia in patients with ALS?

Pneumonia is the most common fatal respiratory complication in ALS. An often overlooked consequence of pneumonia in people with ALS who have adequate or marginal respiratory muscle function is that pneumonia can cause acute respiratory failure, necessitating the consideration of mechanical ventilation. Once mechanical ventilation is started, patients become dependent on the ventilator because of their already weakened pulmonary function.

Pneumonia does this by:

1. Increasing the work of breathing

2. Causing increased secretions that require extra effort to clear from the lungs

3. Increasing the amount of breathing necessary in the presence of fever.

Although pneumonia is often curable with antibiotic treatment, severe pneumonia still claims tens of thousands of lives each year in the United States. Pneumonia in a previously functional patient can often result in the need to consider invasive procedures, ventilation, and the goals of therapy.

How can I prevent pneumonia?

People with ALS who have decreased cough are at increased risk for pneumonia. The following measures are important to prevent pneumonia.

1. Immunization with pneumococcal vaccine and yearly administration of influenza vaccines.

2. Prompt treatment of bacterial infections of the respiratory tract with antibiotics.

3. Careful attention to eating and bulbar function with regard to the risk of aspiration. (See section on speech and swallowing therapy.)

4. Use of assisted cough techniques to augment mucus clearance in the presence of a weak or ineffective cough.

What can be done when weakened respiratory muscles fail to produce an effective cough?

Weakening expiratory muscles can result in an inability to cough and clear secretions and subsequent risk for both aspiration and pneumonia. There are

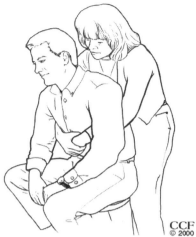

Figure 12-8. Assisted cough technique.

at least four techniques of clearing secretions when expiratory muscles are weak.

1. *Assisted cough.* These techniques are effective in clearing secretions from people who have neuromuscular weakness. The technique of assisted cough involves an abdominal thrust maneuver timed with the cough attempt (Figure 12-8). This technique requires a trained assistant and should not be used in people with feeding tubes or abdominal vascular devices such as vena cava filters.

2. *Cough machine (insufflation/exsufflation).* An insufflation/ exsufflation machine is rarely used but is effective in assisting the cough technique (Figure 12-9). Again, an assistant is often required to time an inspiratory inflation of the lung and then reversal of the machine pressure to achieve a vacuum, assisting cough. Although cough machines are available from many homecare providers, few physicians are familiar with the use of this device.

3. *Postural drainage.* Postural drainage or positioning of the patient to allow gravity-assisted drainage of secretions loosened by percussion to the chest wall is sometimes useful.

4. *Tracheostomy.* A tracheostomy provides a direct access to the major airways (Figure 12-6). Clearance of secretions can be achieved by introducing a suction catheter through the tracheostomy and directly removing secretions from the tracheobronchial tree. A tracheostomy does require a surgical procedure and will make speech impossible unless it can be plugged to allow airflow through the vocal cords. The tracheostomy can also be used to attach a mechanical ventilator to assist weakened respiratory muscles.

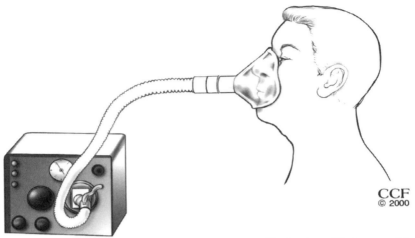

Figure 12-9. One technique for the use of an insufflation/exsufflation machine. Other names include the "in-exsufflator, "cofflator," or cough machine.

Will a tracheostomy prevent pneumonia?

No, not absolutely. However, the answer to this question involves some subtleties in understanding the purpose for tracheostomy tube placement. After the tracheostomy is placed in the airway below the larynx, it can be used (1) to suction the lower respiratory tract in people who may have limited ability to cough, and (2) as an interface for mechanical ventilation. The tracheostomy does not prevent aspiration. It does allow suctioning of the lower respiratory tract to decrease mucus accumulation that may predispose to pneumonia.

What is the role of feeding tube placement in managing problems that relate to pneumonia?

Again, some subtlety in the discussion of feeding tube placement is needed to understand the implications of this question. Feeding tubes (gastrostomy or jejunostomy) are placed in people who cannot safely tolerate nutrition by the oral route. People with ALS who have bulbar weakness often note coughing or choking with meals, which may restrict their ability to eat. Feeding tube placement should be considered if this coughing and choking cannot be controlled by jaw and neck positioning along with altered food consistency, or if there is substantial weight loss as a result of inability to ingest adequate nutrition.

As noted in our previous discussion, aspiration of food particles can cause a pneumonitis itself or predispose to pneumonia. If no food is taken by mouth, this potential is decreased and should theoretically mean a lower risk for pneumonia. However, aspiration of oral secretions, which would be expected in patients considered for feeding tube placement, would still pose a substantial risk for pneumonia. Thus although needed for optimal nutrition in some patients, the placement of a feeding tube alone may not decrease the incidence of lower respiratory tract infections.

How can excessive oral secretions be controlled?

A number of medications have been successfully used to decrease the amount of saliva produced. These are useful for the patient with excessive drooling due to overproduction of secretions coupled with decreased bulbar muscle function, which makes secretions more difficult to control. These medications include: Saltropine, Robinul, Elavil, and others that have significant anticholinergic effects. Their side effects can include dry mouth with tenacious secretions, urinary retention, or gastrointestinal disturbance.

Conclusion: Overall Suggestions and Management Strategies

The following comments summarize a general approach to the pulmonary complications of ALS and their management.

1. I urge all patients to obtain a measurement of respiratory function as soon as the diagnosis of ALS is made and to continue to obtain periodic measurement even in the absence of respiratory symptoms. This will ensure that respiratory complications of ALS may be anticipated and identified as soon as possible.

2. Initiate open and honest dialogue with physicians who have experience with managing the pulmonary complications of neuromuscular diseases.

3. Outline plans regarding treatment strategies for weakness of the respiratory muscles, taking into account realistic expectations of both the burdens and the benefits of the options available. These plans should be discussed *before* measures of respiratory function indicate that a person may experience sudden respiratory failure.

4. Communicate these plans with family and physicians, and document them in items such as living wills or resuscitation orders.

Bibliography

1. Norris FH, et al. Home nursing care by families with severely paralyzed ALS patients. *Adv Exp Med Biol* 1987; 209:231–238.

2. Moss AH, et al. Home ventilation for amyotrophic lateral sclerosis patients: Outcomes, costs, and patient, family, and physician attitudes. *Neurology* 1993; 43(2):438–443.

3. Gelinas DF, O'Connor P, Miller RG. Quality of life for ventilator-dependent ALS patients and their caregivers. *J Neurol Sci* 1998; 160(Suppl 1):S134–S136.

4. Oppenheimer EA. Respiratory management and home mechanical ventilation in amyotrophic lateral sclerosis. In: Mitsumoto H, Norris FH (eds.). *Amyotrophic lateral sclerosis: A comprehensive guide to management.* New York: Demos Publications, 1994:139–165.

5. McDonald ER, Hillel A, Wiedenfeld SA. Evaluation of the psychological status of ventilatory-supported patients with ALS/MND. *Palliat Med* 1996; 10(1):35–41.

6. Aboussouan LS, et al. Effect of noninvasive positive-pressure ventilation on survival in amyotrophic lateral sclerosis. *Ann Intern Med* 1997; 127(6):450–453.

7. Charles RA. Coping with life on a portable ventilator. *Home Health Nurs* 1985; 3:27–30.

8. Bach JR, Wang TG. Noninvasive long-term ventilatory support for individuals with spinal muscular atrophy and junctional bulbar musculature. *Arch Phys Med Rehabil* 1995; 76.

13

Life Support:
Realities and Dilemmas

Mark B. Bromberg, M.D., Ph.D.

Amyotrophic lateral sclerosis (ALS) is a disease of motor nerves. Weakness begins in one area of the body and progresses to other areas. At some point, the muscles of respiration become weak, breathing becomes impaired, and death eventually comes from respiratory failure.

The rate of progression of weakness is gradual. This provides time for patients to reflect on their mortality and gives them the opportunity to make decisions regarding their death. Although death is a necessary consequence of living, it is the one universal experience for which there is no sage advisor available for consultation. Because of the very personal issue of mortality, questions about respiratory failure and respiratory support are uncomfortable topics for people with ALS, their families, and health care providers. This makes counsel and management of respiratory failure one of the greatest challenges for all involved.

The focus of this chapter is on realities and dilemmas. The most important "reality" in ALS is the predictable progression to respiratory failure. The essential "dilemma" is the choice of whether to support respiration artificially with a breathing machine or to pass away as part of the course of the disease. Intertwined with the reality of failure and the dilemma of support are a number of other related issues that affect patients and caregivers. A primary role of health care providers is to give you and your family full information about respiratory failure and artificial respiratory support.

Amyotrophic lateral sclerosis affects every patient, caregiver, and family member in a different way. It is during discussions about respiratory failure that the range of issues in ALS becomes apparent. Health care providers can guide you and your family through the decision process. During this process, the patient's wishes should be held high, but at the same time consideration should also be given to caregivers and family.

This chapter is divided into three sections. The first section discusses the *realities* of respiratory failure. It is important for both patient and health care provider to recognize early symptoms of respiratory failure. Patients learn from a variety of sources that death in ALS occurs from respiratory failure. However, it is our experience that patients rarely understand the mechanism, time course, and physical events that occur with respiratory failure and death in ALS. Having specific information about these difficult issues can help to resolve your fears.

The second section discusses the *equipment* that is used to assist or support respiration. An understanding of the choices and equipment is important for the patient and family in making decisions.

The third section discusses the *dilemmas* of making choices. Assisted or supported ventilation poses dilemmas for the caregivers in the form of increased responsibilities and decreased freedom. The cost of supported ventilation in the home is formidable and can present a financial dilemma. Finally, when a patient is dependent on mechanical ventilation, the decision to discontinue respiratory support as the disease progresses may be the ultimate dilemma for the patient, family, and clinician.

The Realities of Respiratory Failure

This section discusses the symptoms of respiratory failure, how they occur, and how people die from ALS.

Muscles of Respiration

The muscles of respiration are part of the skeletal muscle system. The diaphragm is the major muscle of inspiration. The external intercostal muscles (muscles between the ribs) are the secondary or accessory muscles of respiration. Muscles of respiration, like limb and bulbar muscles, are activated or innervated by lower motor neurons. In ALS these neurons degenerate and die. The loss of motor neurons causes muscles to become weak. The lower motor neurons for the diaphragm start in the upper portion of the cervical spinal cord, segments C3–C5, and travel to the diaphragm in the phrenic nerves.

It is not possible to determine when weakness of the diaphragm first begins. This is due to the fact that a muscle does not become perceptively weak until 40 percent to 50 percent of the motor neurons going to it have died. The delay in weakness is due to what is termed *collateral reinnervation,* the body's attempt to compensate for motor nerve loss. It is a process whereby a surviving neuron grows new branches to reinnervate muscle fibers that have lost their connection after a motor neuron dies. When only a few motor neurons have died, collateral reinnervation can compensate well, and the muscle remains strong. As more motor neurons die, collateral reinnervation can not keep up, and the muscle becomes weak. Weakness will begin earlier in rapidly progressive ALS because muscle fibers are denervated at a faster rate than they can be reinnervated. Although collateral reinnervation is an important compensation process, once it begins to fail, the symptoms of respiratory failure become apparent and progress.

Respiratory Muscle Fatigue

Respiratory failure occurs when the diaphragm can no longer maintain adequate ventilation. An additional factor is muscle fatigue. Normally, the diaphragm never becomes fatigued, even after heavy breathing during exercise. However, in ALS, the diaphragm will fatigue when it becomes weak, particularly if extra physical effort is exerted.

In most people with ALS, the diaphragm tends to weaken only relatively late in the course of the disease, after other muscles have become very weak. For example, a patient who has almost no movement of legs or arms may be able to breathe comfortably when sitting. In these situations, although the diaphragm is weak, it is strong enough to keep up with the patient's reduced level of physical activity. If the patient exerts extra physical effort, however, he may experience fatigue of the diaphragm. One common situation is shortness of breath resulting from the effort of bathing or dressing. Shortness of breath may also be experienced when lying down. In the upright position, the diaphragm moves downward in the chest and does not push the abdominal organs out of the way. In the lying position, however, the diaphragm must work harder because of the resistance in pushing against the organs. Thus, a weak diaphragm becomes fatigued when a patient is lying down, causing a feeling of shortness of breath and the need to sit up.

Oxygen and Carbon Dioxide

The job of the diaphragm is to move air into and out of the lungs. Two things happen in the lungs during breathing: fresh air brings in more oxygen, and the old air gets rid of carbon dioxide. In the lungs, oxygen goes from the inhaled air into the blood and is used by the body's cells for energy production. Carbon dioxide is a waste product of energy production and moves from the blood to the exhaled air.

It is important to understand that there usually is more than enough oxygen in fresh air for the body's needs, even when respiration is shallow from a weak diaphragm. The major problem in ALS is moving the old air out and getting rid of the carbon dioxide. The feeling of shortness of breath comes from an increase in carbon dioxide. Most people can recall contests when they were young to see how long they could hold their breath; the urge to breathe did not come from too little oxygen, but from too much carbon dioxide. As a result, breathing extra oxygen from a tank rarely helps a feeling of shortness of breath in ALS, as it does in other conditions such as heart disease. To relieve the shortness of breath feeling, it is necessary to help the diaphragm (assisted ventilation) or to take over for the diaphragm (supported or artificial ventilation). A weak diaphragm can also be helped by reducing the amount of energy used during activities, such as by resting while bathing or dressing or sleeping in a reclining position rather than flat in bed. When these changes do not relieve shortness of breath, it is necessary to use assisted or artificial ventilation.

Sleep Disturbances

Sleep is a time of particular concern in ALS because a number of changes occur that may affect breathing. One is a change in body position. A person may not be aware that he has turned over onto his stomach during the night, a change that can lead to diaphragm fatigue. A second change during sleep is that breathing naturally becomes a little irregular; if the diaphragm is weak, it may not be able to keep up. The third and most important change that occurs during the period of sleep is the occurrence of rapid eye movement (REM) sleep. The body is in its most relaxed state during REM sleep. All muscles are quiet except for those that move the eyes and the diaphragm. This includes the muscles that help keep the throat open to allow free movement of air. Thus, the work of breathing increases during REM sleep, and the diaphragm may fatigue in people with ALS. When the diaphragm fatigues, not enough fresh air comes in and not enough carbon dioxide goes out. A patient will not go through all the normal stages of sleep but will be "aroused" to a lighter stage of sleep. At the lighter stages of sleep, the muscles that keep the throat open become active and the patient moves more air into and out of the lungs more freely. The patient then drifts into deeper sleep and muscle relaxation. This cycle can repeat many times during the night. Patients will not be aware of these arousals, but they will receive insufficient deep sleep and will experience sleepiness during the day time as a result of chronic sleep deprivation.

Although this situation does not happen to everyone with ALS, it is important to look for signs of disturbed sleep. The first sign may be headache upon waking in the morning. This is presumably due to excess of carbon dioxide from poor movement of air into and out of the lungs during the night. Another symptom is excessive daytime sleepiness, falling asleep during the day when one does not want to. Examples include falling asleep while dressing and eating or while talking to family and friends.

There are several ways to investigate the cause of disturbed sleep in ALS patients when it may be due to respiratory compromise. The physician can order a simple test called nocturnal oximetry, which can be performed in the home. Nocturnal oximetry measures the percentage of oxygen in the blood during sleep. A clip with a sensor is placed on the patient's finger, and a wire goes to a small machine that records oxygen saturation in the blood. The results can be printed on a strip of paper for the physician to review. If there are periods of low oxygen during sleep, called desaturations, the neurologist may recommend additional testing or suggest that the patient try assisted breathing. The additional test is called a sleep study or polysomnogram. This test is usually performed in a special room in the hospital or clinic.

It is important to emphasize again that unless an ALS patient has lung disease, such as emphysema from smoking, desaturations during sleep will not be easily helped with extra oxygen. Oxygen is not the problem—the problem is that air is not being moved into and out of the lungs well enough. The way to treat desaturations is with assisted or artificial ventilation. The neurologist may manage this or have the patient see a pulmonologist (lung doctor).

Measurement of Respiratory Weakness

It is more difficult to measure diaphragm weakness than to measure arm or leg weakness. The most useful test is to measure how much air can be forcefully exhaled. This measurement is called "forced vital capacity" or FVC. A patient will be asked to take in as deep a breath as possible and then blow out as hard and as long as possible—similar to blowing out all of the candles on a birthday cake with lots of candles. To measure the amount of air exhaled, the patient blows into a tube that is attached to a machine called a spirometer. It is important that all of the air go into the spirometer mouthpiece, and a clip may be placed on the nose to prevent a loss of air.

The amount of air exhaled is measured in liters (a liter is a little less than a quart) and is compared against the FVC for people of the same gender, age, and height. This is called the "percent of predicted FVC" (% FVC). Normally, a person starts out with a predicted FVC of 100 percent. As the diaphragm weakens, the % FVC will fall. It is important to understand that the measurement of FVC can be difficult to perform accurately. It takes coordination to place the mouthpiece in the mouth at the right time. It also requires a big effort to blow out all of the air. As a result, % FVC predicted values are not absolutely accurate, and a patient should not be overly concerned about small changes. What is important is a trend of falling values.

Progression of Weakness

Amyotrophic lateral sclerosis is a progressive disorder, and progression of diaphragm weakness is the most important issue. As discussed earlier, diaphragm weakness frequently occurs relatively late in the course of ALS. It is customary to measure % FVC at every clinic visit. For both limb muscles and the diaphragm, the rate of loss of strength tends to be constant for an individual patient. However, it is not possible to accurately predict when respiration will become a problem. Generally speaking, respiratory issues should be discussed at the time the FVC reaches 50 percent of predicted. However, the % FVC is not the only thing to follow, and it is also important to consider the symptoms of shortness of breath that were discussed earlier. As the % FVC falls or the patient has symptoms of shortness of breath, both the realities of respiratory failure and how to manage these realities should be discussed.

Respiratory Failure

Many people with ALS are concerned about how they will die. They frequently worry that they will suddenly choke to death or will suddenly be without air and gasping. It is our experience that most ALS patients pass away peacefully, frequently in their sleep. Choking very rarely causes death in ALS. Aspiration of food leading to pneumonia also is rare. A small number of patients may be anxious or restless or have "air hunger" late in the course of their disease. These symptoms can be managed. If a patient wishes to have respiration supported, machines are available to relieve the symptoms. If a patient does not choose to have respiration supported, medications can be given to make the patient comfortable as death occurs.

Sometimes a patient will be very short of breath and want to have his respiration supported for a limited period of time (several days) to allow him time to put his affairs in order and to say goodbye. Under these circumstances, a patient can go on a breathing machine temporarily. When the patient is ready, he can be allowed to pass away in complete comfort. Medications will be given to make the patient physically comfortable and unaware of his surroundings. Only at that point will ventilator support be withdrawn.

It is useful to have hospice services to help patient care at the late stages of ALS, or any disease. If air hunger occurs with ALS, hospice personnel have experience with relieving the symptoms with medication. In addition, a hospice nurse is always available and can assist the patient and family at any hour.

As this time approaches, it is important to discuss the issues of respiratory failure very frankly with the family and the neurologist, including the options, the patient's wishes, and hospice services.

Assisted and Artificial Ventilation

Although the natural course of ALS ends in death from respiratory failure, it is important for the ALS patient and family to understand that the reality of death can be postponed or prevented by artificial ventilation. This section discusses the various forms of ventilation.

When the diaphragm becomes weak and begins to fail, the only real or effective way to manage respiratory failure is by mechanically assisting or supporting ventilation. There are two general types of mechanical ventilation, invasive and noninvasive. These two types are discussed separately.

Invasive Ventilation

The term *invasive ventilation* is used because a cannula or breathing tube must be placed in the patient's trachea (windpipe). This is also called a "trach" tube. A tracheal cannula is used because it is the only practical and comfortable way to provide air to the lungs 24 hours a day over a long period of time. If artificial ventilation is urgently needed, a temporary tube may be placed in the trachea through the mouth. This is called an endotracheal tube. An endotracheal tube can only be used for about two weeks; after that it is replaced by a tracheal cannula. The tracheal cannula is placed by a surgeon during a simple operation.

With invasive ventilation, a breathing machine automatically provides all the air needed and can completely take the place of the diaphragm. Other terms that are used for invasive ventilation are *artificial* or *supported* ventilation. A patient can live for many years with invasive ventilation and good care.

The breathing machines used for invasive ventilation are also called ventilators (vents) or respirators. They are small devices that are about the size of a bread box. There is a flexible plastic tube that goes from the machine to the tracheal cannula. The controls on the machine are simple, and the machines are reliable. They are powered by household current or a battery and thus are portable. The patient and family usually work with a pulmonologist and a respiratory therapist from a home care agency or through a respiratory therapist from the hospital.

A frequently asked question is "What is it like being on artificial ventilation?" Descriptions from patients who have been on artificial ventilation, although they are not ALS patients, are informative. Initially, there may be panic with intubation and mechanical inflation of the lungs. Because some respiratory muscle function is present when ventilation started, there usually is a period of adjustment during which the natural rhythm of respiration fights with the artificial pattern of mechanical ventilation. In ALS, however, the feeling of air hunger that prompted the artificial breathing machine will disappear immediately, and the patient will feel relief.

Some physical discomfort may occur while on invasive ventilation. Supported ventilation remains permanently "artificial," and the ventilator cannot provide for sighs, gasps, or sneezes, which have been described as part of the "respiratory vocabulary." Because the patient will not be able to adequately cough up secretions from the lungs, someone must suction out the secretions. This requires placement of a small rubber tube inside the tracheal cannula. The rubber tube is connected to a suction machine, and the secretions are sucked up. Suctioning brings relief from the discomfort of secretions but may be an uncomfortable procedure. Although suctioning usually is done infrequently, it may be needed often under certain circumstances, such as when a patient has a cold.

After the initial fears and tribulations of artificial ventilation are dealt with, there is an adjustment period of a different type in which a patient begins to reestablish self-worth, regains control, and begins to think about and make decisions concerning the future. At this time, the reality of all that is involved with artificial ventilation becomes apparent. This transition has been described as "getting on with life." Factors include adjustments in lifestyle and physical living arrangements in the home, reestablishing work and recreational interests, and integrating these with the interests and activities of the rest of the family. The transition phase must be an active and continuous process because more adjustments become necessary as strength and function continue to decline with the passage of time.

Another question is whether an ALS patient will be able to speak while on artificial ventilation. If a patient was able to speak just before starting artificial ventilation, he will not be able to speak right after placement of the tracheal tube. Several weeks later, the first tube can be replaced by a special tracheal tube that allows leakage of air, and a patient can learn to speak with some practice. More commonly, people who need invasive ventilation already have difficulties with speech. The strength to make speech sounds eventually will be lost, and a patient will have to use other means to communicate. These include responding to "yes-no" questions and alphabet boards (see Chapter 10).

Noninvasive Ventilation

Assisted or noninvasive ventilation does not require a tracheal tube. Instead, a mask is fitted over the nose and mouth. The machine does not usually provide all of the air needed but just assists the patient. Noninvasive ventilation is used mainly to relieve symptoms of shortness of breath when the diaphragm fatigues easily, before it has failed. It most commonly is used at night. Another frequently used term for noninvasive ventilation is *bi-level ventilation* or *bi-pap ventilation.* These terms are used because in noninvasive ventilation, air is given to the patient at two levels: a lower level during expiration and a higher level during inspiration. In this way, the patient gets more air for the effort. Strictly speaking, BiPAP® is a brand name for a particular company's model of bi-level noninvasive ventilation machine.

The bi-level ventilator is small and is powered by household current. Plastic tubing goes between the machine and the mask. It is important that all of the air from the machine go into the patient's lungs and that the mask be placed over the nose and mouth. An alternative method is to use soft pads on the end of the plastic tubing that seals against the nostrils. With this device, the mouth is held closed by a strap to prevent leakage of air through the mouth.

The fit of the mask or nasal pillows is most important. Just as there are many different shapes of people's faces, there are many different shapes of masks and nasal pillows. It is important for patients to work with a respiratory therapist to find a comfortable system. This may require several different trials, and a patient may need to alternate between different masks.

A similar question—"What is it like to be on bi-level ventilation?"—is asked about noninvasive ventilation. Patients describe several different sensations. Many people are distressed at having a mask placed over the mouth and nose and may also be distressed at having a stream of air forced on them. However, for many patients, bi-level ventilation improves their sleep and daytime level of energy, and they welcome it. Noninvasive ventilation gives a patient time to adjust to the events of ALS.

Some people have difficulty getting used to bi-level ventilation. Several factors may predict successful use. The most important one is weakness of bulbar muscles. Patients who have weak speech and swallowing tend to have a harder time with bi-level ventilation than those who have good bulbar function. The most important recommendation is that patients "relax" when they first try bi-level ventilation. Because there are two settings (the pressure for the stream of air during exhalation and the pressure for the stream of air during inhalation), it is wise to set these two pressures low when a patient first tries bi-level ventilation and to work up slowly. Some physicians and respiratory therapists let a patient try adjusting the settings themselves to give them control.

Because it can take some time to get used to bi-level ventilation, many neurologists recommend starting noninvasive ventilation early, before a patient actually needs it during sleep.

Can bi-level ventilation can be used to support ventilation full-time; that is, can bi-level be used in place of invasive ventilation? Yes, it can. As patients require more and more time on bi-level ventilation, they can approach full-time use. A recent survey of patients on full-time noninvasive ventilation shows that they are satisfied with this arrangement. However, many people who use full-time noninvasive ventilation eventually convert to a trachea cannula and invasive ventilation.

The Dilemmas of Respiratory Failure

The dilemmas of respiratory failure relate to making decisions about ventilation. No two people with ALS have the same issues or concerns, and no two people will have the same set of dilemmas. However, certain issues are common to all ALS patients, caregivers, and families. This section follows the changes in respiration and discusses the dilemmas and decisions that need to be addressed (see also Chapter 12).

The Choice of Noninvasive Ventilation

Insurance coverage for bi-level ventilation is not a problem for most people with ALS. It is hoped that noninvasive ventilation will make a patient more comfortable, give him a better night's sleep, and perhaps give him more energy or endurance during the day. Early use of bi-level ventilation may extend the life of an ALS patient. Despite these benefits, some patients choose not to use bi-level ventilation. Others try bi-level ventilation but are not comfortable with the mask and stop using it. This is a reasonable decision.

Patients may ask what happens next if they do not choose or cannot use noninvasive ventilation? Not much happens immediately. Most patients are able to continue for some time without any changes. They will continue to be sleepy during the day. They may try different sleeping positions at night, such as sleeping in a reclining chair. They may take more frequent naps. They also will have both good days and bad days. Eventually, they will become short of breath more easily and will have to make decisions about invasive ventilation.

The Choice of Invasive Ventilation

The most important dilemma for a person with ALS is whether to choose invasive or artificial ventilation when shortness of breath becomes uncomfortable. The number of patients who are supported by invasive ventilation is not known, but estimates from a regional survey in the midwestern United States suggest that up to 8 percent of ALS patients are placed on full-time invasive ventilation. It is important to understand that some of these patients intentionally chose artificial ventilation, while others were placed on artificial ventilation during a medical emergency. Choosing to be placed on artificial ventilation or choosing not to be placed on it in an emergency is an important issue for ALS patients and their families to consider.

When patients on artificial ventilation are questioned, the majority report being informed about this issue, but only a few patients chose artificial ventilation in advance. Most patients on artificial ventilation were forced into making a choice, or their families had to make the choice for them, under emergency medical conditions.

In most ALS clinics, arrangements can be made to honor a patient's choice against invasive artificial ventilation if an emergency arises. Without such arrangements, if a patient wishes not to be artificially ventilated, the emergency medical team should not be called. In some communities, documents can be filled out that allow for an emergency medical team to honor a patient's wishes to decline invasive ventilation, and they would then focus on helping make the patient comfortable.

Dissemination of Information About Respiratory Failure and Support

It is hoped that every ALS patient will be able to think about respiratory failure and make a decision about supporting ventilation. It is also hoped that the patient will receive full information from his neurologist or pulmonologist during the decision-making process. It is important that the patient's family be part of the discussion and process. We know from experience that this process is very difficult for a number of reasons.

First, there is only so much information that a patient and family can process during a single clinic visit. Most ALS patients state that they desire as much information as possible from their physicians. However, respiratory failure is a frightening idea early in the course of the disease, and patients may not think that respiratory failure is a real possibility for them. As weakness progresses, however, it is important for patients to request information. Although discussions about artificial ventilation may cause sadness and anxiety, it is important to have detailed information. This includes descriptions of the symptoms and signs of respiratory failure, a description of what it is like to be on artificial ventilation, and an understanding of the manner of death from respiratory failure. Strange as it may seem, this process is often satisfying and may be reassuring to patients as they consider their choices.

Second, it is important to keep in mind that the request by patients for full information also presents a dilemma for the neurologist or pulmonologist. Doctors have personal thoughts and feelings about artificial ventilation, as well as sadness as a patient becomes weaker. These feelings may show through as the physician describes life on a ventilator. A doctor's feelings can influence a patient's decisions. One survey of ALS patients and their ALS clinic neurologists showed that patients were more likely to chose artificial ventilation if their neurologists had strongly positive feelings about it.

Third, patients have difficulty discussing their feelings about artificial ventilation. Only half are able to do so. Patients most commonly talk with their spouse. Although these feelings are expressed less often with their physician, patients generally feel comfortable and in control during these discussions. Despite the fact that a majority of patients seen in an ALS clinic receive information about respiratory failure and support, and half of them discuss these issues, 30 percent prefer to leave care and treatment decisions to their physicians. It is not clear whether neurologists are aware of this preference.

Patient Decision Making

It is important that ALS patients be encouraged to make a decision about artificial ventilation in a timely fashion. An approach used in our Motor Neuron Disease Clinic is to discuss decisions about artificial ventilation in terms of a neutral document, the Durable Power of Attorney for Medical Affairs. We make the argument that all people of legal adult age (older than 18 years old) should designate someone to manage their medical treatment if they should be unable to answer for themselves. This approach shifts the focus from the ALS patient and encourages everyone to fill out a Durable Power of Attorney for Medical Affairs. This document does not require an attorney or lawyer and does not cost anything. Every hospital should have the forms available.

Reaching a decision about artificial ventilation is difficult, and patients should be given permission to change their minds as their experience with ALS grows and circumstances change. The emphasis in our clinic is to keep the patient in control of the decisions. We also stress that there are no "right" or "wrong" decisions with regard to artificial ventilation.

Patient Indecision

When a patient does not make a decision about supporting ventilation, the family and clinician are faced with the dilemma. One clinician's approach is to classify symptomatic treatment in ALS as either "ordinary" or "extraordinary." In this scheme, invasive ventilation is considered an example of extraordinary treatment, and a patient's indecision or "no decision" can be interpreted as a decision against the extraordinary therapy of artificial ventilation. However, many physicians believe that a patient's "no decision" means that the physician must do everything technically possible for the patient. This can result in starting invasive ventilation under emergency conditions.

Stopping Ventilator Support by the Patient

Stopping ventilatory support becomes an important issue for any patient using noninvasive or invasive ventilation. As the diaphragm weakens, a patient will require more ventilator support. For example, if noninvasive ventilation is used just at night, eventually it will be needed during the day. With more experience with noninvasive ventilation, it has become clear that it can be used full-time by some patients. At this point, patients may request invasive ventilation because it is more comfortable.

Weakness in all muscles will progress on artificial ventilation. In the extreme, patients will lose all movement, including the ability to communicate. This is called a "locked in" state. Many physicians believe that this can be a very distressing situation for the patient. It clearly is desirable to know a patient's wishes before he or she loses the ability to communicate.

Some patients consider stopping artificial ventilation when weakness progresses to a certain level. This level varies from patient to patient. For some, it is when communication is no longer possible, while for others it is when a certain goal or event in life has been met. This sounds like a frightening situation, but it is important to emphasize that removing a patient from a ventilator can be done so that the patient is completely comfortable and experiences no air hunger or distress.

Stopping Artificial Ventilation by the Family

The dilemma of stopping artificial ventilation can fall to the family when a patient's wishes are not known and he or she loses the ability to communicate. This is an avoidable burden if the patient makes his or her wishes known in advance.

Dilemmas of the Caregiver

Respiratory failure in the ALS patient also causes dilemmas for caregivers. Most patients on artificial ventilation, either noninvasive or invasive, are cared for at home, which offers substantial psychological benefits compared with life in an institution. As the patient requires more and more time on the ventilator, however, management becomes a full-time, 24-hour job. Most caregivers are spouses, and the overall burden of management falls on them. The task of home ventilatory care usually is divided among several people. On average, it takes 3.5 people per day to care for an invasive ventilator–dependent patient. The average daily time spent by family members in patient care is nine hours, and the balance of care comes from outside personnel if finances permit. Although hiring outside personnel brings relief, it is not without stress. Stresses include finding and interviewing candidates, assessing their level of competence, and determining the reliability of their attendance. Qualifications alone are not sufficient because experienced personnel may be "burned out" from previous work with patients on ventilators.

The impact on the spouse and family is largely hidden from discussion. With the trend for families to assume more of the burden of long-term patient care, questions about the psychological, ethical, and moral limits of their obligation should be considered. Half of the home caregivers in one survey consider the time commitment to be a major burden. The initial enthusiasm frequently wanes, and anger and resentment are common. Anger may be directed toward the patient. Previously established patterns of coping are often used, and family conflicts may become channeled through the patient. Anger also may be directed back to the caregiver. The anger, in turn, often generates guilt, and home caregivers frequently suffer in silence. As a consequence, many caregivers experience ill health.

It is important to note that after living with these difficulties, most caregivers surveyed were happy that their ALS patient chose artificial ventilation. This finding may reflect in part the complex and ambivalent nature of feelings toward the patient. Caregivers' experience with artificial ventilation did impact their attitude toward artificial ventilation, however, and one study showed that only half would choose artificial ventilation if they developed ALS themselves.

Financial Dilemmas

Financing artificial ventilation is formidable. First, it is less costly to care for ventilator-dependent patients in the home than in a hospital. Monthly home costs vary widely, from a low of $500 to a high of $35,000. The major factor affecting cost is the need to hire outside personnel. The major financial concern for the family is the amount of insurance coverage. Data from a survey showed that 83 percent of the monthly costs listed previously were covered by insurance, with more than half of the families receiving full coverage. When incomplete, insurance coverage was usually denied for outside personnel, and the uncovered monthly expenses ranged from $100 to $7,000. The less insurance companies pay for, the more the burden of home care shifts to the spouse and family (see Chapter 26).

Summary

The full spectrum of dilemmas associated with respiratory failure is formidable in both number and complexity. Nonetheless, they can all be managed. ALS patients and families who choose artificial ventilation generally are satisfied with their choice—such is the will and power of the human spirit to deal with and overcome obstacles.

Understanding the full spectrum of dilemmas encourages discussion between patient, family, and health care professionals. A full presentation and open discussion are very important for the well-being of those who choose and those who refuse artificial ventilation.

The reality of respiratory failure in ALS profoundly affects everyone involved with the disease. The dilemmas are shared by all. The opportunity to make decisions regarding the manner of one's death is a unique feature of this disorder. Although these decisions may be frightening, they reflect a control over life, which becomes an important issue in light of the technological advances in medicine. These decisions should be considered the right of every person. In ALS, full information should be made available by health care providers in a neutral manner. Educational materials about respiratory failure and artificial ventilation are available to assist in dissemination of information. Decisions by the patient should be encouraged and supported, and made informally to the family and formally in a document such as a Durable Power of Attorney for Health Care. It is the obligation of health care providers to honor these decisions.

14

Alternative and Complementary Therapies

**Raul N. Mandler, M.D., Joan Werner, B.A.,
Martha Meister, R.N., B.S.N., and Gary LaFontaine, M.Sc.**

Alternative, optional, or complementary therapies (1) are frequently used by people with amyotrophic lateral sclerosis (ALS), often in conjunction with those treatments prescribed by neurologists but often without the neurologist's knowledge. Sufficient controversy exists about the value of alternative therapies, particularly for ALS. This chapter does not endorse or support alternative medicines as effective therapies for ALS. It solely describes common alternative practices used by many ALS patients (2) who are in need of better medical preventive or reparative medications, which so far are unavailable to them.

The words *alternative, unconventional, complementary,* and *unorthodox* are not synonyms and might express quite different approaches. Complementary medicine can be understood as a mere support to scientifically valid treatments. The words *unorthodox* or *optional* confer a negative connotation, an approach that is not in line with current trends in the practice of the medical art of caring for people with ALS, and which is purposely not discussed in this chapter, as it may cause harm to the health and welfare of patients and families. ALS is one of the most devastating diseases of humankind. It results in death within months or years from diagnosis, following a progressive, complete paralysis of extremities, respiratory muscles, and bulbar muscles, with the affected person remaining cognitively intact and thus aware of the incapacitating symptoms. The instinct of preservation leads patients, families, and friends to look for any possible way to preserve quality of life and life itself, often at high emotional and economic costs coupled with relatively low benefit (3,4).

Current Therapeutic Options in ALS

As of 2000 there is only one medication approved by the U.S. Food and Drug Administration (FDA) to treat ALS. Riluzole (Rilutek) has a modest benefit in prolonging survival for a few months. The effects on quality of life have not been established, simply because the scientific studies proving that Rilutek was effective focused mainly on survival as the primary endpoint to detect benefit, rather than on quality of life. Over the last two years, injectable insulin growth factor (Myotrophin) was reviewed by the FDA after a combined study carried out in Europe and North America. With a study design emphasizing quality of life, this research could have provided important information about a rational treatment for ALS based on the trophic factor theory. The lack of approval of Myotrophin by the FDA has upset patients and family members, who harbored high hopes for its availability. Other double-blind, placebo-controlled studies have not proven to be efficacious, including one trial using ciliary neurotrophic factor (CNTF). These negative results in controlled clinical trials have further led patients to seek alternative modes of therapy. However, in contrast with attitudes that preceded the approval of Rilutek, patients and families now actively seek participation in controlled, scientifically based clinical trials of pharmaceutical compounds that have been rigorously pretested in vitro and in animal models of motor neuron disease.

This significant change in philosophy is related to the development of new hopes through rational medications and clinical trials, as well as to several other developments such as the establishment of ALS centers of excellence, those sponsored by the ALS Association (ALSA), Muscular Dystrophy Association (MDA), and comparable associations in many other countries around the world. In parallel, the use of the Internet has brought immediate, available information to patient households. Many user lists are devoted to neurologic diseases, some specifically on ALS (e.g., "ALS-On-Line" of Bob Broedel, a very active, biweekly list). The World Federation of Neurology Subcommittee of Motor Neuron Diseases has a Web page with current information and discussion of recent articles on diagnosis and treatment (www.wfn.als.org). The MDA, ALSA, and several medical institutions also have Web pages that focus on ALS.

Rationale

Any discussion of alternative therapies in ALS can only give direction rather than provide a thorough exploration of various therapies. There has been an explosion of therapies in recent years, many of which are based on natural or organic products, so that any listing cannot be current and would likely be out of date before printing. This explosion must be seen as a positive development, however, because much of it comes from an increasing understanding of the natural balances and needs of the human body. Many of the new therapies also provide viable alternatives to some of the costly and possibly harmful "unorthodox" therapies of the past.

Along with a growing appreciation of a natural approach to the treatment of one's own body, there has been a subtle change in the philosophy of many doctors, who had often been assumed to be opposed to alternative therapy as "quack medicine." Some of this change may be due to the trend toward the use of vitamins and other nutritional supplements as well as physical treatments (e.g., massage therapy) that make good sense and do not counteract the treatments of traditional medicine. Another reason may be the ongoing research into toxic and environmental factors as a cause of ALS. Caution is needed when exploring alternative therapies. It is tempting to assume that information gathered on the Internet is correct and to act on it. Unfortunately, that assumption is not always accurate, and follow-up negative information does not always appear.

As the great Maimonides expressed in his famous medical aphorisms (5), "Do not consider a thing as proof because you find it written in books: for just as a liar will deceive with his tongue, he will not be deterred from doing the same with his pen. There are fools who accept a thing as convincing proof because it is in writing . . ." and then adds, "The truth of a thing does not become greater by its frequent repetitions, nor is it lessened by lack of repetition." So, aside from the obvious admonition of using common sense when pursuing a new therapy, it is extremely important to openly discuss any new therapy, conventional or otherwise, with your doctor before starting them.

Having established these cautionary guidelines, the following is a brief summary of "fashionable" alternative therapies used in ALS, without the endorsement of anyone. More well-controlled scientific studies are necessary to prevent, treat, and hopefully cure ALS.

Medicinal

Antioxidants

Antioxidants remove dangerous, cell-damaging, oxygen-free radicals that can alter nuclear DNA, cell membranes, and cell organelles, including the mitochondria, our cell's "power plants." Vitamins E, C, and beta-carotene are commonly used as antioxidants to prevent the release of free radicals. They are commonly administered by neurologists and ALS specialists; the rationale underlying the administration of these vitamins is based on their inhibition of the production of free radicals, which are toxic to cells in general and to motor neurons in particular. Motor neurons are highly susceptible to oxidative stress, due in part to their limitation of division, their unique structure with a very long axon stemming far from the cell body, and to their particular membrane structure. Cervical and lumbar spinal cord motor neurons have a relative lack of calbindin/calmodulin proteins, which protect other motor neurons that are rarely affected in ALS, such as those that innervate the bladder and the eye muscles. The doses of vitamins vary widely, and no substantial proof of efficacy is yet known. Vitamin E is often administered at 400 mg three times a day with fatty meals to improve absorption. In contrast to vitamin C, vitamin E is lipid-soluble and accumulates in the liver. Theoretically, very high doses of vitamin E might produce toxicity, although some patients have taken very high doses, up to 5 grams per day. Vitamin E should be taken with fatty meals to maximize absorption.

Vitamin C is given at 500 to 2000 mg per day. It is water-soluble. High doses may precipitate diarrhea, but no serious effects have been reported. Beta-carotene is converted to vitamin A in the body, which is then stored in the liver. It is used at 10,000 to 20,000 international units per day.

Direct administration of very high doses of vitamin A may produce serious neurologic side effects, including the syndrome of increased intracranial pressure.

Vitamins of the B group are also used, including B1, B6, and B12. Among a group of 100 ALS patients, we found that three patients had a vitamin B12 deficiency, not ALS. The deficiency was related to pernicious anemia and concomitant alcohol abuse. Treatment with monthly intramuscular injections over the past five years has markedly improved the condition of these initially misdiagnosed patients. The use of very high doses of vitamin B6 (pyridoxine) might produce toxic neuropathy. Vitamin B6 is thought to help in the metabolism of glutamate, an essential neurotransmitter in the nervous system.

Essential minerals, such as zinc, function as coenzymes, assisting enzymes in the removal of oxygen-free radicals.

In summary, the widespread use of vitamin supplements, the relative lack of major side effects, and their moderate price make this form of complementary treatment one of the most popular and safe; it is often supported, if not prescribed, by ALS specialists.

Other antioxidants include allopurinol, a medication that is used to treat gout. It requires a doctor's prescription and may be toxic to the kidneys. Grape seed extract contains oligomeric proanthocianidin complex (OPC), another antioxidant, used in conjunction with vitamins. The recommended dose is 1 mg/kg/day, not to exceed 100 mg total dose. Commercial forms of OPC include the labels proanthocynidin and pycnogenol. Procysteine promotes the production of brain glutathione, a small protein that serves as a major antioxidant and helps preserve cell membranes.

Silymarin (St. Mary's thistle or milk thistle) from the herb *Silybum marianum* exerts antioxidant, antiinflammatory and hepato-protective effects. It is used at 350 to 2000 mg.

Other natural compounds that are used as dietary supplements include calcium and magnesium supplements, potassium, and silicon. Patients also use flaxseed oil and salmon oil, lecithin, bee pollen, and the antioxidant coenzyme-Q. These supplements are usually nontoxic at reasonable doses, although their effectiveness in ALS is disputable [6].

Energy Supplements

The use of the amino acid creatine reflects the new current closeness, even overlap, between scientific-based medicine and complementary therapies. In a recent study entitled "Neuroprotective effects of creatine in a transgenic animal model of ALS," affected animals given a diet high in creatine had the same number of motor neurons preserved as control animals. Mice given creatine in water at a solution of 1–2% lived an average of 26 days longer than those not given the drug, and their muscles remained healthy longer (7). That was twice the benefit observed with riluzole, the only FDA-approved drug for treatment of ALS. Even if creatine had not directly modified the cause of the disease, it might have produced a very effective symptomatic treatment. Obviously, results in experimental animals cannot be directly applied to patients, most of whom have the sporadic variant of ALS, not the genetic form seen in mice. In a small study, 81 patients with muscular dystrophies and other muscle-wasting disorders received 10 g of creatine daily for five days and then 5 g daily for five more days. An average of 10 percent to 15 percent improvement in hand gripping and knee strength was found (8). Although controlled clinical trials are needed to prove the value of creatine in ALS, many patients are already using this amino acid, starting with an induction dose of 5 g four times a day for five days (total dose of 20 g) followed by a maintenance dose of 5 g/day. The written directions read "Mix one heaping teaspoon (5 g) in your favorite beverage daily."

For creatine loading—to be done for no more than 5 days—take four heaping teaspoons per day: one heaping teaspoon at four-hour intervals. Continue this process for four days. Do not exceed the loading level of more than four days in any one-month period. This is due to the fact that some athletes tend to do "reloading" protocols, sometimes on a monthly basis. Using excessive doses may cause kidney disease (9,10). Creatine is widely available in health food stores and is marketed under the ProPerformance label for General Nutrition Centers (11).

Creatine has been used as a performance-enhancing supplement; it has shown beneficial effects on performance during intense athletic activity (12). This amino acid is formed from the amino acids arginine, methionine, and glycine, mainly in the liver but also in the pancreas and the kidneys. It is transported in the blood and taken up by muscle cells, where it is converted to a high-energy compound called creatine phosphate, or phosphocreatine. The average person typically metabolizes approximately 2 grams of creatine a day, and that same amount is normally synthesized by the body, maintaining a creatine balance. The richest source of creatine in food is in meat and fish.

Phosphorylated creatine is an important storage form of high-energy phosphate, the energy source for muscle contraction. Because the FDA does not regulate dietary supplements such as creatine, the compound may not be as pure as would be desirable. It is not known how creatine might interact with Rilutek, vitamins, or other medications. It is hoped that ongoing controlled clinical trials will elucidate the efficacy of creatine in ALS. This alternative medication thus holds promise in the treatment of the disease.

Nonmedicinal and/or Physical Treatments

Acupuncture

This traditional Oriental medical discipline is commonly used by ALS patients. Side effects are minimal when acupuncture is performed by competent acupuncturists who use sterile, disposable needles (13). The acupuncture needle is considered a safe and effective medical device by the FDA and the National Institutes of Health (NIH) (14). For the past years, acupuncturists have carried out controlled studies in which patients were randomly assigned to one of two groups; one group would receive appropriate acupuncture, and a separate group would receive control needling, usually at points inappropriate to the condition being studied, or an inactive surface-electrode device (TENS unit) or other care modality, such as medication, medical device, or physical therapy (15).

Acupuncture has been mainly used in the treatment of acute and chronic pain [16]. It is believed to work by the release of natural endorphins, which are also known to modify the immune response (17). Acupuncture has been found to be effective also in the treatment of nausea, vomiting, and pregnancy-related morning sickness (18). Electric acupuncture has been used in the treatment of peripheral nerve injury (19); a combined treatment of electroacupuncture and manual acupuncture was compared with supportive medication for promoting recovery from trauma-induced peripheral nerve injury. Fifty-four patients with upper and lower limb peripheral nerve injuries received daily, 30-minute acupuncture treatments for one month. Acupuncture points were chosen on the basis of location and extent of nerve injury. Electromyographic (EMG) techniques were used to support the diagnosis of denervation. Improvement was seen in 31 patients (31%) in the acupuncture group but in only 9 patients (7%) in the control group. The authors concluded that acupuncture can enhance the extent of functional recovery from trauma-induced peripheral nerve injuries. Similar controlled studies have not been done in ALS patients. Additionally, the use of a control population might not provide a definite answer because placing needles in "control" areas might also produce positive effects. Many of our ALS patients, especially those with pain syndromes, have used acupuncture and have been satisfied with pain alleviation. In any event, acupuncture does not appear to change the natural history of ALS.

Physical therapy, occupational therapy, and massage therapy have improved the activity and comfort of ALS patients. Massage therapies have also been combined with meditation and holistic approaches aiming at regaining self-control (20). Symptoms related to pain, pseudobulbar palsy, and panic attacks have been alleviated with massage and meditation. These techniques might save precious emotional and physical energy, which can dissipate with stress, as well as with poor diet, fatigue, or smoking.

These complementary, holistic methods, together with moderate exercise, stretching, and good eating habits favor the general well-being of both ALS patients and the general population.

Herbal Remedies

A complete review of specific herbs is impossible because there are more than 20,000 of them (21,22). The use of herbs in the United States dates from the early colonial days, when health care was provided by women in the home, as is still the case in many parts of the world. In the early nineteenth century, as scientific methods became more advanced, the practice of botanical medicine was regarded as quackery. Since the 1960s, there has been a resurgence of the popularity of botanical medicine related to natural health therapies. Recognition of this trend prompted the creation of the Office of Alternative Medicine by the NIH in Bethesda, Maryland, in 1992 (23).

St. John's wort is a good example of the type of herb commonly used by ALS patients for the treatment of depression (23). The herb is found throughout most of Europe and western and central Asia and has been transplanted to most continents. The yellow flowering top contains dianthrones, hypericin, the flavonoid glycoside hyperosid, an essential oil, catechol, tannins, and other substances. It is used to treat melancholia, depression, disturbed sleep related to anxiety and depression, and gastrointestinal disorders related to common neuroses. St. John's wort is used either as an infusion or in the form of capsules, with a suggested dose of 2 capsules three times a day. A bottle of 50 capsules costs approximately $8.00. Results cannot be expected until treatment has been continued for at least a month.

Although regarded by many as benign, St. John's wort does have potential side effects (25). It contains hypericin, a potential monoamine oxidase, which raises concerns for hypertensive reactions resulting from concomitant ingestion of high tyramine-containing foods, such as cheddar cheese and red wines. It also is known to produce photosensitivity (26). High doses produced by brewing a concentrated infusion have produced a peripheral neuropathy syndrome (Latov N, personal communication, 1999).

A wide variety of herbs has been used by ALS patients, including the most popular ones, such as echinacea, garlic (Allium sativatum), goldenseal (Hydrastis canadensis), ginseng (Asian panax), ginkgo (Ginkgo biloba), used by patients with cognitive problems, and valerian (Valeriana officinalis). These herbs have potentially serious side effects. Ginkgo biloba contains ginkgolides, which antagonize platelet-activating factor, and should be used with caution by patients receiving anticoagulant therapies. Gingseng is used to relieve stress, presumably because of its vasodilator and antioxidant properties. Caution should be exercised by people with a propensity to cardiovascular disorders (21). Chamomile is sedative, antispasmodic, and antiseptic (22). Allergic reactions, including edema of the vocal chords with severe respiratory difficulties, may occur because of cross-reactivity with ragweed. Echinacea is potentially hepatotoxic with persistent use.

People with ALS often decide what to take based on recommendations from friends, other patients, and recently Internet sources (27). Unfortunately, there is wide variation in the quality of herbs sold in the United States. ALS patients use various combinations of many of the popular aforementioned herbs but no one in particular. Again, you should consult your ALS specialist about individual regimens.

Summary

Our multidisciplinary ALS centers favor comprehensive approach in the care of ALS patients, based on scientific principles (the *science* of medicine) and communicative principles (the *art* of medicine). We do not endorse expensive, unorthodox, or dangerous methods; rather, we encourage patients to continue participating in well-designed, scientifically based clinical trials, while at the same time continuing to receive quality medical care, especially symptomatic care for respiratory, nutritional, psychosocial, and other dysfunctions that affect people with ALS. Because of our still incomplete scientific knowledge, we accept that our patients may try alternative therapies, provided that they will not be harmful physically or economically and that they will not counteract potentially useful, scientifically proven medications. Open communication is needed. The rational treatment and cure of ALS requires the scientific understanding of its pathogenesis and cause before prevention or cure can be achieved. Well-conducted basic and clinical research is essential to reach those goals.

References

1. Spiegel D, Stroud P, Fyfe A. Complementary medicine. *West J Med* 1998; 168:241–247.
2. Candy D. Real medicine or medicine show? Growth of herbal remedy sales raises issues about value. *The New York Times,* July 23, 1998:D1.
3. Angell M, Kassirer JP. Alternative medicine—The risks of untested and unregulated remedies. *N Engl J Med* 1998; 339:839–841.
4. Eisenberg DM, Kessler RC, Foster C, et al. Unconventional medicine in the United States—Prevalence, costs, and patterns of use. *N Engl J Med* 1993; 328:246–252.
5. Mandler RN, Platt MW, Bennahum DA. History of medicine. Neurologic aphorisms of Maimonides. *Hum Med* 1994; 10:209–214.
6. Blakeslee S. Placebos prove so powerful even experts are surprised. New studies explore the brain's triumph over reality. *The New York Times,* October 13, 1998:D1.
7. Klivenyi P, Ferrante RJ, Matthews RT, et al. Neuroprotective effects of creatine in a transgenic animal model of amyotrophic lateral sclerosis. *Nat Med* 1999; 5:347–350.
8. Tarnopolsky M, Martin J. Creatine monohydrate increases strength in patients with neuromuscular disease. *Neurology* 1999; 52:854–857.
9. Koshy KM, Griswold E, Schneeberger EE. Interstitial nephritis in a patient taking

creatine. *N Engl J Med* 1999; 340:814–815.

10. Pritchard NR, Kaira PA. Renal dysfunction accompanying oral creatine supplements. *Lancet* 1998; 351:1252–1253.
11. Thompson RW. Reply to reference 7. *N Engl J Med* 1999; 340:815.
12. Volek JS, Kraemer WJ, Bush JA, et al. Creatine supplementation enhances muscular performance during high-intensity resistance exercise. *J Am Diet Assoc* 1997; 97:765–770.
13. Kendall, DE. A scientific model for acupuncture. *Am J Acupunct* 1989; 17:251–268.
14. Eskinazi DP (ed.). NIH technology assessment workshop on alternative medicine: Acupuncture. *J Alt Compl Med* 1996; 2:1–256.
15. de la Torre CS. The choice of control groups in invasive clinical trials such as acupuncture. *Frontier Perspec* 1993; 3:33–37.
16. Birch S, Hammerschlag R, Berman BM. Acupuncture in the treatment of pain. *J Alt Compl Med* 1996; 2:101–124.
17. Mandler RN, Biddison WE, Mandler R, Serrate SA. Betaendorphin augments the cytolytic activity and interferon production of natural killer cells. *J Immunol* 1986; 136:934–939.
18. Vickers AJ. Antiemetic actions of acupuncture. *Proc Roy Soc Med* 1996; 89:303–309.
19. Hao J, Zhao C, Cao S, Yang S. Electric acupuncture treatment of peripheral nerve injury. *J Trad Chin Med* 1995; 15:114–117.
20. Horrigan B. Conversations with Dolores Krieger, RN, PhD. Healing with therapeutic touch. *Alt Ther Health Med* 1998; 4:87–92.
21. Corbin Winslow L, Kroll DJ. Herbs as medicines. *Arch Intern Med* 1998; 158:2192–2199.
22. Miller LG. Herbal medicines. Selected clinical considerations focusing on known or potential drug-herb interactions. *Arch Intern Med* 1998; 158:2200–2211.
23. National Institutes of Health, Office of Alternative Medicine. Grant Award and Research Data. Bethesda, MD.: Office of Alternative Medicine. (See: http://altmed.od.nih.gov/oam/research/grants.)
24. Stary F. *The natural guide to medicinal herbs and plants.* New York: Barnes and Noble Books, 1998.
25. Miller S. A natural mood booster. *Newsweek,* May 5, 1997:74–75.
26. Duran N, Song PS. Hypericin and its photodynamic action. *Photochem Photobiol* 1986; 43:677–680.
27. Greenwald J. Herbal healing. *Time,* November 23, 1998:58–69.

15

Clinical Therapeutic Trials

Theodore L. Munsat, M.D.

The development of effective treatments for neurologic disease, or *neurologic therapeutics,* has generally lagged behind drug and clinical trial development in other fields of medicine because of a tradition of therapeutic nihilism that until very recent times has delayed the development of effective ALS drugs. This lack of interest in developing effective treatments resulted from an emphasis on diagnosis and lesion localization rather than treatment. This perspective characterized the practice of most of the founders of modern neurology. For example, the first placebo-controlled trial (a study in which some people are treated while others are given sham-placebo treatment) in all of neurology was not carried out until 1967, more than 10 years after the importance of placebo control was demonstrated in other branches of medicine. There is a general consensus that neurologic therapeutics is approximately 10 to 15 years behind such disciplines as cancer chemotherapy or AIDS, diseases that share many features with ALS. However, after a slow start, neurology has developed an increasingly productive interest in new therapies, as well as in the design of effective trials, and this has certainly been of benefit for those afflicted with ALS.

Of particular importance in this regard is the work done by the World Federation of Neurology (WFN) to develop an international consensus on how to diagnose ALS and how to design clinical trials. This consensus has already resulted in trials that are increasingly scientifically sound, more cost-effective, and, above all, more able to separate treatments that truly work from those that do not. This information can be accessed on the Web site of the WFN Research Group on ALS at www.wfnals.org. This site contains other useful information for those interested in ALS clinical trials.

This chapter deals with certain general issues that are of particular interest and concern if you are considering entering a clinical trial of an experimental drug. Details relating to specific current and future trials are discussed in the next chapter.

Why Are Clinical Trials Necessary?

A clinical trial is not needed when a drug or treatment is so effective that its benefit is immediately apparent to both patient and treating physician. The effectiveness of penicillin for certain infections is often cited as an example where the benefit was so clear and so dramatic when it was first used that a trial was not needed to show that it worked. Unfortunately, most drugs are not that effective. If we were lucky enough to discover a drug that stopped the progression of ALS, let alone reversed the damage, it would be immediately apparent to all within a few months, and an expensive, long, and statistically complicated clinical trial would not be needed. But it is unlikely that such a drug will be discovered in the near future. Rather, we most likely will be identifying drugs that have a modest slowing effect on the course of motor nerve damage such that the benefit may not be apparent to either the patient or the treating physician. This has been the case with riluzole, the first and, to date, the only drug that has been shown to slow the neurologic damage in ALS and the only drug to be approved by the U.S. Food and Drug Administration (FDA) for the treatment of ALS. To obtain government approval for riluzole, a long, difficult, and expensive trial process was necessary to demonstrate its modest benefit.

One might understandably ask why it is necessary to work so hard to demonstrate what is only a modest benefit from a drug when what we really need is something that has substantially greater benefit. It is reasonable to suggest, as many have, that a true cure for ALS must await a more complete understanding of the cause of the disease. However, recent research has revealed that the cause of ALS is much more complex than previously thought and involves several related pathologic processes, not a single one of which could be ameliorated with a single drug. In addition, it is quite likely that different factors are operative for different patients or groups of patients—that is, ALS may be a *family* of related diseases rather than a single disease. Consequently, it is most likely that, as in cancer, the initial effective treatments for ALS will only result in small gains, similar to what we have seen with riluzole. However, it also is likely that if enough small gains are linked together by using combinations of drugs or drug "cocktails," each component of which produces only small benefit, we might achieve significant slowing, if not arrest, of the ALS process. This is exactly the history of the now significant gains that have been achieved in treating both cancer and AIDS. If this reasoning is correct, it then becomes very important to be able to identify drugs that may indeed show only minimal benefit. It is equally important to begin simultaneously testing various combinations of drugs, something that has been disappointingly slow to develop.

The Different Types of Clinical Trials

Clinical trials of new drugs are always preceded by extensive studies in animals to determine whether the drug produces any damage to normal tissue and to determine what doses of the drug might be used in humans. If an *animal model* of the disease is available (that is, a disease that appears to have features similar to the human disease), information about possible effectiveness of the drug in humans might also be obtained. For example, the recent availability of *transgenic* mouse models of inherited ALS may become useful in defining new treatments. Human trials are typically carried out in various stages or phases.

- Phase I trials are often carried out in normal volunteers and are designed mainly to determine whether the drug is safe in humans and what side effects occur with different doses. These trials are done in relatively small groups of subjects. Phase I trials rarely give useful information about whether the drug will be effective in ALS. This information is collected from phase II and phase III trials.

- Phase II trials are typically done in a few centers that specialize in ALS and may be placebo-controlled. These are preliminary trials in ALS patients and have a goal of determining further not only whether the drug is safe but also whether it appears to have a beneficial effect on the disease. If the results of these studies are encouraging, phase III trials are performed next.

- Phase III trials are carried out in many ALS centers and often involve 1,000 or more patients. The goals of these large, placebo-controlled trials are (1) to further determine the safety of the drug in large numbers of different ALS patients, (2) to determine whether the drug is better than placebo or existing best medical treatment, and (3) to prepare a case for FDA approval of the drug so that it can be marketed by the pharmaceutical company that holds the patent.

As you can see, these various steps define a gradual, graded process of bringing a new drug to the patient—a drug that is both safe and effective. Some have argued, with possible justification, that the process leading to drug approval is too slow and too bureaucratic, especially for a disease as serious as ALS. This perspective states that "I'm going to die soon anyway so what difference does it make if the drug isn't fully evaluated?" The most persuasive counterargument points out that unregulated or poorly studied drugs have caused harm in the past and that the mandate and ethical responsibility of the FDA is to make certain that a harmful drug is not approved and to make certain that the drug is indeed beneficial.

After a drug is approved for marketing, the drug company has a continuing responsibility to make certain that longer term use is still safe. This process is often formalized in a phase IV study, which collects information about the drugs safety and benefit over many years.

The Role and Necessity of Placebo Controls

During World War II evaluation of seriously injured battlefront soldiers showed that many experienced little or no pain during the heat of battle. It became apparent that the quality and severity of pain varied greatly depending on emotional state. These observations led to a growing understanding that many physical symptoms could be significantly influenced by a person's state of mind or "psychological" condition. In the middle and late 1950s a series of studies in Great Britain and the United States demonstrated that many patients showed a beneficial response to "sugar pills" if they believed that the pills were of potential benefit. This "placebo response" has been studied in great detail. It is clear that a patient's will to get better—the desire to have a treatment work—may by itself have a powerful effect on his physical, psychological, and even biochemical condition. Some physicians regularly give patients placebo tablets as a form of symptomatic treatment. For example, it has been well documented that people in a clinical trial who are taking placebo do better than those who receive no treatment. As soon as someone begins a clinical trial, important changes in his physical and emotional condition occur, changes that could be attributed to the new drug being tested.

This finding immediately posed the problem of how to determine whether the apparent benefit of a new drug was in fact due to the drug itself or to the placebo effect. The answer was to give one group of patients the active medication and another the placebo—without *anyone* knowing who was receiving which. It is now generally accepted that the "gold standard" for clinical trials is the placebo-controlled, double-blind, randomized trial. *Double-blind* refers to the fact that neither the patient nor the physician running the trial is aware of who is receiving active medication and who is receiving placebo. If the physician knew which patients were in the treatment group and which were in the placebo group, he might manage them differently. If a problem develops that might be related to the medication being tested, the "code" can be broken, a determination made as to whether the patient was taking drug or placebo, and appropriate action taken.

The term *randomization* refers to the process by which patients are assigned to either the treatment group or the placebo group. Patients are assigned by a chance procedure, usually computer-determined, in an attempt to make each of the two groups as similar as possible in regard to gender, age, severity of disease, and so on. When entering a trial, the patient must agree to be enrolled in either of the two groups depending on his assignment, a process that cannot be compromised in order to ensure the scientific effectiveness of the trial. However, it is common practice to allow patients to begin active treatment at the end of a trial if they had been in the placebo group and for patients who had been receiving active drug to continue taking it if they so desire.

The use of placebo controls in trials of new ALS drugs has been somewhat controversial. Most investigators and federal regulatory agencies have insisted on the use of placebo controls in all trials. This position holds that there is no other way to make certain that a drug is truly effective, especially when its benefit is modest. On the other hand, most patients and some investigators maintain that in certain circumstances there may be other kinds of controls that are satisfactory. For example, historical controls might have a role in screening drugs when a fast and inexpensive, but possibly flawed, answer is acceptable. In this situation, the group of patients being treated with the new drug is compared with a similar group of patients who have been seen in the clinic in the past but not been treated with any specific medication. Thus, we use the "history" of untreated patients as a control group. Although this approach has obvious advantages, it also presents major problems because an exact match of treated patients and controls is not possible.

With the advent of riluzole, the situation has changed dramatically and at the same time has become more complicated. It is universally accepted that a physician has the responsibility to make certain that none of his patients are denied effective treatment for their illness. This causes a not insignificant dilemma if placebo is used in a clinical trial when an FDA-approved drug is available. For example, is it appropriate to place patients on placebo and thus deny them riluzole while taking part in the study of a new drug?

Current views on the physician's responsibility to the patient can be traced to the Nuremberg trials, which, among other things, judged the responsibility of Nazi physicians who had performed various medical experiments on concentration camp victims. The judges of this trial established 10 principles of medical research that they believed should determine physician–patient relationships during a research program. This became known as the Nuremberg Code and eventually resulted in important changes in how trials are conducted. In the past, patients typically were expected to be passive, silent, and subservient to the wishes of the physician or researcher. The doctor knew best, what he advised was in the patient's best interest, and he should not be questioned. As a corollary, the general perception was that the important goal was finding effective treatment for human diseases for the good of society in general and that almost any reasonable sacrifice was acceptable with this altruistic goal in mind. The welfare of the individual patient was considered secondary to the welfare of the much larger group of patients in society who had that particular disease.

The Nuremberg Code clearly and dramatically changed this dynamic, such that the individual patient now became the focus. It was suggested and recommended that the physician's primary responsibility was to a specific individual patient and not to a less well defined societal need. The two most important concepts expressed in this Code and now included in every human drug study are (1) the patient must be fully informed about all aspects of the trial, and (2) the patient has the right to withdraw at any time he wishes without penalty.

The principles espoused in the Nuremberg Code were further developed in the Declaration of Helsinki, which was adopted by the World Health Organization of the United Nations in 1964. This document further defined and elucidated the rights of patients enrolled in a clinical trial, again emphasizing that the patient's welfare must always supersede a perceived benefit to society as a whole. It states that "in any medical study every patient, including those of a control group, if any, should be assured of the best proven diagnostic and therapeutic method."

Unfortunately, the rights of the individual patient and the desire to have a scientifically sound research clinical trial at times can be at odds and result in dilemmas that are difficult to resolve. Nowhere has this been more apparent than with the use of placebo. Many physicians carrying out clinical trials in ALS maintain that because riluzole has been accepted by the regulatory agencies and scientific community as a drug that is both beneficial and safe, it is unethical to deny it to any patient who wishes to receive it. This would include patients receiving placebo as a control in a drug trial. This view holds that it is unethical for a doctor to advise a patient that placebo is appropriate because the drug being tested may benefit society as a whole and that the patient has an obligation to act in behalf of this greater good. On the other hand, other investigators have taken the position that the only way to determine whether a new drug works is with a placebo control. They point out that since the benefit from any new drug is likely to be small, testing it against another drug with modest benefit (i.e., riluzole) may hide a beneficial effect.

Some recent trials have been interested in determining not whether the new drug is better than nothing at all but whether the new drug is better than existing treatment. In these trials, the investigational drug is tested against riluzole, which is used as a control. However, random assignment to either of the two drugs is still necessary.

Institutional Protection of the Patient

All clinical trials must undergo careful scrutiny by a special committee before approval for the trial is given. In our hospital it is called the "Human Investigation Review Committee" and is composed of physicians, scientists, lawyers, ethicists, and patient advocates. This committee has the responsibility of ensuring that every clinical trial it approves meets strict scientific and ethical criteria. It ensures that the research is being carried out by competent investigators and that the information obtained will remain confidential. It especially protects the rights of minors and those who are mentally unable to understand the nature of the trial. The committee makes certain that any risks involved are defined and that they are outweighed by potential benefit to the patient. Women of childbearing age are given special attention. It carefully monitors the conduct of the trial once it begins and may order the trial to stop if untoward or unexpected results occur.

Informed Consent

The Nuremberg Code principle, which states that any patient involved in a drug trial must be fully informed about all details of the study, is now incorporated into every clinical trial. This is usually done with an "informed consent" document that is signed by the patient after a detailed explanation of the trial and after ascertaining that the patient does indeed understand his rights and the nature of the trial. People who are ill, especially with a life-threatening disease such as ALS, are particularly vulnerable and often desperate for any possible benefit, As a result, they may unknowingly act against their own best welfare. Sometimes the physician's explanation of a trial to the patient is made in the presence of another person, who acts as the patient's advocate to ensure that he fully understands what he is about to sign. The consent form describes the goals of the study, potential hazards, and what procedures will be required of the patient. It clearly states that the trial participant may drop out of the study at any time with or without explanation. It explains who is responsible for paying for the care needed if medical harm occurs to the patient as a result of his participation in the study. It should contain information about who should be contacted if a problem develops. Consent forms recently have included information about possible physician conflicts of interest that relate to the study, such as receiving payment for enrolling patients. Patients may or may not receive payment for taking part in the study, and this also is described in the informed consent document.

The Patient's Obligations

Although the main obligations of the informed consent process are properly placed on the physician or researcher, it is important to understand that the patient also accepts certain responsibilities when he agrees to enter an experimental clinical trial. Although the patient properly has the right to withdraw from a trial at any time, he should be aware that his full participation and cooperation is essential for the completion of a successful trial. When a consent form is signed, the patient has implicitly agreed to meet all his responsibilities such as obligations to get tests done, have blood samples drawn, make the necessary clinic visits, and so forth. He should not discuss anything about the study with other patients, especially any side effects of the medication received. Above all, he should make every attempt possible to complete the study despite any inconvenience, as incomplete information can result in a serious problem interpreting the study results. Many patients make attempts to find out whether they are receiving active drug or placebo, a course of action that may be harmful to the success of the study.

Clinical Trials and the Internet

As with all new technologic advances, the advent of Internet-based communications has provided both opportunities and dilemmas. The wealth of information related to ALS already on the Internet can be overwhelming and difficult to fully understand. This undoubtedly will increase with the passage of time. It has provided an unprecedented way for both rapid and current data to be provided to patients and their families. Above all, it has allowed patients to communicate with each other and provide not only psychological support but also meaningful and helpful ways to deal with the multiple problems caused by the disease. It has helped them understand that they are not alone with the burden they must bear, and this by itself has a strengthening effect. The Internet has allowed physicians, other health care providers, and voluntary health agencies such as the Amyotrophic Lateral Sclerosis Association (ALSA) and Muscular Dystrophy Association (MDA) to communicate with ALS patients in a rapid and inexpensive manner. It has provided an unprecedented avenue for clinical and basic researchers to communicate research results with each other. There is growing interest in using the Internet to record data from clinical trials; this would markedly reduce the paperwork required and speed the completion of these trials.

Simultaneously, however, it has raised a number of issues that have proven troublesome. Communication on the Internet is essentially unregulated. Anyone can say almost anything they wish, well-meaning or otherwise. This obviously creates the opportunity for a lot of mischief as well as well-intended misinformation. For example, patients occasionally have suggested that they have benefited from treatments that clearly have no therapeutic potential. Undoubtedly, they have experienced a placebo effect. Similarly, claims of benefit have been made by companies selling products that have not been properly studied. Of more concern are claims of benefit from treatments that are potentially dangerous or could intensify weakness already present.

The key to evaluating the validity and usefulness of information provided on the Internet rests with an understanding of the source of that information coupled with an understanding of the disease itself. Every person with ALS and his or her family members should become as knowledgeable as possible about what is known and not known about the cause and treatment of ALS. When reading anything on the Internet, it is essential to find out who wrote it and where it comes from. Information from established voluntary health organizations such as ALSA and MDA is carefully reviewed for accuracy before it is put on the Internet. Similarly, information from established academic health and research centers has been carefully considered before putting it out for the world to see. Patient-generated information has been extremely useful most of the time, but it should be understood that a person with ALS is understandably not an unbiased observer. Be very careful about therapeutic claims made by any company that stands to benefit financially by the sale of its product. Above all, check with your ALS physician about any questionable information you receive before you act. Similarly, be very careful about what information you yourself put onto the Internet. Make certain it will be of true value to other patients or health care providers.

The Future

Therapeutic trials in ALS have suffered greatly from the lack of a "biologic marker" that would indicate whether the disease process is slowed after administration of a drug. Although we have clinical indicators of disease progression, such as change in muscle strength, this is an indirect measure and is relatively insensitive. In diabetes, the blood sugar level indicates the benefit or lack of benefit of a specific drug that is being tested. In AIDS, certain tests can be done on white blood cells to indicate the same thing. Unfortunately, no such test is available for ALS. This has been a major hurdle in understanding whether a new treatment is effective. The entire process of clinical therapeutic trials will be significantly speeded up should such a test become available, and many laboratories are working on the problem.

It is clear that a more perfect understanding of the multiple causes of ALS will eventually lead to more effective treatment. However, as we wait for the further elucidation of this difficult disease, we should not relax our efforts in finding better treatments. The advent of riluzole, the first effective drug for ALS that has a scientific basis, has undoubtedly heralded the beginning of a new age of treatment. The single most pressing need is to begin the process of carrying out trials that simultaneously administer multiple drugs, each of which has demonstrated benefit alone or has a strong potential for doing so. These trials are long overdue.

Although it is not possible to predict exactly when more effective treatment for ALS will become available, it is clear we have recently entered a new era of drug treatment that offers great hope for all those who are fighting the good fight.

Suggested Reading

1. Giffels JJ. *Clinical trials: What you should know before volunteering to be a research subject.* New York: Demos Vermande, 1996.

2. Shuster, E. Fifty years later: The significance of the Nuremberg Code. *N Engl J Med* 1997; 337:1436.

3. Rothman KJ, Michels KB. The continuing unethical use of placebo controls. *N Engl J Med* 1994; 331:394.

4. Hampton JR, Julian DG. Role of the pharmaceutical industry in major clinical trials. *Lancet.* II November 28, 1987; 1258.

5. Bernat JL, Goldstein ML, Ringel SP. Conflicts of interest in neurology. *Neurology* 1998; 50:327.

6. Munsat TL, Hollander D, Finison L. Clinical trial methodology. In: Leigh PN, Swash M (eds.). *Motor neurone disease.* London: Springer-Verlang, 1995.

7. Eisen A, Krieger C (eds.). *Amyotrophic lateral sclerosis: A synthesis of research and clinical practice.* New York: Cambridge University Press, 1998.

16

The Design of Clinical Trials

Robert Sufit, M.D.

Clinical trials underlie the development of any new treatment for any disease. In some diseases a positive effect is relatively easy to measure. For example, within a day of beginning treatment for bacterial pneumonia, the patient generally feels better and the fever breaks. Our ability to treat bacterial pneumonia is helped by relatively easy access to the cause because the patient coughs up material that contains the actual offending organism. Various antibiotics can then be tested in culture against that organism over a day or two. The treatment(s) can be quickly evaluated by assessing whether the patient is responding. However, the diagnosis of amyotrophic lateral sclerosis (ALS) often is not made quickly, and there is no specific test for the disease. Motor nerve cells do not regenerate, and objective strength improvement resulting from any treatment may not occur. It is unlikely that muscle atrophy will reverse. The EMG will still be abnormal. Therefore, the best hope from a treatment aimed at the pathology of ALS is that the disease will stop progressing. Thus, it is quite difficult to tell if a treatment is working, either during its testing in a clinical trial or in a given individual once the treatment has been shown to work in general.

Despite this challenge, or perhaps because of it, there is a continuing effort by scientists, clinicians, and patients to better understand the disease process. The hope is to develop treatments based on this understanding and thus to slow or halt disease progression. This chapter reviews the current state of treatment development. This is accomplished through a series of stages: (1) to explain what accomplishments have been made in understanding disease pathogenesis (its cause) as it

221

relates to treatment ideas; (2) to show how those ideas can be translated to clinical trials; (3) to review the results of completed trials; (4) to inform the reader about what is currently being tried; and (5) to speculate on where the treatment field may be heading. Although this may seem to be a linear process, some of these stages can occur simultaneously as treatment ideas reach maturity. Nevertheless, lessons learned at any of the earlier stages of treatment development will affect the later phases of research. Ideas for new treatments are necessarily speculative and should not be regarded as certain to go to clinical investigation.

Hypotheses of Disease Pathogenesis and Relation to Clinical Trials

It seems logical that the key to developing effective treatments is to better understand the disease. Despite the ultimate development of a similar clinical picture in most people with ALS, the disease has several causes. Between 5 percent and 10 percent of ALS is hereditary, which suggests that there are at least two causes. Of the hereditary causes, approximately 20 percent are the result of one of at least 80 mutations in the gene coding for one type of substance called *superoxide dismutase* (SOD-1). There probably are at least two other gene abnormalities as well.

With that line of reasoning, there also may well be more than one type of sporadic ALS. For example, one thought is that there is difficulty in handling a brain chemical called *glutamate.* We all need glutamate because it is an amino acid building block for proteins throughout the body. It is present in many of the foods we eat. In the brain it is one of the major ways to transmit information from one cell to another. The hypothesis states that ALS arises because the motor nerve cells are exposed to too much glutamate. The hypothesis continues that the cells around the motor nerve cells (and indeed around all neurons), called *astrocytes,* may not be able to eliminate glutamate fast enough once it has done its job as a chemical transmitter. The reasons for astrocyte failure may also be multiple.

Between the hereditary causes and the glutamate hypothesis, it is fairly certain that there are several ways to initiate the disease we call ALS. Moreover, because the disease is currently difficult to diagnose in its earliest stages, it is unlikely that any treatment will be developed in the foreseeable future to prevent the disease from occurring at all, which means that successful efforts to control the disease must focus on slowing or halting its progression.

Disease progression ultimately results in death of a specific kind of cell, the anterior horn cells in the spinal cord, as well as similar nerve cells in the brain stem connecting to the tongue and other laryngeal and pharyngeal muscles, and motor cells in the cortex of the brain. There may be many ways to start the process that leads to cell death, but if we are to treat this disease effectively, we must assume that there is a common factor amenable to treatment. We must examine the pathway(s) of disease progression to develop a rational treatment program.

One idea is that the glutamate hypothesis explains both disease initiation and disease progression. In other words, the motor neurons not only can be damaged by excess glutamate, but also they can eventually be killed by excess glutamate. Moreover, too much glutamate may kill neurons no matter what causes the initial damage. Support for this idea comes not only from experiments with motor neurons but also from neurons damaged by stroke, epilepsy, and Parkinson's disease.

A second view is that molecules called *free radicals* eventually kill the motor neurons. There is no question that excess free radicals can kill cells of all kinds. Free radicals occur frequently in nature, so most living organisms (including plants as well as animals) have developed ways to get rid of them. One way is through the enzyme superoxide dismutase, the same molecule, as mentioned previously, whose gene is involved in some cases of hereditary ALS. There are other free radicals, and there are other enzymes and other methods for cells to handle them. One method is through free radical scavengers such as vitamin E and vitamin C. Beta carotene and coenzyme Q-10 also may function as free radical scavengers. Their advantage is that they are now available over the counter. That easy availability is also a potential disadvantage, however, because it is difficult to study compounds that anyone can take without having a control group.

Yet another idea about how the disease develops centers around what are called *growth factors.* Many nerve cells seem to require a relatively specific factor to remain alive, so the term *growth* may be somewhat misleading. It describes the growth of the nerve cell in culture. A damaged neuron may not make enough of a particular growth factor to keep itself or perhaps its neighbors alive. If a motor neuron is injured, it then fails to make and secrete enough of a growth factor and thus deprives its neighbors of what they need to stay healthy, so the process continues. One such growth factor for motor nerve cells is called *brain-derived neurotrophic factor* (BDNF). There also are molecules called *receptors* that are found on the surface of the nerve cell that respond specifically to BDNF.

A hypothesis supported by fewer investigations is one based on autoimmunity. This concept states that something triggers the body to mount an immune attack on its own tissues, in this case the motor nerve cells. It is not clear whether the evidence for this represents still another mechanism of disease or whether it may simply be the result of the body reacting to damage caused by other mechanisms. In other words, the body may be using the immune system to clean up damage caused by some of the previously described or as yet undescribed causes. Nonetheless, unsuccessful attempts have been made to develop treatments based on this hypothesis.

There may be a problems with some internal proteins called *neurofilaments.* These proteins probably have many duties such as the transportation or at least the guidance of other molecules to their appropriate places. Absence, change, or damage to neurofilaments could thus end up damaging the cell as a whole by many different mechanisms. There are changes in neurofilaments in both animal and human motor neuron disease. However, this damage could well be secondary to some other process. It could be caused by the same process responsible for damaging other cellular constituents such as DNA. Free radicals might be such an agent. Or, there might be an intermediate situation whereby damage to neurofila-ments is not the primary cause of disease but contributes to the death of the motor nerve. This is important because interrupting the pathway of destruction at any point could well slow or halt the disease process. At present there are no known ways to change the neurofilament structure, but research into neurofila-ment biology is ongoing.

Finally, it is entirely possible that there is an as yet unknown mechanism for motor nerve damage. People with the familial form of ALS who have an SOD abnormality seem best explained not only by a lack of normal dismutase activity of that enzyme but also by some toxicity of the abnormal enzyme. In an animal model using abnormal SOD, the mice have normal activities of their own (native) enzyme, and the more copies of the abnormal human SOD they have, the quicker they become sick. This has been called a *toxic gain of function*. At the current time we do not know what that function is, but it seems logical that it is in some way related to the normal function of the enzyme.

All this may seem daunting, but it does allow several avenues for treatment. In addition, if there is a serendipitous clinical discovery that slows the disease process, it could open new doors to similar treatments.

The How and Why of Clinical Trials in ALS

It would seem to be a relatively straightforward matter to test a treatment in ALS. One would give a patient the probable treatment and see if he did not progress and ultimately lived a normal life span. This would be fine if the research community were to stumble upon a treatment rather quickly, and indeed there would be no need to know much about the underlying mechanism of either the disease or the treatment. Reality is quite different.

Many problems with the approach described here are obvious. For example, suppose the patient actually did not have ALS. Or, suppose the patient was one of the 5 percent to 10 percent of patients who progress very slowly. Another prob-lem might be if the patient had a heart attack and died 6 months into the study. It also is possible that nothing unusual would happen. These examples suggest that perhaps one should add a few more patients and perhaps a few different doses. What would happen then would probably be several somewhat different results from the same treatment or perhaps the same result at several different doses. In addition, there still might be patients who had unexpected reactions that seemed not to be related to ALS. Those effects could be side effects of the treatment or they simply could be things that would have happened anyway.

The best treatment would be one that cures all patients without any side effects, but that is unlikely in the near future. Therefore, we are left with treatments that are in some ways imperfect as regards their efficacy or their side effects. To check the efficacy we may well need a relatively large group of patients who among them represent many of the variables that affect the disease and the treatment. How many is enough? One could easily begin to list such variables: age, gender, duration of disease, rapidity of the disease, stage of the disease, sporadic versus familial ALS, dose of the treatment, how long to treat, and so forth.

But that creates another problem. What comparisons do we make? Do we compare 40-year-old women to 80-year-old women to 60-year-old men? How do we get groups large enough to resolve all those differences? And even if we end up with the groups in some response order, how do we know if we have chosen all the correct variables? In addition, is it possible to decide where the cut-off point is for whether the treatment works? Does the treatment work only for the best two or three groups, or does it work for every group? Then there is the issue of side effects. A given group may have more headaches. Is this a side effect of the treatment or is it based on some other aspect of the group such as gender? For example, migraine headaches are more common in women.

The best way out of this dilemma is to do things in a stepwise fashion with the aim of getting a best dose in the group most likely to show efficacy. This group is then divided and tested against itself, with one part of the group receiving treatment and one part of the group acting as the control. The initial part of the testing aims to find out whether there are unreasonable side effects. In this phase I of testing, small numbers of people are given a single treatment, and their responses, particularly with regard to safety, are studied both clinically and in the laboratory. Once the treatment appears reasonably safe (and in potentially fatal diseases there is a little more leeway than in less lethal situations), a larger number of patients can be given the treatment for longer periods and in larger doses. As this testing progresses, a better picture of the side effects will emerge. The best measures for efficacy can be chosen. There is still a need for occasional control patients. When neither evaluator nor subject knows which patients are receiving treatment, it is called double-blind treatment.

The next step is to take what has been learned from these initial phases of testing and choose a large group to test the best dose(s) in the right subjects. At this stage a similar sized control group is needed. Thus, only some of the test group receive the treatment and they are compared with the control group. This is a *controlled parallel group design study.* Patients are chosen from all ages, both genders, different sites of onset, and so forth. One should end up with all groups having *on average* similar ages, gender distributions, sites of onset, and so forth. Variables that are unknown but that could affect the study should also be randomly distributed among the groups. This becomes a randomized, controlled, *parallel group design trial* (RCT).

There are several other aspects of study design. The first is to choose the principal outcome variable before the study starts based on what has been learned from earlier studies. This makes the RCT *prospective* in nature. By chance alone there could be a difference between groups if one looked at enough different variables despite randomization. The only way to eliminate that would be to have impossibly large numbers of test subjects at an enormous cost of both money and time. As in the earlier phase studies, the evaluator and the subject are blinded so they do not bias the outcome. This is a called a *double-blind prospective RCT.*

Some other aspects of a study are not immediately obvious. The duration of ALS is such that we want to get answers quickly for our current patients, and yet the disease is variable enough that too short a period will not allow for separation of the groups. Some of that depends on the outcome variable that is chosen as the primary efficacy measure. If it is survival, most studies are 18 months in length. It takes time to enroll each patient because of the necessities of protecting the patient and making sure they fit the entry criteria. It is impossible to enter all patients on the same day. Thus, there usually is an enrollment period of up to 6 months for most studies. This means that from the day the study starts there is at least a 2-year period before results can be known. Choosing to add even more patients only lengthens that period. A longer period for each patient would allow for fewer patients in each study, but it would take even longer before a conclusion was reached. On the positive side, it would make it possible to test more treatments at the same time for a given patient population. A longer study time per patient would increase the likelihood that a patient would drop out either because he thought something better was coming along or because of a nonrelated event such as another medical illness.

Which patient population should be tested? There are common inclusion and exclusion criteria. Naturally, we want to test a treatment for as many patients as possible. It would cloud the results if patients with primary lateral sclerosis or Kennedy's disease were included in a cohort of ALS patients. Therefore, most RCTs in motor neuron disease include only ALS patients. Some patients who are very early in the disease course but who nonetheless appear to have ALS may end up being excluded from the trial. Someone with drooling and difficulty speaking that develops over three months but who has no other signs of ALS would not meet the entry criteria of most studies. At a later stage in the disease, someone who is already on a ventilator and unlikely to show any slowing of the disease process also would not be a candidate. Other exclusionary criteria typically include patients with other serious illnesses. Any well-designed study involves trade-offs with regard to the population studied, the number of subjects included, and the time frame for the study.

A compelling reason to do an RCT, as opposed to simply opening a treatment to anyone, is the issue of side effects. In organisms as complex as human beings, there simply is no other way to address the issue of whether a given treatment causes untoward events. A few illustrations should suffice to prove this. Suppose several hundred people were treated with a therapy for 18 months and 20 percent of them felt nauseated during that time. Would it be fair to say that the treatment caused nausea 20 percent of the time? One could easily answer that question with a control group. If during that same time period 10 percent of the control group had nausea at one time or another, the treatment was indeed responsible for nausea but only in 10 percent of the patients. Other side effects might occur in both groups 5 percent of the time and not actually be side effects at all. This becomes an even greater concern if the possible side effect is dangerous. Suppose a given percentage of patients developed blood clots in the legs. Is this a problem of the disease, or is it a problem of the treatment? A control group answers that question.

Completed Clinical Trials

Most physicians and patients tend to focus on the current state of knowledge about treatments. When informed about the current state of the art, particularly in a disease such as ALS, the next question often is what else is being thought of and why is it not available now.

There has been an explosion of knowledge about the basic science of the nervous system in the past 30 years. This has led to some of the understanding previously described in this chapter. It also has led to more clinical trials. One such trial was the use of a molecule normally found in the nervous system called a *ganglioside*. Because this molecule promoted nerve cell growth in tissue culture, it was thought that it might help in ALS. Unfortunately, that was not the case, but it does represent the beginning of the concept of using growth-promoting factors in ALS.

A second approach along those lines was to use thyrotropin-releasing hormone (TRH). TRH is also found normally within the nervous system. ALS was treated by delivering TRH intravenously, subcutaneously (under the skin like an insulin injection), and directly into the spinal fluid. Some initial reports suggested a favorable short-term outcome. Specifically, some patients seemed to perform better immediately after the injection. Some patients also had significant side effects. When long-term subcutaneous administration was used, the medication ultimately did not work.

There also were were attempts at dietary manipulation. One example was the administration of branched-chain amino acids to try to reduce the amount of glutamate that was taken into the nervous system. The amino acid L-threonine also was tried. These trials also failed to significantly alter the course of the disease. A significant success of all these initial efforts during the 1980s was that investigators throughout the world began to collaborate. This led to multicenter trials, many of which were multinational. These collaborative efforts also led to standardized ways to assess patients and enter them into protocols.

The explosive growth of cellular biology, including neurobiology, has contributed to the development of biotechnology companies. Many interesting compounds discovered in the laboratory have possible commercial applications. This has led to the development of treatments for health problems such as ALS that affect only a relatively small number of people. There have been several such compounds with specific reference to ALS. One such compound is ciliary neurotrophic factor (CNTF), a compound that promotes nerve growth in the laboratory and benefited some experimental animals with nervous system disease. Therefore, experiments for patients with ALS were undertaken beginning in the early 1990s. The initial safety and dose testing seemed to offer hope, so two larger RCTs were undertaken. Neither of these trials showed any benefit with the agent delivered subcutaneously. Indeed, in one of the studies the patients who received the highest dose seemed to do worse for the first few months of the nine-month study. Most of that worsening seemed to be due to gastrointestinal side effects resulting in excessive weight loss. Delivery of the agent directly into the spinal fluid could avoid that side effect. However, research in that direction is inactive at the current time.

Another naturally occurring growth factor with similar laboratory results is insulin-like growth factor 1 (IGF-1). Two RCTs with IGF-1 delivered subcutaneously were carried out. In the study done in the United States, there was a control group, a low-dose group, and a higher dose group. Using a scale developed to assess ALS progression in general, this study showed a promising slowing in the development of new problems. The study was planned as a nine-month study similar to that of CNTF. Side effects of IGF-1 also seemed modest. A second study, which was done in Europe, failed to show similar results. There also seemed to be a higher death rate in the treated group versus the control group. These two conflicting results have never been adequately resolved. On one side, methodological questions have been raised about the U.S. study, whereas different questions about the European study have been raised by those who believe that IGF-1 works. A decisive third study has not been undertaken. One possible conclusion is that the benefit is too small to show up unless a larger study is done or the study lasts for 12 to 18 months. Such a study seems financially prohibitive. Current laboratory research is still being done on IGF-1. Some of this research is directed at other diseases such as the neuropathy associated with diabetes. If IGF-1 were to successfully treat a different disease, it is conceivable that it might become available to ALS patients through the so-called "off-label" indication. If the drug were approved for marketing for diabetic neuropathy, it could be prescribed by physicians for any patient, including those with ALS.

Another growth factor is brain-derived growth factor (BDNF). It, too, seemed potent in both laboratory and animal studies. Planning for the BDNF trials was on a much larger scale. In the early dose finding studies, almost as many patients were tested as in the RCT for CNTF and IGF-1. The results of the phase 2 study suggested that breathing capacity and survival should be used as outcome variables for the larger phase 3 RCT. Almost 1,200 patients were entered from multiple sites in North America. Many of the investigators thought their patients were doing extremely well, so it came as a surprise that BDNF given at two different doses showed no statistically significant difference in the treated group than in the control group. Side effects were minimal except for excessive diarrhea experienced by some patients. Those patients seemed to have a better outcome. The implications of this are discussed in the section on ongoing trials.

Yet another promising growth factor was glial cell-derived neurotrophic factor (GDNF). The best method of delivery seemed to be directly into the cerebrospinal fluid. This treatment possibility for ALS has been put on hold because of some side effects in early phases of study. There still is some interest in GDNF for Parkinson's disease, so the ALS community may yet hear more about it.

The glutamate hypothesis also generated clinical trials. Initial efforts with glutamate receptor blockers such as MK-801 revealed excessive side effects. One compound that seemed relatively free from side effects was riluzole. This small molecule is given by mouth, thereby making it easier to study than the parenterally administered growth factors. Riluzole was initially tried in France, the home of the parent pharmaceutical company. In a relatively small study with about 150 patients divided into a control group and a treatment group tested over 18 months, there was a survival benefit to the treated group. This benefit was not large, and, moreover, it appeared that only patients who began with speech or swallowing difficulties were helped. Therefore, a large, multicenter, multinational trial was undertaken with 959 patients. These patients were divided into low-, medium-, and high-dose groups, as well as a control group. The study regarded survival as an outcome. This second study confirmed the results of the first. Both the medium dose of 100 mg per day and the high dose of 200 mg per day showed a statistically significant difference from the control group in the percentage of subjects who survived for a given period. The demonstrated difference was approximately three months. The low-dose (50 mg/day) group showed a difference intermediate between control and 100 mg per day, but it was not statistically significant. The principal side effects were nausea and a generalized feeling of weakness. The side effects usually passed within a few weeks, and only a few patients had to stop taking the medication as a result. A common side effect was a blood elevation of liver enzymes, which usually peaked quickly and then lessened. Consequently, riluzole is either withheld or used very cautiously in patients who have had hepatitis.

Several other important factors from this study should be noted. One-third of the patients were deliberately chosen because they had bulbar onset of the disease. In contradistinction to the earlier smaller study, there was no difference between bulbar onset patients and limb onset patients. The difference was demonstrated in groups so that any single patient did not know whether riluzole helped him or her. Other unanswered questions arose. The average time from onset of disease to entry in the trial was almost two years. This was required to ensure that only patients with ALS were entered into the study. Most practitioners would like to start the drug as early as possible in the disease process before the strict research criteria for diagnosis are met. With that in mind, it is difficult to know whether the drug is more effective if one starts the medication at the time the diagnosis is first considered.

There also were no criteria for stopping the medication. Nevertheless, some information exists. Patients participating in the study were allowed to take the medication at the 100 mg per day dose after the RCT protocol was completed but before the drug was approved for marketing. This is so-called "open label" testing. Data collected from this uncontrolled group suggest that the efficacy is maintained for longer than the 18-month trial. Additionally, the drug was made available for a group of patients who had not participated in the trial through what is called "expanded access" or treatment investigational new drug (IND). These patients were followed up primarily to assess side effects. Their side-effect profiles confirmed the results of the RCT. As of this writing, riluzole is the only agent approved by the U.S. Food and Drug Administration for marketing for the treatment of ALS. It is also marketed in Europe and Japan, but it has not been approved by the Health Protection Board of Canada.

No one is quite sure how gabapentin works, but it is possible that it affects glutamate. Gabapentin is currently available, having been approved for marketing for the treatment of certain types of epilepsy. Because it might affect glutamate, it has been tried in an RCT for ALS. In doses of 1800 mg per day it did not show any efficacy at a statistically significant level. However, there was a trend toward efficacy in one strength measure. Arm strength did not deteriorate as quickly in the treated group. That may have occurred through chance alone, however, so a second trial was undertaken. This trial was completed in 1999. Despite the larger doses, the study failed to confirm any efficacy. At this time gabapentin is not being used for ALS treatment.

Ongoing Clinical Trials

The presence of an approved medication has altered the investigation of new agents. The ethically responsible approach continues to be to compare any new agent against current best medical care, and for many patients this includes the use of riluzole. One such clinical trial is actually two clinical trials. An oral compound known initially by its code number of SR 57746A was shown in a small trial to favorably affect breathing capacity and survival in ALS patients. It is thought to work by promoting the production of BDNF in the central nervous system. Two distinct studies were executed. These are multicenter, multinational trials. In one RCT with approximately 1,200 patients, SR 57746A was given at two doses, 1 mg per day and 2 mg per day, compared with that of a control group. Everyone in all three groups took riluzole. The study duration was 18 months per patient. A smaller study with about 800 patients was similarly divided with regard to SR 57746A, but none of these patients started out taking riluzole either because they could not tolerate it or because it was not available in Canada.

SR 57746A has received the name xaliproden. Discussion of the results of both xaliproden trials began in the fall of 2000. Although no peer-reviewed publications have emerged, some measures of efficacy tended to the positive, whereas others were clearly negative. Taking riluzole or not did not appear to affect the results. Thus it appears that there are not sufficient data to warrant general marketing of the drug. As of late 2000, discussions as to further trials are under way.

Another important event has occurred with this study that deserves mention. Clinical trials are undertaken because searching for a single best treatment that would cure the disease would take a prohibitively long time. The implication is that multiple therapies will be used in combination. The trial with the addition of SR 57746A to a treatment regimen that already includes riluzole is the first such attempt. One shortcoming of this trial is that there is no definitive comparison between SR 57746A and riluzole. That is to say, if SR 57746A works, there may not be a clear-cut answer as to which treatment is better used singly.

Two different approaches for BDNF are ongoing to be completed in spring 2001. Because patients with gastrointestinal side effects seemed to benefit the most when BDNF was delivered subcutaneously, a 2nd higher dose subcutaneous trial was planned for 12 months and started in 1999. This trial escalated the dose of BDNF until side effects were achieved or a much higher dose than was previously tried was used. There may well be some problems with blinding, but these problems should not be insurmountable.

The other trial completed enrollment mid June 1999. This is an 18-month trial of BDNF delivered into the spinal fluid through a pump system. Because of the complexity of the delivery system, the trial was designed to look for a much larger effect than those with oral or subcutaneous administration. There were only 90 patients per group. Survival and breathing capacity are the primary outcome measures. Because BDNF is given directly into the spinal fluid, the amount of BDNF administered is extremely low, and there should be no systemic side effects. There probably will be some central nervous system side effects because in the phase I study of 25 patients the higher doses were accompanied by insomnia and in some cases behavior that appeared manic. Results should become available in early 2001. This is, in my opinion, a critical juncture for growth factors. Should both the higher dose subcutaneous and intrathecal (into the spinal fluid) BDNF trials fail to show efficacy, the use of any growth factors for treatment of ALS may well be called into question.

Glutamate antagonism is also undergoing clinical trials. Despite the failure of gabapentin, another drug used in epilepsy is being tried in ALS. Topiramate has a known mechanism of action blocking a specific glutamate receptor that is different from the one affected by MK-801. Topiramate is commercially available; however, a consortium of ALS investigators with both pharmaceutical and NIH support has managed to enroll fully a RCT as of mid 2000. Data from that study should become available in the second half of 2001. Still another trial is also under way. Animals can be affected with motor neuron disease from insertion of the human SOD-1 gene into their DNA. Using these transgenic mice, a small molecule called creatine appeared to slow the loss of motor neurons. This finding stimulated a trial in humans. Creatine occurs naturally in muscle and is available as a food supplement, so patients who are not in the trial may also be taking it, so the trial has taken extra time to enroll. Results probably will not be available until after the topiramate trial.

Speculation on Future Studies

Future trials will continue to be driven by the science coming out of the laboratory. Work done on the basic biology of the nervous system and the molecular pathology of ALS will lead to new ideas. The traditional pharmaceutical firms as well as biotechnology companies will continue to suggest possible new treatments. Compounds called *immunophyllins* could work like growth factors. If intrathecal BDNF proves to be successful, combining it with other growth factors might enhance its effect.

Other ideas regarding regulation of glutamate production or glutamate receptors continue to evolve. Whether these compounds are tried in ALS or in other neurologic diseases first remains to be seen. Nevertheless, once there are more drugs available for other neurologic diseases, patients and investigators can explore their use in ALS.

This approach will also work for possible treatments that are already available as nonprescription items, such as vitamin E, coenzyme Q-10, or alpha lipoic acid. Their testing will not take place commercially. Some of these agents have already been tested in the transgenic mouse model of ALS based on the hereditary human ALS. If these compounds delay or in some way alter the course of the disease, they too, like creatine, can be tested in humans.

Conclusion

The hope of finding effective treatment rests with well-performed clinical trials. This chapter has explained the promise of basic neuroscience, the development of clinical trial methodology for ALS, and the results of clinical trials for glutamate antagonism and growth factors. Patients and investigators continue to be enthusiastic about clinical trials. It is my firm belief that our current programs, plus additional approaches such as free radical scavenging or nerve cell energy enhancement, will result in truly effective treatment protocols.

17

The ALS Patient Care Database

R. G. Miller, M.D., F. A. Anderson, Jr., Ph.D., and the ALS C.A.R.E. Study Group

Over the last decade considerable progress has been made in developing effective disease-specific and symptomatic treatments for ALS. The need for comprehensive management of patients with ALS has seen the evolution of specialized ALS centers involving multidisciplinary teams of health care professionals. Do newly available interventions—alone or in combination—affect the disease course, improve quality of life, and lessen the overall burden of ALS on patients and their families? Does early diagnosis and initiation of a comprehensive management plan correlate with improved care? Although individual neurologists and clinics have monitored individual outcomes, until recently, there was no formal mechanism in place to answer these questions.

Observational databases enable physicians to assess health outcomes and provide answers to questions about optimal patient management. In the past decade, a number of databases have been established in a variety of fields. For example, the *National Registry of Myocardial Infarction* (1) gathers information about the management of patients with heart attacks, and *The Hip & Knee Registry* (2) collects data about the incidence and success of hip and knee replacements. Thus, the *ALS Patient Care Database* was established in response to the need to monitor practice patterns in the management of patients with ALS.

Designing the ALS Patient Care Database

The database is a key component of the ALS Clinical Assessment, Research, and

233

Education (C.A.R.E.) Program, which will include the development of educational programs to improve the care of patients with ALS.

The concept for the database was initially developed by an advisory board of neurologists who specialize in ALS, assisted by statisticians. More recently, nurses and a representative from a national patient advocacy group have joined the project, which is supported by an unrestricted educational grant from Rhône-Poulenc Rorer Pharmaceuticals and cosponsored by The ALS Association. It has also been endorsed by the World Federation of Neurology.

Data Collection

The first step was to design a series of forms that could be used to collect relevant information from patients with ALS, their caregivers, and neurologists. Four forms were developed, as described here.

Health Professional Form

Neurologists who enroll patients in the database are asked to complete a double-sided form that collects information about the duration, severity, and current management of the disease. Neurologists record the date of symptom onset and the date of diagnosis, as well as the diagnostic tests performed. In addition, they rate patient function on a scale of 0–4, including speech, swallowing, walking, and breathing. These functions are evaluated using the ALS Functional Rating Scale (ALSFRS), a validated instrument for this purpose (3). Neurologists also report the use of disease-specific medications, such as riluzole (Rilutek), and other therapeutic interventions, including assistive devices, symptomatic treatments, and feeding tubes.

Patient Form

Patients are asked to complete a six-page form that takes approximately 15 minutes. Table 17-1 lists the types of information collected by this form. Patients are asked to answer questions about the usefulness of various symptomatic medications and to report the degree to which they need assistance in performing the activities of daily living. They are also asked to record how ALS is affecting them emotionally and financially. Patients report whether they are satisfied with their medical care and what the most useful source of information on ALS has been. All of these questions provide insights into patients' perceptions of the impact of the disease on their health and quality of life (QOL). Two previously validated measures of QOL are used: (1) the SF-12, a general health assessment tool (4), and (2) the SIP/ALS19, an instrument designed to evaluate patients with ALS (5).

Caregiver Form

Amyotrophic lateral sclerosis affects not only the patient but also family members and friends. This realization led the ALS C.A.R.E. Program Advisory Board to

Table 17-1. Variables Reported in *ALS Patient Care Database* Quarterly Reports

Patient characteristics (e.g., duration of symptoms, age)
Clinical measures (e.g., ALSFRS score, forced vital capacity)
Type of insurance
Diagnostic criteria
Medications
Feeding modalities
Respiratory interventions
Quality of life
Satisfaction with medical care
Caregiver burden scores

develop a form that collects information from the primary caregiver. Questions include the caregiver's relationship to the patient, employment status, and the effects of caregiving on physical and emotional health.

Completion Form

The Completion Form serves two purposes. In some cases it is difficult to establish the diagnosis of ALS; thus, a neurologist may enroll a patient suspected of having the disease. Should the diagnosis subsequently be ruled out, neurologists are asked to fill out the Completion Form. Moreover, when an enrolled patient with a confirmed diagnosis of ALS dies, neurologists are also asked to fill out a Completion Form. By consulting with the patient's family or other health care professionals involved in the patient's care, the neurologist reports whether death was related to ALS; if the patient appeared to die peacefully; and what interventions, such as respiratory assistance, pain killers (e.g., opioids), or medications to reduce agitation, were used. In addition, information is gathered on whether advance directives were in place and followed.

All forms except the Completion Form are filled out at the time of patient enrollment and at each subsequent follow-up visit. Ideally, follow-up data are collected at least once every six months. Participating neurologists are sent a monthly reminder indicating which patients are due for their six-month follow-up.

Data Analysis and Reporting

Once forms are completed, they are sent to a central data coordinating center where the information is entered into a computer database. The staff at the data coordinating center prepare confidential reports that are sent to participating neurologists on a quarterly basis. The reports include data on a number of issues, including the use of therapeutic interventions, correlation between measures of QOL and functional scores, and patients' level of satisfaction with their medical care (Table 17-1).

The *ALS Patient Care Database* data coordinating center is also responsible for protecting the confidentiality of the data submitted. Neurologists participating in the database are assigned a confidential identification number. They, in turn, assign confidential numbers to the patients they enroll in the database. Caregivers give only their initials when completing forms. Thus, participants cannot be identified.

Benefits of Participation

The overall aim of the *ALS Patient Care Database* is to improve outcomes for patients. By participating, neurologists, patients, and their caregivers can contribute to what is known about ALS and increase the opportunity to identify the optimal management of this disease. The project is an unprecedented opportunity for patients and neurologists to join forces in unlocking some of the secrets of ALS. If every patient with ALS enrolls in the database, it will become a powerful tool to learn much more about this disease.

Collecting and analyzing information on all aspects of ALS from a large group of patients over an extended period of time allows neurologists and patients to look at how their therapeutic decisions impact the patient and the disease. Careful analysis of the data will reveal which therapeutic interventions are helpful and which are not. Neurologists and patients can learn at what point in the course of the disease a particular therapy (disease-specific or symptomatic) or other intervention (e.g., feeding tube, BiPAP) should be started to produce the maximum benefit. In addition, the data allow neurologists to learn more about the disease course and will help them predict what patients may expect as the disease progresses. Because participating neurologists receive reports not only about their own patients but also aggregate data on all patients in the database, they can compare their practice patterns and outcomes with those of their colleagues across North America. Participants can assess whether certain aspects of their management of patients produce less favorable results than the norm. If applicable, they can modify their practice patterns by incorporating those practices that offer the greatest benefit into their management plan.

The information reported by patients provides neurologists with insight into how patients perceive the impact of the disease on their health and life in general. Economic information, such as the type of insurance and out-of-pocket expenses, arms neurologists with the knowledge they need to lobby insurance providers to increase reimbursements and recognize the financial impact of ALS. Similarly, an understanding of the psychosocial and socioeconomic impact of the disease on caregivers provides further evidence of the far-reaching implications of a diagnosis of ALS.

There are certain limitations as to what the *ALS Patient Care Database* can show. It is an observational study that tracks the use of a variety of interventions in routine clinical practice. Since patients enrolled in this database are not randomly assigned to a particular treatment, they are likely to be dissimilar across treatment groups with regard to important characteristics including age, sex, other medical conditions, and so forth. There is also some question as to whether the population within the database is representative of the patient population at large. For example, some clinics may not enroll all of their patients with ALS into the database, which may not reflect the clinic's overall ALS patient population. The majority of patients are enrolled by large, academic ALS centers. Although the demographic data in this database appear to be similar to other large natural history studies (6–8) and to the populations in large clinical trials (9,10) with respect to gender, age, duration of symptoms, and incidence of familial disease, these data represent the results of participating clinics that may not be representative of North American patients with ALS. Efforts are under way to encourage more neurologists in private practice settings to enroll their ALS patients. A broader input will be needed to obtain a representative cross section of practice patterns. Most of the data are cross-sectional at this time; major initiatives to obtain more longitudinal data are under way and will be critical to the success of the database in monitoring practice patterns and outcomes.

Early Results

Some initial demographic and epidemiological findings are shown in Table 17-2. Data gathered to date indicate that the severity of disease varies widely—ALSFRS scores range through the full spectrum from 0 to 40—suggesting that the patients enrolled in the *ALS Patient Care Database* represent a broad patient population. Just over 40 percent of patients enrolled in the database have Medicare coverage (Figure 17-1), and approximately 90 percent are "satisfied" or "extremely satisfied" with their medical care (Figure 17-2). Table 17-3 shows the percentage of patients using services such as occupational and physical therapy and that they found these therapies generally helpful.

Future Directions

As the amount of data available for analysis in the *ALS Patient Care Database* grows, the advisory board will develop articles and educational programs aimed at health care professionals, patients, and their caregivers.

As the number of patients enrolled increases, comparisons between individual

Table 17-2. Demographic and Epidemiological Findings

Variable	Finding mean (range)
Age	60 (20–96 years)
Female	39%
Familial ALS	6.3%
ALSFRS scores	28 (0–40)

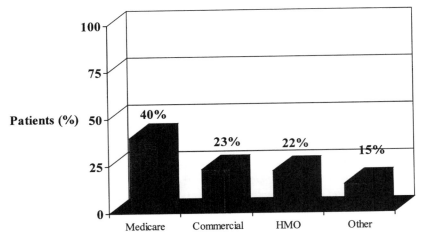

Figure 1. Distribution of third-party payors.

practices and North American benchmarks will become more feasible. The ALS C.A.R.E. Program Advisory Board will continue to provide educational feedback to active participants in the database. Neurologists soon will be able to integrate two powerful tools for defining and refining a standard of care for patients with ALS—the *ALS Patient Care Database* and the practice parameters for managing ALS that have been developed by the subcommittee of the American Academy of Neurology's Quality Standards Committee (11). These guidelines will establish the standard of care for patients with ALS based on an "evidence-based medicine"

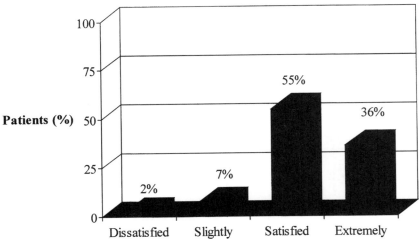

Figure 2. Level of patient satisfaction with health care.

Table 17-3. Services Used by Patients

Service	Patients using service	Find service helpful
Physical therapy	46.2%	83.7%
Occupational therapy	31.0%	79.1%
Speech therapy	21.9%	65.6%
Home nurse	19.8%	84.8%
Dietary (nutrition)	19.0%	83.3%
Social work	17.4%	75.6%
Psychology/psychiatry	11.3%	69.1%

approach, in contrast to the *ALS Patient Care Database,* which provides insight into what is happening in the "real world." In practice, the database will function as a quality check on ALS patient management.

Conclusion

The *ALS Patient Care Database* offers insights into a number of aspects of ALS, including the relationship between disease severity, progression, and the timing of interventions and the impact of the disease on the psychosocial and health status of patients and their caregivers. For the first time, the perception and experience of the patient and the caregiver constitute the core information in a program designed to teach us more about ALS. Health professionals, patients, and caregivers who participate in the database can be confident that the information they contribute will increase our understanding of ALS and improve outcomes.

Acknowledgment. *The ALS Patient Care Database* is supported by an unrestricted educational grant from Rhône-Poulenc Rorer Pharmaceuticals Inc. and by a grant from The ALS Association

References

1. Rogers WJ, Bowlby LJ, Chandra NC, et al. Treatment of myocardial infarction in the United States (1990 to 1993). *Circulation* 1994; 90(4):2103–2114.
2. Fitzgerald RJ, Anderson FA. The outcome assessment of 5,533 patients treated with total hip and knee arthroplasty. In: Program and Abstracts of the 65th Annual Meeting of the American Academy of Orthopaedic Surgeons, March 19–23, 1998, New Orleans, LA. Abstract 377.
3. The ALS CNTF Treatment Study (ACTS) Phase I-II Study Group. The Amyotrophic Lateral Sclerosis Functional Rating Scale. Assessment of activities of daily living in patients with amyotrophic lateral sclerosis. *Arch Neurol* 1996; 51:141–147.

4. Ware JE, Kosinski M, Keller SD. SF-12: *How to Score the SF-12 Physical and Mental Status Health Summary Scales*. 2nd ed. Boston: The Health Institute, New England Medical Center; 1995.
5. McGuire D, Garrison C, Amon R. Relationship of the Tufts Quantitative Neuromuscular Exam (TQNE) and the Sickness Impact Profile (SIP) in measuring progression of ALS. *Neurology* 1996; 46:1442–1444.
6. Mitsumoto H. Classification and clinical features of amyotrophic lateral sclerosis. In: Mitsumoto H, Norris FH (eds.). *Amyotrophic lateral sclerosis: A comprehensive guide to management.* New York: Demos Publications, 1994:1–19.
7. Haverkamp LJ, Appel V, Appel SH. Natural history of amyotrophic lateral sclerosis in a database population. Validation of a scoring system and model for survival prediction. *Brain* 1995; 118:707–719.
8. Rosen AD. Amyotrophic lateral sclerosis. Clinical features and prognosis. *Arch Neurol* 1978; 35:638–642.
9. Bensimon G, Lacomblez L, Meininger V, and the ALS/Riluzole Study Group. A controlled trial of riluzole in amyotrophic lateral sclerosis. *N Engl J Med* 1994; 330:585–591.
10. Miller RG, Moore D, Young LA, et al. Placebo-controlled trial of gabapentin in patients with amyotrophic lateral sclerosis. *Neurology* 1996; 47:1383–1388.
11. Miller RG, Rosenberg JA, Gelinas DF, et al., and the ALS Practice Parameters Task Force. Practice Parameter: The care of the patient with amyotrophic lateral sclerosis (an evidence-based review). Report of the Quality Standards Subcommittee of the AAN. *Neurology* 1999; 52(7):1311–1323.

Appendix

The ALS C.A.R.E. Study Group, in addition to the authors: Walter G. Bradley, DM, FRCP, University of Miami; Mark B. Bromberg, MD, University of Utah; Benjamin R. Brooks, MD, University of Wisconsin; Neil Cashman, MD, Montreal Neurologic Institute; Lora L. Clawson, RN, BSN, Johns Hopkins University School of Medicine; Merit Cudkowicz, MD, Massachusetts General Hospital; Maura Del Bene, RN, MSN, NP-P, Columbia University; Michael Graves, MD, UCLA School of Medicine; Yadollah Harati, MD, Baylor College of Medicine; Terry Heiman-Patterson, MD, Allegheny University; Mary Lyon, RN, The ALS Association; Raul Mandler, MD, Georgetown University; Hiroshi Mitsumoto, MD, Columbia University; Dan Moore, PhD, University of California at San Francisco; Steven P. Ringel, MD, University of Colorado; Jeffrey Rosenfeld, MD, PhD, Carolinas Medical System; Mark A. Ross, MD, University of Kentucky; Michael J. Strong, MD, London Health Sciences Centre; Robert Sufit, MD, Northwestern University.

18

Cultural Effects on ALS

Ann Kuckelman Cobb, R.N., Ph.D.

This chapter examines variations in coping as ALS progresses and relates these responses to cultural context. Five anthropological concepts and five coping concepts are used.

ALS and Other Chronic Diseases

When medical professionals write about coping with chronic illness, they most often talk about conditions such as diabetes, hypertension, arthritis, and cancer. Although each of these is a progressive disease and requires some ongoing adaptation, the progress is often much slower than may be the case with ALS. There usually is time to make an adjustment that may be an effective way to cope for a long time before another adaptation is required. This feature sets ALS apart from most chronic illnesses. A progressive loss of physical function and increasing limitations in social situations demand continuous adaptation by both family members and people with ALS. Although individuals differ in how the disease progresses, patients and families still live with the knowledge that the overall course is usually relentlessly downhill. They must not only cope with current limitations but also deal with future ones.

Coping with ALS can best be described in terms of a spiral (1). A loss is followed by a period of adjustment, then one of equilibrium followed by another loss that calls for another adjustment. This is clearly the pattern in ALS, except that in some cases the losses follow so quickly, one upon the other, that no real equilibrium is reached, and the path is much more sharply downhill. In these instances, coping may simply be a "keeping together" on a day-to-day basis, with little if any respite from the stresses involved.

The Individual and the Coping Response

People generally react to illness the same way they react to other life crises (2). If you are indecisive, you are likely to be indecisive regarding what to do about specific problems that arise in ALS. If you approach things matter of factly and tend to be a problem solver regarding other issues, you probably will have the same basic attitude toward management of ALS. If you tend to be nonconfrontive, to deny that problems exist, you may overuse denial as a coping mechanism. This does not mean that you cannot be helped to adopt a new way of coping. It *does* mean that both clinicians and family caregivers need to know how a person with ALS usually copes with problems in order to build on the strengths of these existing patterns and introduce change when needed.

Social Factors That Influence the Management of ALS

The social context in which coping with ALS occurs includes such things as laws governing decision making in catastrophic illness, levels of technology available in a given society, availability of institutional support services and who pays for them, and federal and state policies regarding management of disability issues in relation to employment (2). These complex issues directly affect how you will cope with ALS. Both national and local ALS association chapters are excellent resources for learning about changing laws and social policies related to ALS.

Cultural Factors That Influence the Management of ALS

Sickness and suffering are universal, but there are differences in how each culture defines and manages a particular illness. This chapter is organized around the anthropological concepts of (1) cultural expectation, (2) reciprocity, (3) belief systems, (4) social networks, (5) social support, and (6) stigma. Each of these is discussed in reference to the way people respond to the progression of ALS. They are related to a variety of coping methods, including (1) information seeking, (2) direct action, (3) inhibition of action, (4) intrapsychic processes, and (5) turning to others for support (3). Aspects of having ALS may violate generalized American cultural values, which can create problems for your family and for the health professionals with whom you work.

Cultural Expectations

Every culture has a set of written and unwritten rules for behavior, which are termed *norms* or *cultural expectations.* Because these assumptions are so widely shared and are so much a part of what we see as "normal" behavior, we often become aware of them only when they are violated. Americans expect people to be responsible for their own actions, to ask for assistance only when absolutely necessary, and to maintain as much control over their own lives as possible. The underlying cultural code is dramatically and painfully laid bare when people with ALS are no longer able to meet these expectations (2).

We also have cultural expectations for "how to be sick." It is acceptable to be ill as long as one seeks proper care, follows directions, and returns to previous social responsibilities within a reasonable length of time (4). We have a low tolerance for prolonged relinquishment of social roles and functions, and people with chronic illnesses violate our expectation that an individual be "productive."

Many people with ALS do continue to be productive. The British physicist Stephen Hawking and the late Senator Jacob Javits are outstanding examples. But we should not overlook the fact that one of the reasons we admire such people is that we share this cultural expectation of being productive—we learn it from birth. Ours is a culture with an emphasis on "doing" rather than "being" (5). It takes tremendous effort on the part of families to help people with ALS continue to "do," and this may be an important part of coping, especially in the early stages of the disease, and depending on what the person's occupational role has been. A mail carrier or an auto mechanic may lose his work role early in the course of the disease as leg and hand function diminish, while someone whose work primarily involves thinking and organizing may continue for some time to feel productive and to be seen that way by others.

Given these cultural expectations, denial of loss of function may occur early in the disease, but eventually people with ALS give up actions either when they cannot do them or when they become dangerous. Giving up an activity can be related to the spiral of loss, grief, and adaptation. A family member in one of our studies said, "It was really a shock the day he could no longer release the catch on his recliner chair to get himself out of the chair. Now he has to wait for someone to come help him, whereas before he could get up and walk every twenty or thirty minutes, and keep comfortable."

As the disease progresses, *direct action* may take the form of simply completing physical care needs. One of our patients said, "It's not like I have any free time. By the time I get up and brush my teeth and have breakfast, sit in my chair, get up and get a drink, three hours have passed! I mean, it takes me THREE HOURS to do this! And it's not that my days go very slowly. I'm just completely occupied with just trying to take care of myself."

This particular person liked to read, but his hands were becoming too weak to hold a book, his eyes were burning, and he was spending all his energy just to complete activities of daily living. We suggested Talking Books, which he initially resisted. But when he found that they were produced more like radio drama than like someone simply reading aloud, he subscribed and found great pleasure in them. Recent enthusiasm for books on tape among busy commuters in the general population may also reduce the stigma attached to their use by people experiencing health challenges. Assistive devices may be readily accepted when they are not specific to the context of illness, as with electric toothbrushes, conference phones, and computers.

As the disease progresses, the person with ALS may need to be given permission to simply "be" and may need assurance that his value as a human being is not tied to what he is able to do. This may be difficult because Americans share the value of the work ethic, but recognizing it as a significant influence can assist in reevaluating how it is expressed and managed.

At the end, people with ALS also may need to be given permission to give up. Again, American culture values the "fighter," the one who does not give in to adversity, and people sometimes feel that they are letting everyone down when they finally feel the need to succumb. They need assurance that it is acceptable to let go.

Reciprocity

Reciprocity is the give-and-take that is an important part of social life. Marcel Mauss's [6] classic study of gift exchange in a variety of cultures concluded that universally, when a gift is given, there is an implied obligation to give something in return. People with ALS may have difficulty with the growing imbalance in exchange that is part of the disease process. People with ALS do change the way they feel about reciprocating over time. Many people with ALS describe an inrushing of care and concern on the part of friends when they are first diagnosed. This may be followed by a dramatic withdrawal, especially as the ability to communicate becomes diminished. Eventually only the most loyal of friends may continue to visit. In these circumstances, it may be fairly easy to accept the early attention and gift-giving, usually in the form of food and favors, especially if the person with ALS has been involved in a community and has "given" in the past. But as the disease progresses and the ALS person is forced to become more and more dependent on caregivers, it is sometimes difficult to accept help and gifts and to feel that he or she has anything to give in return.

Some patients manage to *reciprocate* rather well over a long period of time. Early in the disease, when physical functions are not too inhibited, the person with ALS may take on household tasks usually performed by a spouse or children. As functional abilities deteriorate, many patients design assistive devices to help caregivers in managing their care. They continue to *take direct action* by using their thinking abilities, combining this with another coping mechanism, *turning to others*. Although they may no longer be able actually to hold a pencil and write, they may accept the help of someone taking dictation.

During the final stages of the disease it is most difficult for people with ALS to feel that they *reciprocate,* that they have anything to give. The coping mechanism of *intrapsychic processes* may be the only one possible at this point. They may need to refocus their attention or reappraise the situation so that they may see themselves in some way as giving. Some patients are able to do this by continuing to use their cognitive abilities, such as by dictating letters of encouragement to others. For some, even this will be difficult. What may be helpful to people in advanced stages of ALS is reassurance that, even in very difficult chronic illnesses where there is the assumption that no reciprocity occurs, family members do report that their ill relative gives, even in small ways.

Belief Systems

Beliefs and values are two of the major components of culture, and religion is sometimes listed as a coping mechanism by those who write about chronic illness. If focused on health issues, belief refers to what people think is the cause of their illness, how it should be treated, and the way they judge the success of the treatments received. As a culture, we share a general belief in science and the scientific treatment of disease, and expect a cure [7]. When dealing with a chronic illness for which there is no curative treatment within the scientific system, people may search for and experiment with many forms of alternative treatment. Our patients have used chiropractic, macrobiotic diets, various forms of intravenous injections, snake venom, and perhaps many others that they have not told us about. We have assumed a nonjudgmental stance about such treatments in order to keep the lines of communication open and so that we may know whether there is any perceived benefit from these treatments. Recent changes in attitudes toward "alternative," "complementary," or "integrative" therapies may make it easier for patients and family caregivers to explore their questions about non-mainstream treatments with health care providers or to find providers who are willing to listen.

One of the *intrapsychic processes* used for coping with ALS may be a well-developed and tightly interconnected set of beliefs about cause and cure. In some instances, this may be totally secular, such as the belief that there is a biological deficit—some missing element—for which taking megadoses of certain vitamins seems a reasonable treatment. In other cases, people with ALS may believe that the illness is a punishment from God or that God "punishes those whom he loves" and consequently may feel that, regardless of what professionals do, the possibility of healing is in the hands of God.

Professionals in a clinic setting may see this belief as a form of denial. But denial can be an effective way of coping, especially in the short term. For example, one of our patients wrote a beautiful letter just before her death. In it she said that she still was hoping for a healing, but if that did not happen and she got to heaven and found that there was a healing committee, she was going to ask right away to serve on it. Her belief in God and in the possibility of a miraculous healing sustained her to the end. Another patient placed her faith in medical science, hoping until the very last for a cure that would be beneficial to her, even when to the objective observer the atrophy had advanced beyond any possibility of reversal.

The concept of *belief* systems, then, encompasses more than just religious belief. It can include the interlocking set of explanations for cause, treatment, and cure that people with ALS use throughout the course of their illness. Sometimes they are different from beliefs that professionals have, but if they are logical and consistent for the patient, they can function as a major coping mechanism from diagnosis to death. They are connected to all five of Cohen and Lazarus's [3] coping strategies: it is on the basis of what people believe about their illness that they *seek information, take direct action, inhibit other actions, use various intrapsychic processes,* and *turn to others for assistance.*

Social Networks

The concept of *social networks* and coping by *turning to others for assistance* are closely related. If we define *social networks* as the web of relationships an individual has, social *support* is the outcome patients receive by turning to people in their network for assistance. In preindustrial societies, every individual had kinship, friendship, or work relationships with essentially every other individual in the community. In our culture, however, people may have networks that are very small in structure or that may be limited, as in a work relationship. It is the depth and intensity of relationships that largely determines the kinds of help that friends and relatives are willing to give, how often they can be expected to be called on for help, and over what period of time.

It is important to evaluate the quality of the social network early in the course of ALS because it can help to predict how well you will be able to continue over time to cope with the increasing demands for care as the disease progresses. Your social network is a potential source of physical and psychological respite that family caregivers will require as the disease progresses.

One example of a person with an extensive network was Mary, who moved with her husband to Kansas City so that they could live in a residential community made up of church members. Her husband became employed as a caretaker for the church, and they attended services every Sunday, with Mary continuing to edit the church newsletter for a long time. They were in close physical proximity to family, church members, and work associates, and they were able to make contributions in which they could maintain some reciprocal balance, at least for a time.

In contrast, our local ALS chapter has worked with some people with ALS who not only live alone but also have few close contacts of any kind. In one instance, George, an impeccable, articulate, African-American man who had always lived alone, managed for as long as he could, mostly with the help of ALS society volunteers and auxiliary home care workers. When this was no longer feasible, he was welcomed back to Texas by his extended family, who cared for him until he died several months later. In other cases, people have had to enter long-term care facilities when they were no longer able to care for themselves. There also are instances in which a person's primary social network, that is, spouse and children, dissolves in the face of the stresses that ALS produces. Family caregivers can expand their social network and often find support through local ALS chapters.

Support Groups

Members of support groups are alike by virtue of surviving some kind of difficulty, which often comes on rather suddenly and is not, in essence, solvable. Members have a shared life experience, and the interaction in such a group revolves around how to deal with this life problem. What is therapeutic about these kinds of groups is that the affliction is reframed in such a way that those afflicted become, in some sense, healers. The participants become empowered by group sharing and problem solving. They learn how to deal with day-to-day problems; they can see themselves, at least within the group, as "special" rather than "different"; they are given an opportunity to reciprocate with new members, to offer them the wisdom of their experience in dealing with the affliction.

ALS support groups serve all these functions. For most people with the disease, the group calls into play most of the five coping mechanisms discussed in this chapter.

In the early stages of ALS, the support group acts as a resource for those who are *seeking information*. Although your physicians and nurses may intend to provide information at a pace you can handle, this is extremely difficult in the short time allotted to a typical medical appointment. People also need time to absorb the impact of the diagnosis, and you may not be ready to ask questions until some weeks after the clinic visit [8]. You probably will find it helpful to know there is a support group with a library of information as well as volunteers with whom you can talk.

As the disease progresses, you will learn a variety of helpful *direct actions* you can take, and in the group you also may learn what kinds of *actions* need to be *inhibited* to conserve energy and to preserve your relationships with each other. People often go to the group for just this kind of practical advice, but they find that the *intrapsychic processes* involved in coping with ALS also form a significant part of the exchange. For example, in one support group meeting, efforts were made to assist participants in dealing with the death of an individual who was particularly important to the group. A suggestion was made to break into small groups and "get our emotions onto the table" by looking first at the three emotions of grief, fear, and frustration; then, "on a more positive note," to look at acceptance, hope, and support. This kind of sharing of feelings is an important aspect of coping, which, of course, becomes more and more difficult as the person loses the ability to communicate.

It is important that the facilitators in ALS support groups (as well as caregivers in hospitals, clinics, and homes) allow the time needed for patients to spell out or use other means of communicating what they have to share if they have lost the ability to speak. This loss is one of the most traumatic aspects of having ALS, and the only place the ALS person is given adequate time to fully express a thought may be in the support group. One patient said, "My family tries, but by the time I've gotten across what I want to say, the conversation has moved on to something else." This may be less true when the person with ALS is talking one-on-one with someone, but in a group they often feel like "the silent ones." Not to allow time for them to speak in their own way is to deny their basic humanity. The orientation to time in American culture reflects a culture in a hurry. "Time is money," and it is necessary to become aware of how ingrained these attitudes are and the ways in which they manifest themselves if people with ALS are to really be helped in coping with the disease as it progresses. Many surviving spouses have continued to remain associated with the ALS group for extended periods after the death of a family member. They do an invaluable service in sharing their accumulated wisdom of this traumatic life experience.

Stigma

Every culture has culturally determined standards for physical beauty and norms of behavior. Because ALS causes atrophy of certain muscles, there are changes in the physical appearance of people who have the disease. Speech also changes because the muscles of the tongue are affected. Some people fear going out in public because gait may be unsteady in the early stages of the disease and there is a danger of injury from falling. Besides the concern of physical injury, there is the social *stigma* involved with the belief that others may think they are inebriated.

The emotional lability often seen in people who have the bulbar form of ALS violates our cultural norms, which dictate when it is appropriate to laugh or cry. People who cannot control this emotional expression may withdraw from social interaction because of the *stigma* they feel this causes. This emotional lability decreases as the diseases progresses, but difficulties with chewing and swallowing also may cause people to avoid eating in public places, which causes further isolation. Some families cope with this by inviting to their home friends who are sensitive to the effects of changes in body function and self-image. Coping with your self-image is an ongoing challenge for the person with ALS throughout the course of the illness.

Conclusion

It is difficult to have a terminal, progressive, degenerative disease such as ALS, which has no known cause or cure, and which sometimes progresses so rapidly that there is little time to recover from and adapt to one loss before another must be confronted. It is difficult to be chronically ill in a culture that stresses individual achievement, responsibility, and productivity, when the disease robs people of the ability to function in these ways and causes physical changes that add to a feeling of stigma. Health professionals, family members, and friends need to recognize that these are value patterns that we learn almost unconsciously throughout our lives and that recognizing them is an important step in evaluating how they affect the way we deal with people who have ALS. The kinds of coping required of both family members and people with ALS over the course of the disease are numerous and varied.

References

1. Scott, DW, Oberst, MT, Dropkin, MJ. A stress-coping model. *Adv Nurs Sci* 1980; 3:9–23.
2. Cobb, AK, Hamera, E. Illness experience in a chronic disease—ALS. *Soc Sci Med* 1986; 23:641–650.
3. Cohen, F, Lazarus, RS. Coping with the stresses of illness. In: Stone GC, Cohen, F, Adler, NE (eds.). *Health psychology: A handbook.* San Francisco: Jossey-Bass, 1979.
4. Parsons, T. Definitions of health and illness in the light of American values and social structure. In: Jaco, EG (ed.). *Patients, physicians and illness.* 2nd ed. New York: Free Press, 1971.
5. Kluckhohn, R, Strodtbeck, F. *Variations in value orientations.* Evanston, IL: Row, Peterson, 1961.
6. Mauss, M. *The gift.* New York: Norton, 1967.
7. Young, A. The relevance of traditional medical cultures to modern primary health care. *Soc Sci Med* 1983; 17:1205–1211.
8. Beisecker, AE, Cobb, AK, Zeigler, DK. Patients' perspectives of the role of care providers in amyotrophic lateral sclerosis. *Arch Neurol* 1988; 45: 553–556.

19

The Caregiver's Experience

Ann Kuckelman Cobb, R.N., Ph.D., JoAnn B. Reckling, R.N., M.A., Ph.D., and Karen J. Fernengel, R.N., Ph.D.

Students working on a Ph.D. in nursing at the University of Kansas focused on the experience of caregivers for people with ALS. Although the primary goal of the class was to teach methods of data collection and analysis, important issues related to family responses to the progression of ALS and their ways of coping and of caregiving were identified that may be of assistance in your own situation.

We found that the ways families coped with ALS could be grouped into five categories:

- "Taking It"—Experiencing an awareness of unanticipated, uncontrollable, and/or unknown events from which an ALS caregiver has no escape

- "Staying Afloat"—Surviving: Tolerating the situation and attempting to maintain normalcy, but efforts to maintain balance occur in the face of continuous conflicting tensions, and with a sense of impending crisis

- "Losing Ground"—Experiencing loss, as, for example, in relationships, self-control, privacy, tolerance, and own's own health

- "Regrouping"—Regaining a degree of control either by getting physical and/or informational assistance from outside, and/or spiritual and/or emotional assistance from within or without

- "Holding Together"—Doing what you can with what there is. Making the most of the situation at hand, understanding it, accepting it, and adjusting to it

MODEL OF THE ALS CAREGIVERS' EXPERIENCE

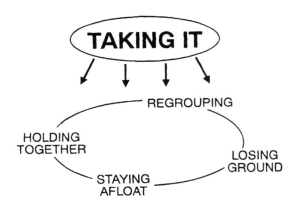

We labeled the first category *Taking It* because the phrase was often used by our respondents. *Taking It* was defined as experiencing an awareness of unanticipated, uncontrollable, and/or unknown events from which an ALS caregiver has no escape. *Taking It* had two subcategories, *Taking It In* and *Taking It On*. The first was defined as an awareness of feelings, thoughts, and sensory perceptions associated with experiencing the unanticipated, uncontrollable event. The second refers to committing to the situation, making the continuing choice to stay, to help, knowing that one does not really know what it will be like. This category of *Taking It* is related to the other four categories, which represent a cyclic process that families go through as ALS progresses.

Holding Together describes the optimum link in the process, when caregivers are managing relatively well. *Staying Afloat* implies managing and attempting to keep things normal, but with a feeling that a new crisis could happen at any time. *Losing Ground* describes the caregiver's ongoing experience of loss. When *Regrouping* occurs, there is some regaining of a sense of control, using devices such as physical or informational assistance from others and spiritual or emotional assistance from within or outside of oneself. If *Regrouping* is successful, even on a temporary basis, *Holding Together* again occurs. *Taking It* is a process that caregivers experience repeatedly in connection with the other categories as new changes take place. As an ongoing process, this cycle may repeat itself several times within a single day. In the larger context, it characterizes the overall pattern of the experience of ALS caregivers and patients in managing ALS over time.

Before discussing these coping strategies in detail, let us say something about hope. Several years ago, Dr. Cobb conducted a videotaped interview with Keith Worthington, an ALS patient and founder of what has become the Kansas City chapter of the ALS Association. Keith was then on a respirator. One of the things that came out very clearly in that interview was his statement, "It is very important to have a physician who does not subscribe to the 'no hope' school of thought." There was, in the 1980s, an ongoing argument in the literature about the relationship between hope and denial—when is hope a form of denial, and does denial keep patients from seeking appropriate health services? Consensus seemed to be that denial, at least at certain stages in an illness, can be a positive coping mechanism, that is, it can help to preserve hope and prevent despair (1,2).

The other concept we wish to bring in is the concept of courage. Shelp discusses courage as a moral virtue in the patient–physician relationship. It seems clear, however, that courage is a virtue required of all parties in the ALS encounter—patients, family members, and professionals of all types. Shelp defines courage as ". . . the disposition to voluntarily act, perhaps fearfully, in a dangerous circumstance, where the relevant risks are reasonably appraised, in an effort to obtain or preserve some perceived good for oneself or others, recognizing that the desired perceived good may not be realized" (3). But courage refers not only to *action;* it also may apply to *enduring.* The essence of courage is the mastery of fear for the preservation of good. In Shelp's definition of courage, risk implies vulnerability, and the ultimate vulnerability is death. Sickness causes one to come face-to-face with death and to find meaning in a situation in which meaning is threatened. Caregivers can help to impart that meaning. Shelp states that physicians tend not to disclose their doubts to patients and colleagues so as to sustain an image of strength, superiority, or power. He suggests that a better image is that of a "sustaining presence," which allows for strength and weakness; this implies that one wants to help, is loyal to the other party, and is honest about one's limitations. The sustaining presence of caregivers can convey that the patient is affirmed by others and is therefore worthy of self-affirmation. We "learn of courage as [we] abide by patients when there is little or no more [we] can do" (3). If courage is a moral virtue relevant to the patient encounter, encouragement can be thought of as a way of enhancing coping in ALS.

Taking It

We defined *Taking It* as experiencing an awareness of unanticipated, uncontrollable, and/or unknown events from which an ALS caregiver has no escape. Examples of such events are the diagnosis delivered to the ALS patient, the fear it engenders, situations in which everything happens at once, loss of yet another function by the patient, loss of sleep for the caregiver, and so on. Needless to say, the person with the disease undergoes a similar experience. The subcategory *Taking It In* is the awareness of feelings, thoughts, and sensory perceptions associated with this response. People in this situation said, "Life has changed drastically," "Neither of us realized what we were getting into," "Very traumatic, unbelievable."

Taking It and *Taking It In* are clearly apparent in the early stages of ALS, when the patient and family have just been given the diagnosis and are faced with the task of processing just what it may mean to them, their relationships, their work, and social roles. One caregiver said, ". . . when they told me 'amyotrophic lateral sclerosis,' I thought, Doc, what are you talking about?" At this point, *intrapsychic processes* of denial of the full consequences of the disease may be necessary to maintain hope. When patients or family members say, "Neither of us realized what we were getting into," this screening of reality acts as a protective device for the moment. Wright and Shontz (4) see this as a dimension of hoping in which one achieves a hopeful attitude by intentionally keeping the future undifferentiated in the face of a threatening reality. It is the "one day at a time" attitude, and health professionals and others need to support and validate such statements (5).

Taking It On means committing to the situation, making the continuing choice to stay, to help, knowing that one does not really know what it will be like. One caregiver interviewed for the study was a 72-year-old woman whose 41-year-old son had ALS. The son was separated and eventually divorced, so his mother and her retired husband took on the responsibility of caregiving as the disease progressed. They had been looking forward to retirement, but they willingly came to their son's assistance when the need became apparent. What they had not bargained for was caring for the grandchildren as well. The woman told us, "They have three children and when [husband] and I decided to come we didn't realize that three children would be part of our responsibility too, at times, because they only live a mile from our house, and, of course, they are the light of [son's] life, each day that he can see them." This couple made a continuing commitment to stay, despite this unanticipated additional burden. The respondent said, "You do have to adjust your thinking and your doing in many ways. [Husband] and I are both seventy-two, so it's been an adjustment for both of us, but we're so happy we can do it and wish we could do more."

This example is very much like what Shelp (3) is describing when he speaks of courage. Freedom of choice is one dimension of courage, and although it seems as if patients and families have no choice, we have known family members who chose not to stay. Those who do, who take on the responsibilities and the risks to their own health, are exercising moral courage. Patients have less choice, but they exercise courage in living each day and in facing their own death and finding meaning in it. Health professionals, too, must have the courage to *Take It On*—to be that "sustaining presence," to affirm the selfhood of the ALS person even as abilities decline, even when the professional is challenged by knowing there are no specific curative treatments to offer. Both professionals and family caregivers, like the patients, must be willing to endure, to admit our limitations, making the continuing choice to stay.

Once one has *Taken It On*, coping mechanisms such as *information seeking* and *direct action* are called into play. Professional caregivers must be sensitive to patient and family readiness to learn more about ALS (6) and the readiness to seek help through the coping mechanism of *turning to others for support*, such as through participation in support groups. Going to the first support group meeting may be a significant act of courage for people with ALS. That is, they know they will be seeing other people in more advanced stages of the disease, and the risk is one of being robbed of hope. People with ALS sometimes come to support groups, at least initially, as a way of giving something to the family caregivers, whom they recognize as needing a night out, time with people who also are enduring the stresses of caregiving. The risk to their own self-image as they see the effect of the disease on others is high, but so, too, is the possibility of increasing hope when they realize that their own assets and abilities compare favorably with those of others. One thing both professional and family caregivers can do is to help the person with ALS recognize remaining abilities by reviewing and valuing their physical strengths and interpersonal skills and pointing out the ways they still fulfill their social and family roles (5).

Staying Afloat

Staying Afloat is defined as surviving: tolerating the situation and attempting to keep things normal, but efforts to maintain balance are constantly challenged by conflicting tensions, and there is a sense of impending crisis. One of our respondents said, "You keep hoping he isn't going to get worse, but on the other side of your mind, you know that he is." This "hoping" statement is another example of what Wright and Shontz (4) refer to as "the unpromising future," a version of living in the present as a way to maintain hope. It might also be seen as a pattern of "hoping against hope" (7). The feeling of "just surviving" may be most acute in the early phases of the disease, when you are trying to become accustomed to growing physical and social limitations and to the severity of the illness. It also characterizes more advanced stages of the disease, when there are tremendous demands on physical, emotional, and financial resources and a growing awareness of reaching the limits of these resources. One woman in her thirties whose 34-year-old husband experienced rapid deterioration from ALS and was in advanced stages said, "My problem is . . . with two small children and trying to take care of the house and the yard and the car and the bills and the doctor visits and the kids being sick, and, you know, running one to soccer, and . . . I can't do it all. I have been, but I'm ready to go crazy . . ." She was attempting to maintain normalcy but was barely *Staying Afloat,* aware that finances and her own personal resources were stretched to the limit.

Losing Ground

Losing Ground describes the experience of loss as, for example, in relationships, self-control, privacy, tolerance, and one's own health. Both people with ALS and their caregivers experience these losses. Relationships alter as communication and other physical abilities decrease with the progress of the disease. There may be a reversal of roles between spouses and a loss of self-control and tolerance in the face of almost impossible demands. Ironically, two of the coping methods that may be useful in these circumstances—*direct action* and *turning to others for support*—have the undesirable effect of invading the privacy of both the person with ALS and caregivers when care is given at home. Caregivers seek and receive help from a variety of care providers such as nurses, home health aides, volunteers, and friends. Yet, for all the assistance they both want and receive, they suffer from the loss of privacy when helpers come into their home. One caregiver said:

> *"I feel like I have a revolving door. I have no privacy. Every time I turn around somebody is coming in. I just had to finally accept that. I haven't liked it, but I've had to accept it. My home is just not my home anymore. We leave the garage door up all day. And they [care providers] know to just walk through the garage door and come in through the family room door and there we are. People are coming and going all the time, somebody is always coming or going. And . . . you cannot take care of him alone . . . you give up your privacy . . . you give up the control of your own life."*

It can be viewed as an act of courage on the part of family caregivers to allow this invasion of what is in some sense a sacred space for the good of another—the person with ALS. Similarly, professionals who take themselves into the home setting where they are without the normal sense of control afforded by a clinical context are also exercising moral courage. They are that "sustaining presence," willing to risk a certain amount of vulnerability, willing to affirm the selfhood of the person with ALS by continuing care when cure is not possible.

In relation to *Losing Ground,* what sets ALS apart from other chronic and/or terminal illnesses is the rapidity with which losses can occur and the relentlessly downward course of the progress of the disease. Scott, Oberst, and Dropkin (8) presented a model of coping based on the metaphor of the "recurring spiral," in which there is a loss, followed by grieving of the loss, then attempting new coping responses, and reaching another temporary equilibrium. Wright and Shontz (4) identify mourning as an aspect of hoping, but with ALS in some cases the losses follow so quickly one upon the other that there is no time for mourning, and no real equilibrium may be reached. One respondent said, "It has progressed so fast in [husband] that we've never had any time to adjust to it before he loses something else. He's losing everything all at once." When the progress of the disease is not so rapid, there may be time to give vent to the realistic and deeply felt sorrow when Losing Ground, providing an opportunity for *Regrouping* to occur.

Regrouping

Regrouping involves regaining a degree of control either by getting physical and/or informational assistance from outside and/or spiritual or emotional assistance from within or outside of oneself. Examples are obtaining assistive devices, getting information and supervision in using equipment, benefiting from reassurance, sharing in support groups. *Regrouping* is the category most clearly related to coping. It is action-oriented and may include *information seeking, direct action, intrapsychic processes,* and *turning to others for support. Inhibition of action* may also take place when regrouping involves preventing the person with ALS from carrying out activities that he or she can no longer do safely without potential harm to self or others. *Regrouping* is the attempt to reach a state of equilibrium in the spiral of loss, even if only for a short period of time. One respondent reported obtaining outside assistance through hospice services:

> *"We also have a hospice nurse who has been a godsend. I rejected this in the beginning very much . . . But . . . I just can't say enough for her. She comes twice a week and takes J's blood pressure and last winter he was on the verge of a cold and she got some [medication] for him right away. She's just a delightful person, and she puts my mind at ease. If he's not breathing just like we think he should be, she checks his lungs and reassures us."*

Holding Together

Holding Together is defined as doing what one can with what there is; making the most of the situation, understanding it, accepting it, and adjusting to it. In our model, it is the closest concept to a state of equilibrium or balance. It is a more positive state of coping than *Staying Afloat.* The feeling component of *Holding Together* includes the perception that one really is making the most of the situation. The doing component includes such things as willing self-sacrifice, loving, giving, grieving together, and being able to support other caregivers. *Holding Together* has both a descriptive meaning and a metaphorical meaning. Metaphorically, the emphasis is on "together," that is, the ALS patient and family are at a place where they are not being pulled apart by the demands of their situation. In a sense, they encircle one another, forming a kind of mandala of support that gives a sense of enduring together, with a margin of strength left over to give to others in similar circumstances.

Holding Together is most likely to occur when the progress of the disease is slower and there is some time to adjust to changes. It is also affected by the type of resources available to the family. Caregivers who were caring for a spouse, had grown children, were retired, and were financially comfortable were most likely to feel that they were *Holding Together.* In contrast, the young mother of two small children, whose 34-year-old husband was in advanced stages of the progression of the disease and was being cared for by her at home, and who was running out of funds, was barely *Staying Afloat.* She was using coping methods such as *turning to others for support,* but she had the sense that such support was not unlimited. She also attempted to *inhibit* her husband from lying in one position in the knowledge that his skin was beginning to break down, but she was frustrated in this by his refusal to cooperate. She understood that his action was one small way of continuing to assert himself, but she foresaw further crises for both of them if he persisted. Eventually, shortly before he died, she took *direct action* by placing him in a nursing home when she could no longer both provide direct care to him and manage the needs of their two small children.

When families are *Holding Together,* there is room for active hoping. There is some time and energy to review with the ALS patient her or his remaining assets and abilities. Active intervention can be undertaken both by family caregivers and by health professionals. Another aspect of hoping in which all care providers can be actively involved is in encouraging the person with ALS to see the illness as an opportunity for personal growth (5). It is not so much a matter of telling the person that such growth is possible, but rather supporting and reinforcing his own insights. Kim (5) gives an example: the patient might say, "Through my loss of muscle coordination, I learned to take time in doing tasks and the experience of ALS taught me to discover other sides of myself." To support such a statement is to reinforce hope.

With regard to courage, Shelp (3) states that one of the duties of a physician the relief from suffering through imparting meaning to a situation where meaning is threatened. Shelp goes on to say that how that is done is an open question, but that doing it well may require greater energy and creativity than performing well in physical diagnosis and treatment. To quote him:

> *"In the experience of sickness and suffering the weak and strong are bound together in a therapeutic alliance. Rather than being abandoned, the sufferer is a central concern. The one who suffers may be supported in his or her sickness as a means of affirming his or her place in the community. Alternatively, his or her decision to endure no more may be respected and he or she may be assisted in dying as a means of affirming those cherished powers that gave life meaning but that now are gone" (3).*

Summary

This chapter describes, primarily in the words of the family caregivers interviewed, the experience of caring for a person with ALS as the disease progresses. Families go through a cyclic process over the course of the disease, from *Taking In* the diagnosis and its consequences; through *Taking It On,* committing to stay without really knowing for certain what that entails; through the hard times of barely *Staying Afloat;* and then *Regrouping* through a variety of coping methods until there is a little space of adjustment that we have called *Holding Together.* This cycle may repeat itself several times in a single day—from getting up in the morning committed to doing whatever needs to be done that day; to perhaps facing a barrage of unanticipated demands and crises; finding at least some temporary solutions or help; and maybe finding a little breathing space in the day where one has time for oneself. On a given day, the cycle may feel more like a continuous spin. Through it all, both patient and family caregiver may call on the several coping methods discussed. The elements of hope and courage are continuous themes in coping with ALS. Your health care team will hope with you. As for courage, we agree with Shelp (3) that "Courage is required of those who choose a profession that embodies care and concern. And 'encouragement' is properly one of [health professionals'] duties." Physicians and others who provide a "sustaining presence" will help you to do the same.

> *"Sharing in another's life does not consist of burdening the other with requirements. Rather, it consists of eliciting the recognition of personal values and capacities that may go unrealized otherwise. Eliciting courage is not the same as imposing values and norms. For [health professionals] it is assisting patients in not letting fear overtake them so that the opportunities present in sickness and dying are not lost to them and others. As 'sustaining presence,' the [health professional] shares responsibility for the process and the results. No one bears it alone. Learning to live includes learning even in dying. Without courage the evils in the context of sickness and dying go unchallenged." (3)*

Let us be courageous and hopeful together.

Acknowledgments. The authors acknowledge the contributions of Valerie McCann and Jane Berg, who assisted in collection and initial analysis of data.

References

1. Wright BA. The question stands: Should a person be realistic? *Rehab Counsel Bull* 1968: XI:291–296.
2. Herth K. Development and refinement of an instrument to measure hope. *Schol Inq for Nurs Pract* 1991; 5:39–51.
3. Shelp EE. Courage: A neglected virtue in the patient-physician relationship. *Soc Sci Med* 1984; 18:351–360.
4. Wright BA, Shontz F. Process and tasks in hoping. *Rehab Lit* 1968; 29:322–331.
5. Kim TS. Hope as a mode of coping in amyotrophic lateral sclerosis. *J Neurol Nurs* 1989; 21:342–347.
6. Beisecker AE, Cobb AK, Ziegler DK. Patients' perspectives of the role of care providers in amyotrophic lateral sclerosis. *Arch Neurol* 1988; 45:553–556.
7. Morse, JM, Doberneck, B. Delineating the concept of hope. *Image: J of Nurs Schol* 1995; 27: 277–285.
8. Scott DW, Oberst MT, Dropkin MJ. A stress-coping model. *Adv Nurs Sci* 1980; 9–23.

20

Sharing the Experience of ALS: Patient and Family Support Groups

Marlene A. Ciechoski, M.S., R.N.

This chapter addresses the purpose and structure of ALS support groups and the questions, issues, and considerations people may have when deciding whether to participate in such a group.

The diagnosis of ALS is an emotionally overwhelming event to the entire family. Because of limited knowledge of the disease, people may turn to an ALS support group to seek helpful information.

The concept of support groups for disease-specific problems is not new. Historically, support groups have formed in response to people's needs to become educated and to share data, feelings, and resources with others who are living a similar experience. The supposition is that people who share common problems have something valuable both to teach and to learn from each other.

Since the early 1980s ALS support groups have been formed in various areas of the country and facilitated by health care professionals or lay volunteers. In addition, people with ALS have come together on the Internet. Although the Internet affords a contemporary opportunity for people to seek and explore ideas and receive feedback, it differs in respect to the humanistic exchange of feelings and physical presence that bring people closer together, minimizing the aloneness and distancing expressed by many people with ALS.

Whether small or large, support groups are developed to identify potential resources and especially to create a caring atmosphere for one another. Groups may choose to have a scheduled agenda of meetings and topics. The core is always to connect people who are faced with ALS and who would benefit from opportunities to share challenging experiences. Joining a support group holds anxiety for most people because it acknowledges the reality of the diagnosis and its ramifications for one's life.

For the recently diagnosed individual, ALS is tension-producing, depressing, and threatening, and it has a remarkable effect on one's sense of self. The diagnosis brings with it several inevitable questions. Who am I now that I have ALS? Am I the same person or a different person since my diagnosis? Where do I fit in, or *do* I fit in? What is to become of my loved ones and me? What about my work, my interests, my friends? As people begin even cautiously to obtain information about the disease, they quickly learn of its debilitating and progressively fatal course.

Most people approach a support group with both interest and caution. Support groups have often been a curious subject largely because of unfamiliarity and inadequate information as to their purpose. When considering a support group, a number of questions and concerns often emerge—Is "support group" another term for group psychotherapy? How much self-revelation is expected? How will an individual be affected by others who are more slowly or more rapidly progressive in their ALS?

People have their own agenda as to why they attend a support group. They may want information about ALS chapters or centers, adaptive equipment, home care, research, or clinical drug trials. People with ALS want to achieve a sense of connectedness with people in similar life circumstances. In the new and strange world of ALS, every individual needs a reference group of people who intimately understand what he may be experiencing.

Comfort in attending a support group is best achieved when people know what to expect. No one needs to be surprised or feel apprehensive about going to a group meeting. Most people have similar questions about a support group. Who facilitates the group? What is this individual's background with ALS? Where does the group meet? How frequently do they meet? How accessible is the meeting place? Is there a scheduled agenda or an open forum for discussion? What is expected of me? Am I required to talk to the group, or can I be a listener? Do people get angry or tearful? Are my family and friends welcome to attend? Will I be singled out in any way?

Not only does a person diagnosed with ALS have to respond to the physical, emotional, social, and economic impact of the disease, but also he is faced with a life-threatening diagnosis and eventually dependent existence. These concerns and others may prompt one to seek out an ALS support group. People often ask what is required of them to participate in such a group. Actually, the answer is courage. It takes a lot of plain old guts to bring one's self to a meeting of people who share this devastating disease.

Let's picture a coming together of a group of people with ALS to explore forming a support group sponsored by a local ALS chapter. The ALS chapter issues an invitation with a specific time and location to meet. The designated professional facilitator is responsible for setting a comfortable environment and tone for the meeting while warmly greeting and introducing himself. Name tags are helpful to make getting acquainted easier. Refreshments may be provided. The facilitator is mindful of comfortable seating, room temperature, ease of movement for individuals with mobility problems, and accessible restroom facilities. The facilitator explains the relationship between the support group and the local ALS chapter and/or center. He also provides information about services and programs.

The facilitator will ask the participants to introduce themselves to the group. Adequate time should be allowed for people to have an opportunity to tell the group a little about themselves. People may want to tell where they live, when their initial symptoms occurred, what the pathway to their eventual diagnosis was, and what specific problems they may be experiencing. Some may use this time to communicate anger, frustration, fear, hope, or expectations. Still others may focus on what resources are medically available to assist them. Participants may also introduce family and friends accompanying them because they are an important part of the ongoing life of the group.

Group participants share a curiosity about the facilitator's experience working with people with ALS. The facilitator should have expertise in conducting support groups and a working knowledge of ALS. Sensitivity to the dramatic ways in which ALS affects peoples' lives is essential. It is not a necessary prerequisite for a facilitator to have personal experience with ALS, but it is vital that he have a commitment to the group and its mission.

The facilitator promotes discussion in response to peoples' questions. For example, some members may believe that they would like an open program to present issues that are important to them. Others may see the group as having a formal agenda of speakers and topics related to ALS. Still others may want a combination of both. The interests, needs, and concerns of the participants most appropriately should determine the content of the support group. Experience has taught that the more involved members are in the design of the group, the greater their desire to make the group a success. Even minor considerations that are decided on by the group help foster a sense of collective planning and participation. The facilitator continues to convey a very special sense of purpose to the group. He maintains awareness of the level of tension and supports each and every question or concern, thereby imparting a great sense of emotional comfort and security. Creating a safe haven for group members is paramount to helping you feel less anxious about their participation.

At the end of what generally is a two-hour session, a date and an agenda for the next meeting are developed. Hopefully, people will leave with a sense of accomplishment and eagerness about having formed a new group. The facilitator may communicate to the group early on his or her availability to respond to some individual questions after the group if necessary. However, questions about the group should be encouraged to be expressed within the group setting. A day or two following the meeting, the facilitator may choose to call the participants in an attempt to identify any personal post-meeting issues or questions that might have arisen.

In subsequent meetings, the facilitator supports an active working phase. The facilitator encourages expression of new or continuing problems relative to speech, swallowing, mobility, or emotional distress. Members may feel uncomfortable if they or others cry or express anger or frustration within the group. The facilitator provides reassurance that such feelings are acceptable and understandable. In fact, most people are likely to have similar feelings. In some cases, these emotions may be related to bulbar symptoms. The facilitator may use this as an opportunity to explain pseudobulbar symptoms and their effect on emotions (see Chapter 24).

As the group continues its educational process about ALS, members will more than likely begin to share their personal responses to living with the disease. Although each person's role in the group has a somewhat different nature to it, every individual's role is valuable. Some may be creative thinkers, while others may use their gift of humor, sensitivity, or spirituality. Each person is a knowledgeable mentor to other members.

The facilitator addresses the group as a strong and sturdy network of people who are interested and concerned about each other. Emphasis is placed on the collective insight, skills, and talents of the participants. The facilitator acknowledges the importance of each individual's continuing membership. He provides a thoughtful and guiding presence, while supporting the group's ability to identify and address shared problems. In a sense, the facilitator supports the group's autonomy while guiding it through decision making and expressions of feelings, especially with regard to the changing circumstances of each member and the group as a whole. The working phase of the group is continuous and adapts and changes as the interests and needs of the group change.

The social life of the group may expand beyond the two-hour meeting. Networking outside the group often continues through the exchange of telephone numbers, mail, E-mail, or visits between meetings. Group members may choose to celebrate and acknowledge various events, such as birthdays, anniversaries, or holidays.

In an ALS support group, themes of change and loss are constant. The death of members is an ever-present reality in the life of the group. People may end their group participation because of the degree of disability they are experiencing, and new members join. It is important that the group continue to focus on its mutually shared concerns and be flexible and allow for this ebb and flow. The facilitator supports the group to invite new members warmly and to process the loss of other members. Veteran members of the group are essential contacts for the introduction, support, and orientation of new people. For instance, a veteran member can provide comfort and support by sharing his own initial experiences with an obviously anxious and tearful new member.

The impact of ALS is felt not only by the individual but also by his family and friends. A support group that includes patients and their loved ones provides an excellent opportunity to address many issues experienced by the family unit. In a group setting, people may express concerns that they may be reluctant to speak about otherwise. Such discussion is a significant way to identify different views as well as the strength of the family as a whole.

Each person needs an opportunity to speak freely about his or her experiences, and the facilitator needs to be sure that no one member dominates the conversation and that adequate time remains for others to speak also. However, on occasions when one or more individuals find their own concerns so overwhelming that they monopolize the group, other members appear to accept and understand this particular need.

Participants in a support group are most comfortable when they are in agreement and share similar responses to situations. However, this tranquil state is unrealistic in the sense that as individuals we all have interests and needs that may differ from other members in the group. Although the success of a support group may be seen by some as dependent on the degree of harmony among the members, its real measure has to do with its ability to resolve conflict and allow the freedom of expression for each individual's point of view. At times, members demonstrate anger with each other or with the facilitator and may express this either directly or indirectly by their words or behaviors.

The facilitator may choose to address conflict. In fact, it is quite healthy for the group to deal with problems, rather than to use passive-aggressive behavior or to discontinue participation without explanation. But if the group is unable to do so, the facilitator may need to intervene with information or comments about the problem and possible solutions. When group members are in conflict with the facilitator, hopefully the facilitator will not respond from a personal perspective but rather will help the group focus on the origin of the difficulty. The ability of the group to deal with conflict shows a strong bond and trust with each other.

In continued meetings of support groups, a broad spectrum of problems are likely to be a part of any one meeting. Typical issues presented include tenuous living situations, in which the physical environment of the home presents obstacles to the patients' mobility, and people may discuss alternative arrangements. Accessibility in the home with regard to bathing, toileting, and meal preparation often are important topics for discussion. Risks associated in living alone with ALS or with family members require identification and remedy. These may include use of stairs, access to the outside, or quick evacuation in an emergency situation.

At other times, the group may express criticism regarding the health care delivery system, inadequate government response in terms of support for research, or complaints directed at health care providers. Sometimes people convey unrealistic expectations or a sense of entitlement because of their diagnosis. Emotionally charged issues, such as feelings of dependency, isolation, and depression, may emerge.

Decision making about care and treatment is a significant component of a group's agenda. Whether to have a feeding tube, use of Bi-PAP, ventilator support, and hospice care are profoundly important issues to the group. The option of accepting, refusing, or discontinuing care will inevitably directly or indirectly promote discussion about death and dying.

The theme of loss does not exclusively refer only to death. Loss for people with ALS comes in many forms: the inability to walk without assistance, difficulty with lack of speech, or problems with eating safely by mouth. Losses such as the inability to shake hands with a new acquaintance or to put one's arm around a loved one are devastating. Holding and physically expressing love to one's partner has a profound effect on a person's self-esteem and, in some cases, the relationship. People with ALS have too much experience with losses, major and minor, and are constantly called upon to accept change and find different means to make up for what they can do no longer.

In the group setting, these types of losses have an impact on both the individual and the group. For example, members whose speech is compromised or nonexistent may require alternative communication devices. Other members may struggle in an attempt to understand the person with dysarthria or difficult speech. To an outsider, an ALS support group may seem to involve rather frightening circumstances. Some members may require suctioning while attending a group or may be on a ventilator or may need to be fed by a feeding tube. The facilitator must prepare the group for these circumstances, and to their response to seeing them, by explaining the various procedures. If a group member finds it too difficult to remain in the group when another individual is doing these things, his response should not be criticized. The facilitator needs to support all responses to the events occurring in the group.

The death of a member has a profound impact on other members and often shows itself in expressions of sadness, or even in denial of the meaning of the loss of the individual. People see their own eventual demise in the deaths of people with whom they have had emotional ties while participating in the group.

Family and friends who have been a part of the group may choose to return to a meeting following the death of their loved one. This often represents their own continuing grief work and helps effect closure with the other group members. It allows the group to acknowledge the loss of the person and the meaning it holds to others, both individually and collectively. Generally, surviving family may want to attend one or perhaps two meetings. However, the facilitator must be sensitive to any request for continued participation, and assist the family with the transition to a bereavement counselor or to a grief and loss support group.

With the death of members, the facilitator assists the group in their attempt to cope with their losses. This may be accomplished through a period of silence when deceased members are remembered, sharing thoughts of the deceased person, or perhaps a poem or prayer among the members and the facilitator. Spirituality experienced as a calm and heartfelt sense of sharing among members of the group strengthens a sense of trust and mutual understanding. Some groups may designate a portion of meeting time to spiritual expression. Others may feel uncomfortable if spirituality is placed in a religious context. The members and facilitator should discuss these concerns as they have others. A skilled facilitator continues to observe and identify themes and interactions among the group members. When it appears that the group has difficulty expressing itself, the facilitator assists in the identification of concerns and makes suggestions as to their resolution.

Quality of life and end-of-life considerations are ongoing concerns that a group explores. The degree to which these issues are verbalized are greater or lesser depending on the group members need to address them. The facilitator recognizes that these topics are provocative and a source of great anxiety. Group members are keenly aware of changes in other members and may need assistance in coping with their response to new circumstances. A skilled facilitator continues to observe and identify themes and interactions among the group members. When the group has difficulty expressing itself, the facilitator assists in identifying problems and makes suggestions to promote discussion.

Periodically, the group and the facilitator allow time to evaluate what the group has accomplished, where it would like to go, and its influence with regard to informing, educating, and supporting its members. A group needs to reflect on its success as well as the concerns it wishes to further address. The life span of a group may be many years because new members continue to join. A support group is not rigid but reflects the changing life circumstances of its members. The group experience exists solely for the support and benefit of its members, and as such participants feel pride, responsibility, and ownership for the unique involvement that they have with each other.

Participants in a support group develop a significant bond with the facilitator. She may be seen as a resident expert regarding ALS, as an ally in struggles experienced by group members, as a mediator between patients and health care providers, as a liaison between support group members and an ALS center or chapter, or as a trusted and significant friend. The facilitator and the members benefit from discussion of shared expectations or differing expectations of each other. The availability of the facilitator before or after meetings is important for members to know. The role and commitment of the facilitator to the group necessitate that she have available a consultant and mentor with whom to discuss the content and process of the group. Of course the facilitator informs group members that confidentiality is respected and identifies anyone with whom she may discuss the group and seeks member's approval for this. The facilitator benefits from the experiences of a consultant/mentor in developing insight into her behavior and its effects on the group. This mentoring relationship gives the facilitator an opportunity to evaluate the effects of intervention in the group as well as growing in understanding and experience as to the group's progress.

The facilitator of the group may leave it for any number of reasons, personal or professional. The group and the facilitator deal again with change and loss. It is most desirable if the facilitator plans for such change with the group. For example, the new facilitator may attend a meeting of the group while the departing one is moving toward termination from the group. This allows for a greater sense of continuity and stability.

An ALS support group addresses the myriad of challenges related to this catastrophic life event. The group affords opportunities to:

- Become more knowledgeable about ALS.

- Discern accurate and more complete information about the illness.

- Identify the important role of the national voluntary organizations, such as ALS Association and MDA, and the ALS centers, which provide clinical care to individuals and families.

- Connect people with local ALS chapters or MDA centers and their programs of services including transportation, adaptive equipment, and assistive communication devices, among other resources.

- Inform people about current and future ALS research and clinical drug trials.

- Educate patients and families about various levels of decision making relative to feeding tubes, BiPAP®, ventilator support, and hospice care.

- Identify various resources, public and private, which may provide helpful assistance.

- Provide information about adjunctive/alternative therapies.

- Discuss end-of-life care issues.

- Sustain a sense of hope through mutual sharing.

Ultimately, an ALS support group is a significant opportunity for people with ALS, their families, and friends to enhance knowledge, facilitate change in care and treatment, and serve as a model for caring, compassion, and advocacy for people with ALS. The unfolding of the group through discussing concerns regularly builds a network of strong relationships and a sense of feeling and bonding with each other that is extraordinary in its scope and nature.

Acknowledgment. Special acknowledgment and affection are extended to Francine Grabowski, M.S., R.D. CDE, whose assistance in the preparation of this manuscript has been vital.

Suggested Reading

1. Biegel DE, Song LI-u. Facilitators and barriers to caregiver support group participation, *Journal of Case Management* 1995; 4(4):164–172.

2. Boise L, Heagerty B, Eskenazi, L. Facing chronic illness: The family support model and its benefits. *Patient Education and Counseling* 1996; 27(1):75–84.

3. Carlson R. *Don't sweat the small stuff . . . and it's all small stuff.* New York: Hyperion Press, 1997.

4. Carlson R, Shield B. *Handbook for the soul.* Boston: Little, Brown, 1995.

5. Cheng WC, Schuckers PL, Hauser G. Psychological needs of family caregivers of terminally ill patients. *Psychological Reports* 1994; 75 (3):1243–1250.

6. Earl L, Johnston M, Mitchell E. Coping with motor neurone disease—an analysis using self-regulation theory. *Palliative Medicine* 1993; 7(4 Suppl):21–30.

7. Feenberg AL, Licht JM, Kane KP. The online patient meeting. *Journal of the Neurological Sciences* 1996; 139:129–131.

8. Feigenbaum D. *Journey with ALS.* Virginia: DLRC Press, 1998.

9. George H. Gallup International Institute; Spiritual beliefs and the dying process, a report on a national survey. Conducted for The Nathan Cummings Foundation and Fetzer Institute, Princeton, NJ, October 1997.

10. Hatchett L, Friend R, Symister P. Interpersonal expectations, social support, and adjustment to chronic illness. *Journal of Personality and Social Psychology* 1997; 73(3):560–573.

11. Hutchinson J. *May I walk you home?* Indiana: Ave Maria Press, 1999.

12. Keeling DI, Price PE, Jones E. Social support: Some pragmatic implications for health care professionals. *Journal of Advanced Nursing* 1996; 23:76–81.

13. Larsen LS. Effectiveness of a counseling intervention to assist family caregivers of chronically ill relatives. *Journal of Psychosocial Nursing* 1998; 36:26–32.

14. Lynne J, Harrold J. *Handbook for mortals.* New York: Oxford University Press, 1999.

15. McDonald ER, Wiedenfeld SA, Hillel A. Survival in amyotrophic lateral sclerosis: The role of psychological factors. *Archives of Neurology* 1994; 51:17–23.

16. Monahan DJ, Hooker K. Caregiving and social support in two illness groups. *Social Work* 1997; 42:278–287.

17. Pennix BW, van Tilburg T, Boeke AJ, et al. Effects of social support and personal coping resources on depressive symptoms—Different for various chronic diseases? *Health Psychology* 1998; 17:551–558.

18. Ruppert RA. Psychological aspects of lay caregiving. *Rehabilitation Nursing* 1996; 21:315–320.

19. Schreurs KMG, de Ridder DTD. Integration of coping and social support perspective: Implications for the study of adaptation to chronic diseases. *Clinical Psychology Review* 1997; 17:89–112.

20. Tausig M. Caregiver network structure, support and caregiver distress. *American Journal of Community Psychology* 1992; 20:81–96.

21. White NE, Richter JM, Fry C. Coping, social support, and adaptation to chronic illness. *Western Journal of Nursing Research* 1992; 14:211–224.

21

Meditation and ALS

Gian Domenico Borasio, M.D.

*With all your science can you tell
how it is and when it is
that light comes into the soul?*

Henry David Thoreau (1817–1862)

John had been a successful manager before contracting ALS at the age of 48. Yet the very first time I saw him (he had come to our ALS clinic to ask about possible enrollment in a clinical study) he struck me with a calmness and a peace of mind that was all the more remarkable since at that time, almost four years into the disease, he was unable to move his arm or legs and was completely dependent on outside help. His speech, however, was still almost unaffected. I asked him about his feelings about the disease, and he said "You know, at the beginning I was shattered. My business, my career, my life plans—I had to give it all up. It was terrible. I went into big-time depression. Suicide seemed a reasonable option, since I did not want to become a burden to my wife and family. At that point, a friend pointed out that Buddhist philosophy and meditation might help me. I was quite skeptical, but willing to try anything, and I gave it my best shot. Now I am totally dependent on others for help (the thing I dreaded most) but I would say, strange as it may seem to you, that my quality of life is actually better than before the disease started. Then, I didn't have time for anything, I was constantly rushing and stressed. Now, I have time for myself, and what is even more important, I can make use of this time and live in it."

271

One possible reaction to this account might be to doubt John's mental sanity. How could anybody with a clear mind say that he is happier *with* ALS than *without?* Yet John showed absolutely no signs of psychosis or delusions. He was perfectly at ease, and one could sense that he was actually trying to make everybody else in the room feel comfortable, too. On one occasion he made it clear that he was indeed not feeling "happier" in the common sense of the word. His physical disability, his breathing problems requiring non-invasive ventilation at night, and the fear of losing his speech sooner or later were all things he was painfully aware of. "But," he said "that is exactly what it is all about: awareness. At least now I am aware of what is happening to me, while before I wasn't. Therefore, now I can enjoy even little pleasures much more than before."

It should be said that John and his family were quite well off and that he could afford first-class, round-the-clock, professional nursing help. However, this was not nearly enough to explain his remarkable inner balance. I had seen plenty of other patients with equally good economic resources who were unable to come to terms with their disease. John was the first patient I knew who had turned to meditation as a way of coping. He was also one of the first ALS patients in Germany to receive noninvasive ventilation (NIV) and had pushed for starting it even before developing signs or symptoms of chronic respiratory insufficiency because he thought that this might delay the onset of respiratory problems. (Incidentally, this is still an open clinical question today, and he might very well be right!). He was on NIV for almost five years, and during this time he helped a lot of ALS patients overcome their fears of NIV (and of percutaneous endoscopic gastrostomy as well) by talking to them about his own experience, either in person or on the phone.

John stopped NIV voluntarily when he was in need of ventilation for most of the day because he did not want to go on tracheostomy. We arranged for him to spend his last days in a hospice institution to make sure that he would receive appropriate medication to relieve his terminal dyspnea. To the surprise and awe of the entire hospice team, after having said goodbye to his wife and family, John simply slipped into sleep, from there into coma, and died peacefully a few hours later. Even through his death, John spoke to the world around him. The collaboration of our ALS clinic with that particular hospice, who had been reluctant to accept ALS patients, especially if ventilated, has been excellent ever since.

Although John's personal development was certainly exceptional, he is by no means alone. Helga, a 49-year-old ALS patient, recently told us that she had been meditating before the disease started but had actually intensified her practice since then. She had struck us before with her pragmatic, no-nonsense approach to the disease, and I had previously noticed during a patients' meeting that she had a very positive influence on other patients. Starting next year, Helga will lead a patient support group and will also offer some initial help with meditation techniques.

In the wonderful book by Mitch Albom, *Tuesdays with Morrie,* which many of you have probably read, there are no fewer than four references to "meditation teachers" as playing an important part in Morrie's last years of life. Again, Morrie was certainly an exceptional person with a deeply rooted love for and under-standing of humanity long before he contracted ALS. However, it is notable that he thought it important to devote a considerable portion of his limited remaining life span to learning and practicing meditation. I can only assume that this was part of what led him to that remarkable serenity in the wake of his disease's progres-sion that has inspired innumerable readers of the book and that strongly reminded me of John's attitude.

What Is Meditation?

It may be helpful to first point out what meditation is not—it is not a relaxation technique. It is not an exotic Far Eastern ritual that can be properly practiced only by Buddhists or Zen monks (in fact, there is a new but strongly growing tradition of meditation practice within, for example, Christian communities). It is not going to change any of your symptoms of ALS, much less stop the disease from progressing. But it may change the way you look at your disease and your life.

The tradition of meditation goes back for at least 2,500 years and probably much longer. Although best known from Buddhism, where it plays a central role in religious practice, elements of meditation are present in all great religions, most evidently in their mystical currents, like the Hinduist Sadhus, the Islamic Sufis, the Jewish Hassidim, or the Christian medieval mystics.

There are innumerable definitions of meditation—some pragmatic, some poetic, some cryptic—but they all fall somewhat short of grasping its essence. One of the most compelling definitions of meditation is *just being there*. Another definition is simply *mindfulness*. James H. Austin, M.D., author of *Zen and the Brain* says: "[Meditation] becomes a way of not thinking, clearly, and *then of carrying this clear awareness into everyday life.*" As far as technique goes, the Zen master Dogen (1200–1253) says: "Free yourself from all attachments . . . think neither of good nor evil, and judge not right or wrong. Stop the operation of mind, of will, and of consciousness; bring to an end all desires, all concepts and judgements." The Tibetan master Jamyang Khyentse Rinpoche (1896–1959) once said: "Whenever you end a thought and before you start the next one, isn't there a little pause, a gap? Well, prolong it! This is meditation."

Meditation cannot be defined fully with words—it has to be experienced. If you try it, at first you may notice that you become more aware of what is going on, less attached to your thoughts and emotions, and more "centered." Gradually, you will realize that all reasons for pain and anxiety, as well as all sources of joy and happiness, are within yourself. Ultimately, the practice of meditation may lead to the blossoming of love and compassion both for ourselves and for others.

There are several different kinds of meditation practices, all of which adhere to the same basic principles: transcendental meditation, mindfulness meditation, Ti-betan meditation, Zen meditation, and many others. This chapter will not teach you how to meditate. If you are interested, a number of excellent books are listed at the end of the chapter (many of which are also available as audiotapes) to which you can turn for an introduction. I would particularly recommend the book by Jon Kabat-Zinn entitled *Full Catastrophe Living,* a title that can be fully appreciated by ALS patients and their families. This book describes the Stress Reduction Program at the University of Massachusetts Medical Center and contains a working program that can serve as an initial guideline to test whether meditation may be of help for you.

Some reasons why meditation might be particularly useful in ALS are outlined in the next section—but beware of any theoretical considerations, because it is *your* life and it is only *you* who can decide what is good for you and what is not. However, there certainly is no harm in trying. Just one piece of advice: if you want to try it out, do it like John—give it your best shot. Do not feel frustrated if you do not see any immediate or short-term "results" or "improvements in well-being"—stick to it for a while. Meditation requires persistence.

Why May It Help in ALS?

People face a radical change in their life's perspective when they are told that they have ALS. Any long-term plans or goals have to be abandoned or reshaped. Adapting to ALS often requires going through a painful phase of depression and denial before coming to an acceptance of the disease. Time is limited, and death becomes a reality that has to be dealt with. This is true for every one of us, but most people postpone confronting the issue of death and dying until it is too late. All great traditions have emphasized the importance of integrating death into our lives (a particularly beautiful example is *The Tibetan Book of Living and Dying* by Sogyal Rinpoche). Herein lies one of the chances of ALS.

Why should people with ALS invest their precious time for something as time-consuming and demanding as meditation practice? The answer is that they should not unless they really want to. At the beginning of the disease, patients are often most concerned with the quest for a cure. As the disease progresses, they find themselves having, as one person put it, both too little time and too much time. Too little time left before death, yet too much time because most of the usual activities cannot be performed anymore. The loss of physical functions and independence leads to anger and frustration. On the other hand, meditation does not require any physical ability. All it requires is an intact mind, some time, and a firm commitment.

As mentioned previously, one of the central aspects of meditation is *letting go* or "non-attachment." We are constantly in the process of clinging to certain pleasurable aspects of our lives, especially when we are in danger of losing them. Meditation can help us to release and let go and to accept things as they are. This is possibly the most difficult psychological task in ALS, but those individuals who succeed in it (whether by meditation or by other means) are rewarded with a quantum leap in their quality of life.

Meditation has no immediate "goal" other than making us aware of the beauty and preciousness of the present moment. This is of particular importance in a disease like ALS, in which the life span is limited but the potential for awareness is not. In a disease such as Alzheimer's dementia, for example, survival times are considerably longer than with ALS. However, Alzheimer patients experience a rapid deterioration of their memory and personality. Many of them are completely different people within six months of disease onset and have all but lost the ability to communicate with the outside world within a few years. In contrast, people with ALS retain their full intellectual, emotional, and social skills throughout the disease. However, this capacity is a two-sided sword. It may bring out constant anguish about the future course of the disease and eventually lead to the development of a nihilistic attitude ("nobody can help me") and even to requests for physician-assisted suicide. On the other hand, it may also be used for the person's benefit to develop adequate coping strategies and maximize the quality of life for the remaining life span.

Richard, a 55-year-old ALS patient, and his wife had been discussing his advance directives with us for two hours. He had late-stage ALS, he could barely speak, and his breathing capacity was markedly impaired. He refused tracheostomy and asked that he be given morphine in the terminal phase, which he felt to be impending (he was right). At the end, I asked him if he had any further questions. He then said, quite unexpectedly, "When am I going to be cured, doc?" It took me a while before I could reply: "Medicine cannot *cure* ALS today. But when you realize that your most important qualities as a human being, your personality, your emotions, your intellect, your memory, your ability to give and receive love, are not and never will be diminished by ALS, then you will have made a big step toward *healing*." He smiled and said: "Then I am healed already, doc." He died peacefully in his sleep a few weeks later.

A Word of Caution

What has been said so far by no means implies that meditation is the right approach for all or even most people with ALS. Which coping strategy is the "right" one for any particular patient (or caregiver) is all but impossible to determine in advance. You have to try it out. It is your life, and never let anyone else tell you what you should or should not do. What professionals can do is point out several alternatives that have already helped others so that you can choose which way you want to go. Meditation undoubtedly has helped some. This chapter had no other purpose but to inform you of that. If you think that it might be good for you, go ahead and try it. Later, if you could spare a few moments to tell me about your experiences (positive and negative), please do so by using the e-mail address below—your experience might help other patients in the future.

Please send any comments you might have on this chapter or accounts of your own experiences with meditation and ALS to Dr. Borasio at the following e-mail address: Borasio@lrz.uni-muenchen.de

Suggested Reading

(The books marked with an asterisk are also available as audiotapes.)

1. *Albom M. *Tuesdays with Morrie: An old man, a young man, and life's greatest lesson.* New York: Doubleday, 1997.

2. Austin JH. *Zen and the brain.* Cambridge: MIT Press, 1998.

3. De Mello A. *One minute wisdom.* New York: Image Books, 1988.

4. De Mello A. *The way to love: The last meditations of Anthony De Mello.* New York: Image Books, 1995.

5. Enomiya-Lassalle HM, Ropers R, Snela B. *The practice of Zen meditation.* London: Thorsons, 1993.

6. Gaffney P, Rinpoche S. *Glimpse after glimpse: Daily reflections on living and dying.* San Francisco: Harper & Row, 1995.

7. *Hanh TN. *Being Peace.* Berkeley: Parallax Press, 1988.

8. *Hanh TN. *Touching peace: Practicing the art of mindful living.* Berkeley: Parallax Press, 1992.

9. *Hanh TN. *The miracle of mindfulness: A manual on meditation.* Rev. ed. Boston: Beacon Press, 1992.

10. *Kabat-Zinn J. *Full catastrophe living: Using the wisdom of your body and mind to face stress, pain, and illness.* New York: Delta, 1990.

11. *Kabat-Zinn J. *Wherever you go, there you are.* New York: Hyperion, 1995.

12. Longaker C, Rinpoche S. *Facing death and finding hope: A guide to the emotional and spiritual care of the dying.* New York: Doubleday, 1997.

13. Meister E. *Selected writings.* New York: Doubleday, 1995.

14. *Rinpoche S. *The Tibetan book of living and dying.* San Francisco: Harper & Row, 1994.

15. *Suzuki S. *Zen mind, beginner's mind.* Weatherhill, 1972.

22

Living with ALS: Quality of Life Issues

Patricia L. Andres, M.S., P.T., Brenda J. Thornell, A.S., P.T.A., and Linda T. Skerry, A.S., P.T.A.

Quality of life has been defined as an evaluation of all aspects of our lives, including, for example, where we live, how we live, and how we play. It encompasses such life factors as family circumstances, finances, housing, and job satisfaction. This chapter describes some of the ways that ALS affects quality of life and offers suggestions for how health care providers can improve the quality of life for people with ALS.

Receiving the diagnosis of ALS changes everything for you—profoundly and forever. This disease touches almost every aspect of life—from basic physical functioning to financial planning, from personal relationships to a changed sense of spirituality. People learn not only that will they die but also that their remaining few years will likely include losing the ability to walk, speak, swallow, or perform even the most personal of self-care activities. A long-term future has been denied, and the short-term future is filled with the anticipation of which muscles will fail next.

Families must deal with the relentless, escalating physical needs of the person with ALS while adjusting to the realization that their loved one will soon be taken from them. Family roles often change. The provider often becomes the cared-for and the child becomes the caretaker. Frequently, families pull together and become stronger. Occasionally, families are weakened by the stress.

Sensation and cognition are unaffected because ALS is a pure motor disease. Patients who suffer pain do so as the result of avoidable secondary complications such as frozen shoulder syndrome. Additionally, it is common for casual acquaintances to wrongly assume that a person has diminished mental capacities when they observe slurred speech, drooling, and facial weakness.

Despite the physical decline, the lives of many people with ALS paradoxically become enriched in some ways. Typically, after initial struggles with denial and anger, they become more introspective, philosophical, caring, and tolerant. ALS has been called the "nice guys" disease. This disease, which drains one's physical strength, somehow often enables inner strength to emerge. The courage and dignity of people with ALS is inspiring. People faced with death often use the precious time remaining to find meaning in their lives and to enrich their relationships with others. A tenderness often emerges as their priorities change. This fatal disease, which leads to a decline in one's physical quality of life, simultaneously can become a life-enriching experience.

The physical, emotional, and social effects of ALS are as diverse as the people who experience the disorder. The following case studies illustrate some of the diverse challenges of ALS.

Case 1

J.S., a married 38-year-old father of two young children, enjoyed tennis and sailing. He was a self-employed as a carpenter and had very limited private insurance coverage. He was diagnosed with ALS about six months after first noticing twitching in his arms and difficulty with his tennis game.

J.S. no longer played tennis because his game had deteriorated to the point where it had become a frustrating experience. He had trouble holding nails and tools and was unable to carry heavy equipment. He frequently cut himself shaving and had to switch to using an electric razor. He had difficulty unlocking doors with standard keys, especially on cold mornings.

During his first visit to our ALS clinic, J.S. experienced painful cramping in limbs during strength testing. We showed him how to gently stretch his muscles to relieve painful spasms. A medication was prescribed to lessen the muscle cramps. The physical therapist instructed him in self-range of motion (ROM) exercises for his shoulders and legs to avoid future muscle and joint stiffness. In discussing his previous high level of physical activity, the suggestion was made to avoid excessive fatigue and to delegate heavy lifting to his coworkers.

We made the following suggestions to ease his morning self-care activities: (1) purchase an electric toothbrush with a large grip, (2) use a pencil grip for writing and eating utensils, (3) purchase a rocker knife for cutting food, and (4) use a molded plastic extension for his car and house keys. Informational brochures from the Muscular Dystrophy Association (MDA) and the ALS Association (ALSA) were given to him, along with a discussion of the services provided by these nonprofit organizations.

While driving in to the city for his next clinic appointment, J.S. was unable to retrieve the change out of his pocket at the tollbooth. He was observed in the waiting room trying unsuccessfully to unwrap a piece of candy for his very impatient four-year-old daughter. His wife reported that he had been depressed and irritable. There had been several episodes of blowing up at his wife, children, and friends. He had to take several days off from his job for medical workups and second opinions. He had trouble sleeping. Although he kept his diagnosis a secret for fear of losing clients and his workers, people noticed changes in his work habits and asked a lot of questions. He expressed anger because he was not eligible for a clinical trial.

Both J.S. and his wife were allowed to express their views openly during their clinic visit. Every effort was made to be supportive and nondefensive as they expressed their anger and frustration. We again suggested that they contact the MDA and ALSA to join a patient or family support group.

J.S.'s gait had become unsteady. The physical therapist demonstrated the use of a wheeled walker that would maintain balance while allowing him to walk at his normal pace. He rejected the walker, stating that he was not ready for any "handicapped equipment." Both he and his wife had attended several support group meetings and found them to be both informative and very comforting. They met a couple from a nearby community who were experiencing similar challenges and were forming a close bond with them.

One year after the diagnosis, J.S. no longer sailed, and his arms were too weak to safely drive a car. He could barely feed himself and needed help with most other activities of daily living (ADLs). News of his diagnosis had leaked out from his wife a few months previously. Two of his best workers stayed with him, but the others left. He had few new contracts and was unable to work at the sites. His financial situation had worsened. His wife had to accompany him on job estimates to drive and to help with the writing. He was beginning to limp, and he tired easily. The previous winter he had fallen while skating with his daughters. Because of severe arm weakness, he was unable to break his fall and hit his head, requiring several stitches. He wore sweat pants most of the time because he could no longer manipulate a zipper, even with a ring attached to the zipper pull.

At a recent clinic appointment, J.S. finally accepted a prescription for a wheeled walker. Despite the fact that his arms were too weak to lift the walker, he was able to rest his hands on the grips, which were modified with an extra-thick coating of foam. The walker had large wheels for use outdoors and folded for easy transport in the back seat or trunk of a car. J.S. was able to walk longer distances using the walker, and his wife was less worried about him falling.

Within 18 months after diagnosis, J.S. had little use of his arms. He needed total assistance with all ADLs. His walking was very unsteady. He ambulated short distances after being helped up and having his arms placed on a walker that was modified with forearm supports. His business had been dissolved, and he was receiving a small disability check. His wife worked part-time at home as a typist. His former employees built a ramp for him over the front steps. The physical therapist arranged to get a wheelchair from the MDA loaner closet that had easy-off wheels to make car transport manageable for his wife. The therapist reviewed safe transfer assistance techniques with his wife to avoid injury to either one of them. His wife was instructed in passive range of motion exercises, especially for his shoulders. A tub transfer bench with a back was recommended along with a hand-held shower head.

Two years after the diagnosis, J.S. was nonambulatory. A Hoyer lift was used to transfer him from bed to chair or commode. His speech was slightly thick, with decreased volume. He required oxygen at night and at times during the day for shortness of breath. He was unable to tolerate lying flat and usually slept in his recliner all night. The physical therapist instructed his wife in correct positioning techniques to avoid pressure areas and to comfortably support his limbs, trunk, and neck.

Less than three years after first noticing twitching in his arms, J.S. passed away at home surrounded by his family and close friends.

Case 2

L.T. was a 72-year-old married grandmother who maintained homes in both New England and Florida. Her husband was retired from his executive job with a large bank. They had Medicare and excellent supplemental insurance coverage. They enjoyed frequent visits from their five grown children and 11 grandchildren. The patient first noticed a problem with choking, especially on thin liquids. She had an irritating sensation of built-up secretions in the back of her throat. Her friends noticed that her speech on the phone was slurred. Her best friend actually con-fronted her with the accusation of an alcohol problem.

After several visits to various physicians and extensive medical work-ups, L.T. was diagnosed with ALS about one year after noticing the first symptom. By the time her diagnosis was confirmed, she had to use a thickener in her liquids and had dropped several foods from her diet, including chicken and crackers. At this point, her speech was slow and gravelly. Casual acquaintances often had to ask her to repeat herself, especially on the phone. Her gait was normal, although she tired easily while shopping. Her arms felt fine except for some occasional twitch-ing in her biceps. Despite current good functional strength, we instructed her in daily self-range of motion exercises for both shoulders to avoid future shoulder pain and stiffness. We also advised her to engage in an enjoyable light aerobic exercise such as walking, swimming, or biking to maintain cardiovascular fitness. The therapist carefully advised her to build up her activity slowly and avoid excessive fatigue.

Two years after her first symptom, L.T. had lost 20 pounds and needed a gastric feeding tube. She also had a portable suction machine to handle mucus secretions in the back of her throat. She had seen a speech and language patholo-gist and had a voice synthesizer. She had teletypewriter (TTY) service through the telephone company. She received home care nursing visits three times per week to check the gastric tube, and she had a home health aide to assist her with bathing.

She also had received six visits from a home care physical therapist to assess the home environment and instruct her in independent gentle conditioning exercises to maximize muscle and cardiovascular fitness, while avoiding strenuous exercise.

At this point, L.T. had significant weakness of her arms and early signs of foot drop. We provided her with a wheeled walker because of her fatigue and unsteady gait. On the clinic's recommendation, she was fitted with custom-molded plastic ankle-foot orthoses to avoid toe drag and stabilize her legs while walking. Using the wheeled walker and ankle braces, she was able to continue her daily routine of walking around the mall.

At her clinic appointment L.T. was, as always, surrounded by her husband and several of her children. She came with a lengthy printed message to the neuro-muscular team that usually included a funny story. She continued enjoying her nightly martini, although now it was fed directly into the gastric tube. Her pulmonary function had decreased significantly, and her physician discussed options regarding supplemental oxygen and ventilators.

A year later, L.T. needed a customized three-wheel cart to maintain her ability to go to the mall and be outside with her family. She was fitted with a Freeman executive collar to maintain proper head position and provide support during transport. She used oxygen at night and had an electric hospital bed because she could not tolerate lying flat. Her husband had the bathroom redesigned to include a walk-in shower stall. Her arms became significantly weaker. She needed help for most ADLs. The voice synthesizer was becoming more difficult to use.

Four years after diagnosis, L.T. required oxygen all the time. She walked only a few feet with a wheeled walker and assistance. Her family members had all been instructed in positioning techniques and range of motion exercises to keep her muscles and joints comfortable. Hospice care was started approximately three months before she died at home.

Summary

There are at least three major ways that health care providers can contribute to the quality of life of people with ALS. First, painful secondary complications of the disease usually can be prevented by appropriate education. In general, people with ALS should not be in pain. Early and continued education in self-range of motion exercises or assisted ROM exercises usually prevents frozen shoulder syndrome. Proper stretching can ease painful muscle spasms for those who experience significant spasticity and muscle cramping. Learning proper body mechanics and efficient techniques for transfers, positioning, and ambulation can prolong safe mobility and prevent injury to both the patient and the caregivers. Proper medications can aid in sleeping, prevent drooling, regulate bowel function, and improve breathing.

Second, prescribing adaptive equipment and durable medical equipment (DME) based on your individualized needs can greatly improve comfort and safely prolong independence. Such simple devices as a built-up fork, rocker knife, or plastic key extension can enable a person with ALS to maintain independence for a prolonged amount of time. Problem solving with health care providers about each individual's challenges and frustrations often can lead to creative solutions to make people with ALS more comfortable and functionally independent.

Careful ordering of equipment such as wheelchairs and walkers will reduce the need to make frequent changes in prescriptions, which can be financially and psychologically difficult. For example, if you need an ambulatory device, anticipation of future decline should be considered. It may be less emotionally traumatic to use a wheeled walker rather than progress to a cane, crutches, and finally a wheeled walker. In considering a wheelchair order, it is important to look down the road and consider the need for a high-back recliner if the person with ALS is at risk for developing neck weakness. Proper seating and cushions can prevent skin breakdown. Correct positioning when sitting places the upper extremities in an optimal position to maximize functional mobility, ease breathing, and support the trunk and neck.

The amount and expense of equipment that will be needed during the course of the disease varies greatly depending on your rate of disease progression, available financial resources, and each individual's unique perspective. For example, J.S. was reluctant to use equipment, whereas L.T. and her family had the resources and mind-set to want anything that would make her more comfortable.

The third, and usually most important, way that health care providers can impact your quality of life is by the bond of understanding that should be established between the members of the health care team and the family. A bond of trust is usually formed based on your understanding that these highly trained specialists know what is coming next and will listen and assist you to make choices that hold your quality of life in the highest regard.

23

Psychological, Social, and Spiritual Factors

Evelyn R. McDonald, M.S.

Socrates said, "There is no disease of the body apart from the mind."
This means that the activities of the mind (one's thoughts, emotions,
and psychosocial and spiritual experiences) and the physical body
are not separate, walled off entities but are interconnected, each
continually influencing the other, creating human beings who are
unique in their responses to all of life, including illness.

Each person with amyotrophic lateral sclerosis (ALS) has his or her psychological, social, and spiritual well-being challenged every step of the way, which can
affect the critical issues faced by the individual and the family. This chapter examines the relationship between ALS and the psychosocial-spiritual dimensions
of patients, their spouses, and their health care practitioner.

Much of your experience of living with ALS is related to factors over which
you have no direct control. No patient or family member can control the age
at which ALS is contracted, its severity, or how rapidly the disease will progress.
The ALS Patient Profile Project shows, however, that patients and family
members do have control over a number of other factors and that these factors
can substantially influence quality of life and, in some cases, survival rate as
well.

The ALS Patient Profile Project studied 144 ALS patients and 123 of their
spouses or primary caregivers in three metropolitan areas of the United States—
Seattle, San Francisco, and Philadelphia. Entry criteria for patients consisted of a

confirmed diagnosis of ALS made by a neurologist and the absence of diagnosed dementia or known alcoholism. Every three months for a year and a half, participants in the study completed 10 standardized psychological tests and a data form that asked questions about demographics, medical history, lifestyle, and participants' attitudes and beliefs about themselves and their lives. In addition, researchers interviewed each patient to evaluate physical function and the extent to which ALS had progressed.

Patients in the study ranged in age from 25 to 82 years. Two-thirds were men, 79 percent were married, and 60 percent had completed at least some college. The average age at which participants were diagnosed with ALS was 55 years. Patients participating in the study had ALS from one month to 30 years, and the severity of their disease ranged from barely perceptible functional impairment to extreme functional impairment and almost complete paralysis.

Caregivers and spouses who participated were between 19 and 78 years old. Three-fourths were women, and 60 percent had completed at least some college. Approximately three-fourths of the spouses had been working before their mate's diagnosis of ALS, but nearly one-fourth had stopped working to care for the person with ALS by the initial interview.

The ALS Patient

An initial question was whether people with ALS had a characteristic personality pattern that was different from patterns in populations with other illnesses or "normal" populations not suffering from illness. In an attempt to answer that question, each person's psychological, social, and spiritual condition was evaluated by measuring 10 different aspects: depression, hopelessness, perceived stress, expression of anger, loneliness, degree of control over health care issues, life satisfaction, sense of purpose in life, social support, and coping style.

When their average scores were compared with scores from a normal, healthy population, only minimal differences were found. The ALS patients exhibited more depression (60% had some level of measurable depression compared with the 16–20% that is typical of the general population), and they had a more external health locus of control—that is, they wanted others to make decisions for them and tell them what to do in regard to their health care and treatment options. Neither depression nor an external health locus of control is unusual in patients with chronic disease.

The surprising finding was that approximately one-fourth of the patients in the study were, on average, mildly depressed or not depressed at all. These patients were not lonely. They wanted to be involved in decisions regarding their care and treatment. If they perceived stress, they confronted it effectively. They expressed anger appropriately, maintained a sense of hope, and felt their lives had purpose. These qualities led to a sense of psychospiritual well-being and a high quality of life.

Quality of Life

The study also found that, as a group, those patients who experienced psychological well-being had higher quality lives and longer survival times during the study than patients who experienced psychological distress, regardless of disease severity, time since diagnosis, or age. In fact, only 32 percent of the patients expressing psychological well-being died during the course of the study, while 82 percent of those with psychological distress died. The risk of mortality for patients with psychological distress was 6.8 times greater than for those with psychological well-being (1). Patients with psychological distress had an increased risk of dying and decreased survival time.

Those patients who experienced psychological well-being exhibited a high quality of life, regardless of the severity of their illness. Quality of life cannot be measured simply by evaluating physical function. There were people in our study who lived rich and active lives despite being severely debilitated by ALS. High quality of life is also a function of an individual's perception and is reflected in a sense of psychological, social, and spiritual well-being, even in the face of severe physical handicaps. There are ALS patients who travel with wheelchairs and portable respirators, coach football, direct video productions, oil paint, or explore the nature of the universe. They do all this despite profound physical limitations.

One of the powerful experiences of working on this study was meeting people whose physical functioning was extremely limited but whose spirits soared. There was a young woman who could not speak, walk, or feed herself, yet she managed to infuse her family with love and laughter.

The life of Stephen Hawking, the well-known British physicist whose physical function has been severely limited by ALS for many years, reminds all of us that physical disability in no way limits one's ability to contribute to humanity.

Quality of life was closely related to the "spirit" of a patient. In our study, 37 percent of the people with ALS found that some aspect of their lives actually improved after they developed the disease, in ways that ranged from having closer relationships to finding increased appreciation for life. This leads to one of the most important conclusions of the study: that anyone living with ALS has the potential to lead a life of quality, despite the profound physical limitations imposed by the disease. As a widow recently said, "Some aspects of this disease were hell. I would never choose to go through the experience again, yet I learned so much that has helped me in life, that I am grateful for." ALS may seem hopeless because there is no cure, but there is hope—because positive psychological patterns, attitudes, and ways of coping can lead to greater psychological well-being and a higher quality of life.

Response to Physical Challenges

A person's psychological, social, and spiritual well-being is not determined solely by the physical aspects associated with progression of ALS, but they are related in a number of ways.

Mode of Onset

One might suspect that patients with bulbar onset (affecting speech or respiration) would have a lower level of psychological well-being than those with spinal onset (affecting the arms or legs). Yet the type of onset was not directly related to psychological, social, and spiritual status. Many patients experienced fear and anger. For some it was over losing the ability to communicate clearly. For others it centered around the apparent or imminent loss of independence. Such a loss could be a major adjustment for the 66 percent of the patients in this study who described themselves as fiercely independent before the onset of ALS. Only 18 percent considered themselves fiercely independent at the time of the study. Regardless of the mode of onset, patients with unresolved anger and fear were often reluctant to participate in family or social functions and generally experienced a decrease in psychological well-being. This was where a good social support system came into play. If the patient had even one person with whom he or she could vent the anger, experience the grief of loss, or name the fear, then he or she could often regain a sense of well-being. Some individuals would see a counselor during these times to help them identify and accept their feelings.

Age

Older patients (those over 65) showed higher levels of depression and hopelessness than younger ones, indicating more psychological, social, and spiritual distress. It is possible that ALS did not cause this depression or hopelessness but rather exacerbated a state that existed before onset of the disease, especially if the patient had already been facing end-of-life issues.

End-of-life issues can be difficult to discuss, and their importance cannot be overstated. Throughout years of interviewing and being with people with ALS, I have seen the increased fear and loneliness that comes from avoiding these discussions. One couple had never mentioned the word death between them. When I first visited them, the husband was in an advanced state of ALS; an awkward silence hung in the air. Each of them was very angry and very lonely; then a hospice nurse got them to talk about their fears. For the first time in a couple of years they cried together and shared not only their fears but also their love for each other. On the next visit, there was a new closeness between them, and they were eager to share their insights with me.

In addition, many older patients voiced concern about being a burden on their spouses, particularly when a spouse had physical limitations or a chronic illness. Couples found creative solutions for relieving this sense of burden. Sometimes family members set up a rotating schedule of visiting to allow the caretaking spouse time away from the home. At other times church members became a care-team and actually spent one day a week caring for the person with ALS. Perhaps the greatest challenge was for the healthy spouses. They often felt guilty about taking time for themselves, believing that they shouldn't go to a movie or out with a friend. This type of rejuvenation is important because it renews not only the spirit but also the body, and in addition provides new experiences for conversation.

Severity of Disease

As one might expect, there was a relationship between psychological, social, and spiritual status and the severity of illness. Mildly ill patients had higher levels of well-being than moderately or severely ill patients; in particular, mildly ill patients were less depressed and perceived less stress. There was no difference, however, between psychological, social, and spiritual status in moderately ill and severely ill patients. Furthermore, for most people psychosocial-spiritual well-being did not necessarily decline during the 18 months of participation in the study. Although some patients did show increased distress, an equal number experienced an increase in well-being, and the majority remained at the same level of distress or well-being throughout the testing period.

Length of Illness

It is particularly enlightening to observe the study's findings about patients' psychological, social, and spiritual status in relation to the length of time they had been ill. The current assumption is that most ALS patients will die within three to five years after diagnosis and will have increasing feelings of depression, hopelessness, and perceived stress and an ever-decreasing purpose in life. Many patients had experiences like the woman whose neurologist recently told her, "You have a horrible disease, and if you're planning a vacation take it now, for soon you won't be able to."

However, studies now report five-year survival rates ranging from 18 percent to 42 percent, with many individuals surviving far longer than that (2–4). One study found that, "Other factors, such as the patient's will to live and the support of his family, play significant roles in extending his life" (5).

Of the 144 ALS patients who entered our study, 31 percent had already survived longer than five years. Overall, these long-term survivors exhibited greater psychological, social, and spiritual well-being than those with ALS for a shorter period of time, even though one of five was severely affected by the disease. Most saw a physician only rarely or had not seen one for years. "Why should I," many asked, "when the doctor told me I'd be dead years ago and there was nothing more he could do for me?"

These patients demonstrate that there is hope. Some cases of ALS progress very slowly and may even reverse, although this is extremely rare. In addition, there are patients with a normally or even rapidly progressing disease who maintain a healthy psychological, social, and spiritual status and have a quality of life far beyond what one might expect.

Rate of Decline

One factor that can strongly influence a patient's psychological, social, and spiritual well-being is rate of decline. In a patient whose disease is progressing rapidly, changes can occur so fast that there may be little opportunity to integrate the loss of one function before another is confronted. The phase of healthy denial of the disease, which can give an individual time to integrate the diagnosis and call upon her inner resources to deal with it, is not available to individuals who every day experience themselves losing more functional abilities.

What about the individual whose disease is progressing more slowly? It is commonly assumed that these patients experience greater psychological well-being than those who are declining rapidly. In our study, an unexpected finding was that patients who were moderately affected by ALS and who had had the disease 1.5 to 5 years were, as a group, in a state of psychosocial-spiritual distress that was exceeded only by that of severely ill patients who had had ALS less than 1.5 years. The surprise was that these moderately ill patients were in such a state of struggle. Could this be a critical time for psychological intervention? This distress was characterized by high levels of depression, hopelessness, and perceived stress and by low purpose in life. Patients in such distress need support from their families and their medical team.

This seems to be a crucial time that often goes unnoticed. It is a time when loss of abilities and changing roles may have the most devastating psychological-spiritual affect. Patients at this point could benefit from seeing a counselor or perhaps beginning to take a mild antidepressant. Family members can assist by helping the patient experience herself as a vital and important part of the family.

Use of a Respirator

As ALS progresses, the patient, spouse, family, and health care provider must face the question of whether to use a ventilator as a treatment to prolong life. Many health care providers have strong feelings (either pro or con) about respiratory support. They may forcefully encourage it or they may refrain from discussing it, depending on their personal belief. Their view often is based on experiences with a few patients or on their projection of what they themselves would do in that situation. Of the ALS patients we evaluated, only 24 percent said they would be willing to use a respirator. Little information has been available about how individuals on ventilators fare psychologically; however, while the prevalent assumption is that life on a ventilator must be psychologically distressing, research supports what could seem like the opposite conclusion (6–7); life is not without meaning and purpose for everyone in this situation (8).

Eighteen patients (12%) were on respirators when they entered our study. Contrary to expectation, as a group they were not more psychologically distressed than other ALS patients. They had similar levels of depression, loneliness, hopelessness, and perceived stress, and they considered their lives to have purpose and meaning. In addition, they had a more internal health locus of control than ALS patients who did not need ventilation. Although one might assume that only those individuals with a strong family support system would choose ventilatory support, we observed that patients electing to be placed on respirators included those who were dependent on hired caregivers as well as those with tight-knit families.

Being on a ventilator does not condemn a patient to a miserable life, devoid of purpose and isolated from friends and family. In fact, quite the opposite was true for many of the 18 patients in our study. Working with their families and health care practitioners, many of these individuals found life more satisfying than before they went on the respirator, one reason being that ventilatory support allowed them to leave the house and participate more fully in life.

Response to Nonphysical Challenges

In addition to physical challenges, ALS places other severe stresses on the patient and family. How these are dealt with ultimately affects the patient's quality of life and sense of well-being.

Isolation

Individuals with ALS often experience ever-increasing isolation from family, friends, events of the world, and nature. Many have decreasing numbers of visitors just at the time when they are less able to get out of the house. This was true for 40 percent of the patients in our study.

One of the most effective ways to decrease the sense of isolation is to have a good support system. The more people involved in a support system, the greater the support is thought to be. However, many participants in the study expressed satisfaction with their support system even though it involved just a few people. The number of people involved does not seem to matter as much as whether the patient perceives that support is being offered.

The family and friends of a person with ALS can be supportive in many ways. As functional abilities decrease, some people lose their sense of purpose in life. Those who continue to participate in activities with their family, friends, and coworkers relate that their lives still have purpose and meaning. The family can find ways to involve the patient more in their lives, no matter how severely affected he may be by ALS. This may include making the extra effort to take him on family outings, seeking his input on family decisions, keeping him apprised of happenings in each family member's life, and discovering how his many gifts can still be given.

Another way to decrease isolation is to keep channels of communication open. Nowadays we are using the Internet to keep in touch with family and friends and to "talk" with other people with ALS. The most challenging time comes when speech is severely affected. Patience and creativity on the part of family and friends is crucial at this time. One family learned Morse code (the father with ALS already knew it) to keep open communication lines. In another family the wife and home care nurse could easily read the patient's lips and became his voice.

Embarrassment

Living in a culture that values physical perfection, a person with ALS may feel embarrassed or ashamed by the condition of his body and therefore be reluctant to appear in public. For many people, the main social event is a visit to the clinic or doctor's office. Some patients stopped going to church (16% in our study), and only a small percentage (19% in our study) participated in support groups.

Reassurance of one's attractiveness was the best way to overcome this sense of loss. It is important to remember how people like their hair fixed or if they enjoy wearing fingernail or toenail polish, putting on make-up, or shaving (or letting the beard grow). These are just a few suggestions on how to help someone continue to feel good about his or her appearance. All of this takes time, yet it can add immeasurably to quality of life.

Loss of Traditional Roles

Over time people with ALS may no longer be able to function in roles that once defined their lives and their sense of purpose. The "breadwinner" can no longer work; the person accustomed to cooking can only watch someone else do it. A patient may begin to question her competence as a spouse, parent, friend, or lover, and family relationships may become a source of stress rather than support.

Several couples did not want to fall into the "patient-caregiver" roles. They worked to maintain their husband-wife partnership. This meant that intimacy was important. Once again, creativity surfaced. Perhaps they could no longer make love as they used to, but they could still touch, kiss, and hold one another. Another important aspect was including the ill partner in decision making. The more this was done, the less was the pain of loss over changing roles.

Financial Worry

Worries about money often increase dramatically when someone has ALS. Being a burden on others can be the most difficult aspect of the disease; this was true for 12 percent of the patients in the study.

There were no easy answers to dealing with this worry. The most effective strategy was communication. It would often lessen if the patient felt informed about and included in financial decisions. However, there were times when the well partner thought it would be detrimental for the person with ALS to be aware of their overall financial picture. The irony of this situation was that the patient would often confide how he knew finances were bad but did not want his spouse to know that he knew. This need to protect each other can add strain and burden that decreases quality of life and increases stress and anxiety for everyone.

Loss of Genuine Leisure

Most participants in our study also felt that their lives were devoid of leisure, despite the fact that they watched an average of four hours of television every day. Evidently no part of the day was experienced as leisurely, that is, devoted to having fun and participating in activities that would truly distract them from their disease.

Ingenuity was the answer. One family instituted joke time. On Monday nights they would gather together simply to tell jokes, relate stories, or sing funny songs. Even when Dad could no longer communicate, he still enjoyed these evenings. Another couple had a time every week when they invited friends in to see a movie, and, of course, popcorn was provided.

The Role of the Spouse

Amyotrophic lateral sclerosis is a disease that affects the entire family and can have profound physical and psychosocial-spiritual consequences for the well spouse in particular. As a group, the psychosocial-spiritual profile of spouses was similar to the norm for the general adult population except that they had higher depression scores (although much lower than patients had) and experienced a greater degree of loneliness. Many spouses were clearly experiencing psychosocial-spiritual distress. Approximately 15 percent felt profoundly hopeless and were moderately to severely depressed, 23 percent experienced a high degree of loneliness, and 47 percent perceived a high degree of stress in their lives.

Isolation

Many spouses curtailed their volunteer work and church or community activities to stay home and care for the person with ALS. The number of spouses doing volunteer work decreased from almost half before diagnosis to a third at the time the study began. The percentage of those not attending church almost doubled. Such changes can lead to a sense of isolation and loneliness, loss of sense of self, and resentment toward the ill spouse. Fortunately, most spouses reported that they had an outlet for their emotions and were able to have some amount of time alone.

One of the best ways to decrease isolation is to have a community of family and friends on which to draw. The experience of ALS can bring family and friends closer. While some friends may drift away, many others may want to deepen their friendship. Any number of friends can become an integral part of the family life, lending their skills to design and implement assistive devices, being there to listen, and relieving the spouse from the demands of physical care so that he or she can have some personal time. This type of partnership greatly diminishes a sense of isolation.

Loss of Traditional Roles

Many changes take place over time in the spouse's daily life. When the patient's traditional roles in the family alter with the decrease in functional ability, these roles must be taken on by the spouse or other family members. Careers may need to be suspended. Wives may have to undertake everything from managing household finances to mowing the lawn for the first time in their lives; husbands may find themselves chief cook, dishwasher, and child-rearer. Everyone in the family system will probably experience changes in the roles they play.

It is vital to talk about the experience of these changing roles. Open communication is one way to keep this from being a burden or from feeling as if unwanted demands are being placed on you. If you, as the healthy spouse, can keep your wife or husband in the decision-making process, this will increase the sense of partnership and decrease the experience of isolation.

Financial Worry

A reduction in income coincided with soaring medical costs for many families, which greatly increased the occurrence of financial difficulties. Before the onset of ALS, only 3 percent of the spouses described themselves as "very worried" about money, whereas 18 percent were "very worried" after its onset. Some spouses (9% in the study) took on a job to meet their family's financial obligations, often at a time when they were increasingly needed at home.

Many spouses sought financial advice from a lawyer or trusted financial consultant. It was also important for a number of families to work with the social services department of the hospital. Both of these strategies lowered the stress related to financial worries.

Loss of Genuine Leisure

A number of spouses spoke of their sense of guilt whenever they engaged in an activity they enjoyed. On the other hand, several people spoke of their sadness that their spouses were no longer doing things they enjoyed, such as playing tennis, going to their reading club, or participating in church activities. Once again, communication is the key. Spouses can share their experience of playing tennis, going to a movie, or having dinner with a friend and thus enable their ill spouse to be part of the adventure.

The Spouse-Patient Relationship

Many factors affect the spouse-patient relationship during the course of ALS. These include changes in roles, differing experiences of the disease, the tendency for the patient and the spouse to experience emotional difficulties at different stages of the disease process, dissimilar perceptions of the patient's illness experience, and the presence or lack of family support.

Loss of Traditional Roles

The changes in roles necessitated by the decreased functional abilities of the person with ALS can lead to an unrecognized and unacknowledged shift in the relationship between spouse and patient—from that of husband-wife to that of caregiver-patient. The husband-wife relationship needs to be nurtured and maintained for the psychosocial-spiritual well-being of both patient and spouse.

The couple can accomplish this by having other people help with physical care and by continuing to enjoy previously shared activities, such as seeing movies, playing cards, watching sunsets, having sex, or going to the park.

Couples who reported having high-quality lives despite ALS said that living was the center of their lives—not ALS. We found that couples who were successful in living fully and maintaining their relationship saw the disease as a shared experience and were able to communicate well enough so that resentment, guilt, or other negative emotions did not build up over time.

Experiences of the Disease

The stressful aspects of living with ALS may be quite different for the patient than for the spouse. Eighty-three percent of the spouses listed health issues as their major stressor, as opposed to only 55 percent of the patients. Many patients (12%) were most concerned about financial matters, while only a few spouses (2%) listed finances as their primary stressor. It is easy to see how communication difficulties can arise when the spouse wants to talk about the patient's health at a time when his attention is focused on financial concerns, or when the spouse is preoccupied with coping with the disease while the patient is wanting to focus on living, not on his illness. In fact, relationships themselves were a major stressor for many patients (18%) and spouses (12%).

As a group, the spouses in the study were more lonely than the patients. The spouses, having given up such previous activities as pursuing a career, luncheons with friends, or competing on a bowling team, often felt house-bound. At the same time they were reluctant to leave the house because the patient could not. This sense of loneliness and isolation sometimes escalates to resentment and guilt. It is important for the spouse to maintain activities with friends to help lessen the experience of loneliness. The patient who encourages his spouse to take time away often finds that the spouse has more to give to him, not less.

Spouses may want to be more involved in the health care plan than the patient does. A spouse sometimes tries to talk with a patient about his research into ALS and cannot understand why his ill partner does not want to know more about the disease. Or the spouse may want an in-depth explanation from the physician of all the phases and complications of ALS that her ill partner will probably encounter, along with a discussion of the various forms of supportive treatment available, while the patient has no interest in participating in this process. The opposite also may be true: the spouse may simply want to be told what to do to help his partner without taking part in any decision making. Such different approaches to illness are simply part of human nature; respecting these differences is a key to maintaining a loving husband-wife relationship.

Timing of Psychosocial-Spiritual Distress

One of the most important findings in our study was that patient and spouse often experienced psychosocial-spiritual distress at very different stages of the illness. The couple may expect to experience the stress of ALS in the same manner at the same time—that is, if the patient is depressed and lonely, he may assume that his spouse is having similar feelings.

Sometimes this is true, but many times the patient may be experiencing distress while the spouse is not. Or the patient may be feeling a sense of well-being and be unaware that his spouse is feeling hopeless and lonely. Such differences can lead to friction or misunderstanding. It is essential to acknowledge to your spouse and health care professional how you are actually feeling, and it is equally important for the spouse to refrain from assuming how the person with ALS is feeling and "talking" for him to the health care professional. It is also important to be sensitive to how your spouse is feeling. Friction and feelings of isolation can develop if you and your spouse are having very different emotional experiences and have not developed skills in listening to and understanding each other. Learning the art of listening can increase understanding, tolerance, and love. The help of a qualified counselor can be invaluable in such a situation.

Differing Perceptions of the Patient's Experience

The spouse often perceives the experience of the person with ALS very differently from how he or she experiences himself, which can complicate your whole realm of mutual understanding and communication. Spouses in our study tended to rate their ill partner's level of life satisfaction lower than the ill partner rated it—a very interesting finding. Spouses' ratings of the patient's self-acceptance and acceptance of help often were very much lower than the patient's own evaluation. Spouses also thought that patients were more worried about money than patients themselves reported. Furthermore, the spouses believed the patients were not as honest in communicating how they felt as the patients reported they were.

Many dynamics can play a role in these differences. For example, the patient may be in denial, not ready to acknowledge or accept the current reality of her life. In addition, both patient and spouse may perceive their partners through the filter of their own emotional state—which, as noted earlier, may be quite different from that of their mate. It is important to remember that rarely can one individual accurately know the psychospiritual state of another. Too often, we project how we think we would feel if we were in that particular situation. It is easy to project feelings of hopelessness, depression, anger, and guilt onto others, but it is important to remember that these feelings do not have to be the baseline from which we live each day.

Relationships with Health Care Professionals

Health care professionals can be an important part of your "wellness team." Even though they cannot alter the progressive disability encountered in this disease, they can provide symptomatic treatment, and they can help you and your family maintain a high quality of life throughout the illness. This can happen in many ways. Nearly 60 percent of the patients in our study had some degree of depression, for example, but many severely ill people are happy or only mildly depressed. Depression can be assessed and, if appropriate, the patient can be offered counseling and/or antidepressant medication. Alleviating depression can greatly improve the quality of life. In addition, it is becoming increasingly clear that alleviating depression enhances the body's immune system, thus contributing to slowing the rate of decline in many diseases.

The better the patient and spouse can communicate their desires, the better assistance the health care team can provide. For example, you both can express how active a role you want in planning for care. Do you want to be told what to do, or would you like to be an active part of the decision-making process? How much information does each of you want about ALS, drug trials, and support groups?

A patient and spouse may want different levels of participation. If the person with ALS has a high external health locus of control, she may not want to be given multiple options for symptomatic support or treatment; rather, she may want the health care team to be directive, telling her the course of action to be taken and demonstrating how she can most accurately follow instructions. On the other hand, if the patient has a highly developed internal health locus of control, she will often study the disease and learn about options for experimental treatments or alternative therapies. Telling her what to do without giving her information and options may lead to conflict between the health care professional and the patient. She wants the health care professional to be a team member who facilitates decision making but recognizes that the patient will have the final say. The level of involvement is not the point; what matters is that there is clear communication and mutual respect.

There are many things that those who wish to play an active role in their health care can do. Both patient and spouse will benefit by preparing beforehand for their visit to their primary physician or clinic. You might list your concerns and questions and, if you are attending a clinic, make a separate list for each team member (the dietitian, the speech therapist, etc.). When you are well informed, you will be able to grapple more effectively with difficult questions about life support and other treatment options. You can also make your needs known to the health care team and offer suggestions. For example, you might want a medication to dry up secretions, or a patient and spouse or whole family might want a referral to a counselor to learn better techniques for coping and communicating.

If you and your spouse do not feel a rapport with their primary physician or are not being accepted as part of the team, you can change physicians. The late Dr. Forbes Norris, a leading ALS neurologist, reminds us to "never forget that the patient is in charge throughout the illness."

The spouse can also ask the health care team for assistance for herself. At times a spouse may need counseling, psychotherapy, or treatment for depression. The health care team can also explain available home care options, such as hospice care, respite care, and home health aides. Family members or even friends can be trained to care for the patient. This can help a spouse to avoid feeling trapped or abandoned. In addition, the spouse can also ask where to seek financial assistance, apply for disability, and locate needed assistive devices.

Leading a High-Quality Life

People with ALS and their families can do more than merely cope. As the ALS Patient Profile Project clearly shows, it is possible to maintain a life of quality and dignity even in the face of massive physical, mental, emotional, and spiritual challenges. Those who managed to establish and maintain psychological, social, and spiritual well-being had a lower risk of dying and a longer survival time than patients who experienced psychological distress.

For some patients and their families, maintaining a sense of well-being may evolve naturally in the process of learning to cope with the disease. For others, it may be a step-by-step process of understanding and discovery requiring extensive support from family, friends, and the health care team. For people suffering from ALS, there seem to be eight keys to developing or sustaining the sense of well-being associated with living a high-quality life. These include:

1. Maintaining a sense of hope—hope not necessarily in the sense of believing that "They'll find a cure," but in knowing what research is happening, in participating in clinical trials when possible, and most of all in recognizing that life can still be meaningful and rewarding in spite of nearly overwhelming obstacles.

2. Drawing on your own inner strength and maintaining a sense of purpose and meaning.

3. Sustaining or developing a nurturing support system.

4. Shifting from a focus on the effects of ALS to a focus on sharing a life that is meaningful to you, your family, and the other people who are important to them.

5. Developing an understanding and respect for others and communicating thoughts and feelings effectively with them.

6. Maintaining and creating family and social activities in which the person with ALS can participate.

7. Enlisting the support of the health care team.

8. Maintaining a willingness to seek treatment or counseling if needed for patient, spouse, or family.

Amyotrophic lateral sclerosis affects every facet of life for everyone involved; individually and collectively you must meet physical, mental, emotional, and spiritual challenges. The ALS Patient Profile Project allowed us to scientifically examine the ways in which people meet those challenges. We came to understand the important role of psychological well-being in establishing and maintaining a high quality of life for the person with the disease, his spouse, and the family. This knowledge can help you understand why tensions may develop and why it is vital to communicate about them. In addition, it can expand and enhance the care provided by health care professionals.

References

1. McDonald ER, Wiedenfeld SA, Hillel A, Carpenter CL, Walter RA. Survival in amyotrophic lateral sclerosis: The role of psychological factors. *Arch Neurol* 1994; 51:17–23.
2. Rosen AD. Amyotrophic lateral sclerosis: Clinical features and prognosis. *Arch Neurol* 1978; 35:638–642.
3. Mortara P, Chio A, Rosso MG, Leone M, Schiffer D. Motor neuron disease in the province of Turin, Italy, 1966–1980: Survival analysis in an unselected population. *J Neurol Sci* 1984, 66:165–173.
4. Caroscio JT, Mulvihill MN, Sterling R, Abram B. Amyotrophic lateral sclerosis: Its natural history. *Neurol Clin* 1987; 5:1–8.
5. Mulder DW, Howard FM. Patient resistance and prognosis in amyotrophic lateral sclerosis. *Mayo Clin Proc* 1976: 51:537–541.
6. Moss AH, Casey P, Stocking CB, et al. Home ventilation for amyotrophic lateral sclerosis patients: Outcomes, costs, and patient, family, and physician attitudes. *Neurology* 1993: 43:438–443.
7. Bromberg MB, Forshew DA, Iaderosa S, McDonald ER. Ventilator dependency in ALS: Management, disease progression, and issues of coping. *J Neuro Rehab* 1996; 10:195–216.
8. McDonald ER, Hillel A, Wiedenfeld SA. Evaluation of the psychological status of ventilator-supported patients with ALS/MND. *Palliative Med* 1996; 10:35–41.

24

Quality of Life Issues and Treatment Goals

Maura L. Del Bene, M.S., R.N., NP-P

"The manner in which an individual faces life-threatening disease and obtains support from others reflects the shared beliefs and values of the particular culture, society and treating health care team" (1).

People with amyotrophic lateral sclerosis (ALS) face challenges of muscle weakness that are continually symptomatic and progressive. The course of illness requires constant adaptation to interventions needed to control symptoms, organizing the health care team and family system for support and care, and adjusting the family and health care team's roles as the disease progresses. For example, at the time of diagnosis, the neurologist is the primary team member in the patient's plan of care, but when respiratory weakness begins, the primary care provider may be the pulmonologist, and the family may need to take a more active role in the person's care because of symptoms of fatigue and the use of medical support to assist with the respiratory weakness.

As a progressive terminal disease, ALS may create an undercurrent of anticipatory grief and a sense of impending doom. The disease reduces quality of life (QOL) and impairs the ability of both patient and caregivers to carry out a medical-psychosocial plan of care. The optimal care of people with any progressive disease includes attention to both psychosocial and medical needs, with the goal of maintaining or improving QOL (2).

Although promoting and maintaining quality of life for people with ALS is a primary concern of health care practitioners, only a few studies have assessed how people with ALS define quality of life (3).

There is no adequate test to assess quality of life in ALS. The available QOL tests do not include the patient's perceptions (4). They are broad and not individualized for people in different stages of the disease, do not distinguish among the physical symptoms of ALS that affect QOL scores, and do not identify factors that respond to specific interventions. To assess an individual's quality of life, it is essential to understand the perceived stressors of living with the disease as experienced by each patient and caregiver.

Effects of Disease on Quality of Life

Any chronic progressive illness has a profound effect on both the person with the disease and his or her family (5). The ultimate stress of living with illness results from several factors, including the disease, the individual's unique approach to life, and the influence of the multidisciplinary health care team (6).

The assumption is usually made that specific medical or psychosocial stressors (as identified by patient and caregiver) may lead to symptomatic discomfort from the illness. Addressing these stressors through specific interventions may therefore increase your capacity to adapt to the disease and participate in your plan of care.

Symptoms of ALS cause severe physical disability because of general muscle weakness and psychological distress related to the progressive, terminal nature of the disease. How these symptoms influence you as an individual is unique and personal, and dealing with them requires critical assessment of your own disease-related stressor.

Quality of Life

Quality of life is a multidimensional concept that includes physical functioning, psychosocial well-being, socioeconomic condition, emotional well-being, family functioning, symptom distress, and spiritual well-being (7). Most important, however, it is a subjective statement of the positive or negative attributes of your life. The following section identifies the dimensions of quality of life in ALS and the development of a plan of care.

Dimension of Physical Functioning

The physical symptoms of ALS have a major effect on QOL. The pattern of weakness is unique for each person, and dealing with them presents one of the greatest challenges to those diagnosed with ALS. Changes in physical functioning affect not only your personal independence but also your perception of self and how you participate in social, personal, and professional activities.

It is widely believed that the multidisciplinary model of care in an ALS center provides the highest level of coordination to promote functioning and independence. These interventions affect a person's ability to participate in various aspects of life for a greater period throughout the disease course (personal observation).

Dimension of Psychosocial Well-Being

The psychological impact of ALS affects all aspects of QOL. It affects your ability to cope with and adapt to the progression of the disease. It includes depression, anxiety, emotional lability, and changes in interpersonal relationships.

Although health care professionals assume that depression and anxiety are very common in any disease of a progressive nature with no known cure, this is not necessarily true in ALS (8). Symptoms of depression may include sadness, anxiety, loss of interest, loss of pleasure, and decreased appetite. For a formal diagnosis of clinical depression, according to the *Diagnostic and Statistical Manual of Mental Disorders IV (DSM-IV)*, these symptoms must be pervasive, present more days than not, and present for most of the day. In a study of depression and ALS now being conducted at the Eleanor and Lou Gehrig MDA/ALS Center, only 10 percent of patients meet these criteria for clinical depression (8).

Most people with ALS express sadness in response to progressive loss of physical functions. They have an uncertain future and often avoid discussing the terminal stages of the disease. This is not depression, but rather is considered a reactive mood syndrome, a normal reaction to a distressing situation. An evaluation by a mental health professional (psychiatrist or mental health nurse practitioner) may assist you and your health care providers to distinguish between depression and reactive mood syndromes and thus determine appropriate intervention. Mood symptoms, when serious, can be treated aggressively with psychopharmacologic drugs. Untreated clinical depression can severely affect the ability to adapt and cope and adversely affect participation in the plan of care.

The emotional responses of the person living with ALS often change in different phases of the disease. The ability to adapt throughout the disease is of utmost importance to everyone concerned with managing the disease.

Emotional lability is often confused with depression. Emotional lability is a syndrome of ease of laughing or crying that is not in concert with one's mood. Also referred to as "pseudobulbar affect," lability is a neurochemical response seen in people who have upper motor neuron signs, and often with dysarthria and dysphagia. For example, talking about the birth of a grandchild is often emotional, yet the individual experiencing lability will cry inconsolably and appear distraught, although they may in fact feel happiness and report no feelings of sadness. Emotional lability also applies to laughing. Emotional lability may have a negative effect on social or professional activities. Tricyclic antidepressants in low doses often provide effective treatment.

Dimension of Social Functioning

Interpersonal relationships may be one of the most important factors in maintaining quality of life at any stage of ALS. The support a person with ALS requires and receives from family members, friends, and health care professionals varies in different stages of the disease. Maintaining open communication, establishing trust, and accepting the assistance of others are all essential components. It often is these relationships that serve as the foundation on which an individual's ability to adapt, cope, and face the challenges of ALS is built.

Patients and family members often benefit from participation in family-based therapy to assist the family as a unit to understand preillness coping mechanisms and how to apply these mechanisms in the presence of illness. This functional form of short-term therapy can facilitate communication and increase your understanding of how your family unit as a whole can cope with the disease. Most important, it can help mobilize the family to maintain a sense of normalcy and develop a mutual support.

Dimension of Spiritual Functioning

A personal yet important aspect of life that can easily be overlooked is the spiritual dimension. As a form of coping, spirituality draws from the attitudes, beliefs, or practice that animate your life. Spirituality does not necessarily imply a belief in God or participation in structured religious activities.

Spirituality affects not only coping with illness but also the decision-making process throughout a disease. In a study of 46 individuals with ALS, Murphy and colleagues (9) found that people with a higher degree of spirituality were more likely to have completed advance directives, were less likely to have gastrostomy, were less fearful of death and dying, were less likely to participate in support groups, and were more likely to choose a natural death than the intervention of mechanical ventilation (9). Most important, spirituality may play an essential role in easing the adaptation to a serious diagnosis and the transitions of life that occur in the dying process.

Dimensions of Socioeconomic Issues

The financial issues of ALS can be devastating. They are one of the outstanding problems within health care in the United States (10).

Specialized equipment to meet the growing needs of the patient is often not recognized as medically necessary by insurance companies. For example, an augmentative communication device can enhance QOL, allow some people to continue working, help participate in the medical care plan, and foster interaction with family, friends, and caregivers; however, it is not allowed by most or all insurance companies.

Managed health care has dramatically changed the climate of living with illness. Insurance support and services to individuals living with ALS is less than optimal. ALS care is defined by insurance companies as "custodial" because improvement is not expected. This definition is an immediate barrier to receiving home care services. The need for home care services is often high for ALS patients. The increasing difficulty with activities of daily living and the need for supervision and safety are not covered under the terms of custodial care. Families are faced with the stress of balancing the personal needs of the patient, the financial costs of private home care, and the necessity of the primary caregiver to continue working to maintain income.

This type of dependency usually is not incorporated into the average person's planning. Long-term care insurance may be helpful, but only a small percentage of people invest in this form of insurance. Purchase of such a policy is impossible after the diagnosis has been made. Medicare is accessible only after two years of disability, and even then home care eligibility falls under the custodial terminology and is therefore limited. Medicaid (for only the individual diagnosed) is an option but requires a limited amount of assets.

Dimension of Disease Management

Multidisciplinary teams of ALS practitioners are located throughout the United States in ALS specialty centers. The centers may be sponsored by the Muscular Dystrophy Association, the ALS Association, or independent ALS Foundation, or they may be independent practices. ALS families need to evaluate local resources and consider the following attributes of the center: years of experience in ALS, availability of a multidisciplinary team, participation in clinical trials, and general support to the patient and family.

The comprehensive medical and psychosocial care provided at experienced ALS centers affects QOL. Knowing when, where, why, and how often to accept or implement recommendations for medication, clinical trials, rehabilitation, respiratory support, or feeding tube placement is best accomplished in this multidisciplinary setting.

One of the benefits of the ALS center is continuing education about disease progression and management. The patient and family can maintain a level of control by participating in the management of symptoms. This is done through regularly scheduled meetings with the ALS team and ALS educational support groups.

Role of the Health Care Team

The unique manner in which ALS starts and progresses in each person is an essential component in assessing QOL. The health care practitioner must have a keen understanding of ALS pathology, prognosis, and critical pathways to provide optimal symptom control. Understanding the financial and psychosocial resources of the patient and his or her family system is also integral to the team's holistic understanding and care of the patient, as well as the educational program to promote informed decisions.

Working within a context of palliative medicine (see Chapter 28), the plan of care is geared toward alleviating symptoms, as well as achieving and maintaining your maximum physical and psychological well-being. Within the ALS center, you will interact with several members of the health care team on any given day throughout the course of the disease.

You need to understand the goals of each intervention offered by the team, and the information should be woven into the comprehensive plan of care. Counseling and discussion of how this plan may benefit you throughout the disease will result in a better ongoing relationship and your increased participation in the care process.

The ALS nurse clinician acts as the bridge between disciplines within the multidisciplinary team. She coordinates the recommendations made by members of the health care team in relation to your specific needs, promoting integration of the team–patient relationship. This results in positive patient outcomes and higher QOL.

If you do not understand an intervention, you are less apt to accept it and therefore less likely to benefit from it. People with ALS and their families have developed a sophisticated Internet connection, where a broad base of information is available about symptom management and treatment of the disease. The Internet now offers an option for self-navigation through the course of ALS. The health care team can validate new information and answer your questions based on information obtained on the Internet in relation to your particular problems, available interventions, possible benefits, and QOL.

It is crucial that the health care professionals who work with you understand and predict your capacity to adapt. They can then knowledgeably and deliberately select those interventions that will increase your adaptive capacities. Only in this way can individualized, appropriate care be effectively and economically provided to you in a way that affects the quality of your life.

References

1. Starr P. *The social transformation of American medicine: The rise of sovereign profession and the making of a vast industry.* New York: Basic Books, 1982.
2. Murphy PL, Del Bene ML, Albert, SA. Multidisciplinary integrated psychosocial and palliative care. In: Younger DS (ed.). *Motor disorders.* Philadelphia: Lippincott, Williams & Wilkins, 1999.
3. Swash M. Health outcome and quality of life measurements in amyotrophic lateral sclerosis. *J Neurol* 1997; 244 (Suppl 2):S26–S29.

4. Miller RG, Anderson F. Assessing quality of life in ALS: Comparison of the Short Form-12 Health Survey with the ALS Functional Rating Scale, forced vital capacity, and ALS Quality of Life Index. Poster Presented at the International MND/ALS Conference. Glasgow, Scotland, 1997.
5. Shaw MC, Halliday PH. The family, crisis and chronic illness: An evolutionary model. *J Adv Nurs* 1992; 17:537–543.
6. Leidy N, Ozbolt J, Swain MA. Psychological processes of stress in chronic physical illness: A theoretical perspective. *J Adv Nurs* 1990; 15:478–486.
7. Dibble SL, Padilla GV, Dodd MJ, Miaskowski C. Gender differences in the dimensions of quality of life. *Oncol Nurs Forum* 1998; 25:577–583.
8. Rabkin JG, Wagner GJ, Del Bene ML. Resilience and distress among amyotrophic lateral sclerosis patients and caregivers. *Psychosom Med* 1999 (in press).
9. Murphy PL, Albert SA, Weber C, Del Bene ML, Rowland LP. Impact of spirituality and religiousness on outcomes in patients with amyotrophic lateral sclerosis. 1998. *Neurology* 2000 (in press).
10. Newby NM. Chronic illness and the family life cycle. *J Adv Nurs* 1996; 23:786–791.

25

Legal and Ethical Issues

Susan J. Stagno, M.D.

The fact that you are reading this book probably means that either you have amyotrophic lateral sclerosis (ALS) or care for someone who does. It also is likely to mean that you are interested in learning all you can about the disease, its management, and what you can do to help yourself or someone else.

Amyotrophic lateral sclerosis can be a devastating diagnosis because there currently is no available cure and the disease slowly erodes a person's physical function. However, much can be done to ensure a good quality of life with ALS and help one maintain as much control as possible. It is important to know that you have rights and can control the decisions made about management of your illness.

This chapter focuses on the legal and ethical issues important for patients with ALS, such as advance directives (the living will and durable power of attorney for health care), decision making, patient rights, forgoing interventions such as ventilators or feeding tubes, as well as assisted suicide and euthanasia. Relevant information about the law is included in each section. However, the information in this chapter should not be substituted for or regarded as legal advice.

Many of the legal and ethical concerns regarding the care of people with ALS arise in the context of end-of-life decisions. Therefore, this chapter discusses death and dying. If you are not yet comfortable with this aspect of ALS, you may want to reserve this chapter for a later time.

Adjusting to the Diagnosis

The first and most important thing to do when being told you have ALS is to be certain that the diagnosis is correct. Because the prognosis associated with ALS is so poor, it is crucial to be sure that the symptoms that brought you to the attention of a physician are in fact due to ALS. The clinical features and diagnostic process are described elsewhere in this book. Once the diagnosis has been ascertained, it will be important to learn as much as you feel comfortable with to better understand the disease, its process, and the decisions that will need to be made over time.

Gathering Information About ALS

It is not uncommon for a person to react to a diagnosis such as ALS with fear, sadness, anger, and panic. These are perfectly normal reactions to hearing bad news. A useful way to deal with these feelings is to get information about the disease and its management, especially the things you can do about it and the choices you can make. People tend to feel most anxious when they do not know what to expect or do not have enough factual information. By gathering this information, you will be able to decrease your anxiety, deal more effectively with your health care providers, and be more in control of the course of your illness. Chapter 32 of this book provides a compendium of information and resources regarding ALS support groups, treatment programs, research organizations, and other education materials.

Your Relationship with Your Doctor

The relationship with your doctor is crucial as you plan, make decisions, and outline goals of treatment. Some people would like to have their doctor make most of the major decisions because the doctor is experienced and knowledgeable about the disease, its progress, and the options available. However, most people with ALS want to have as much information as possible and want to be active participants in medical care decisions. They also want to discuss with their health care provider issues such as life-sustaining therapies, including the use of mechanical ventilation and cardiopulmonary resuscitation (1). Most people would like to be in a relationship with their doctor that is more of a partnership. The person who is ill is interested in being a recipient of the physician's experience, knowledge, and expertise, as well as taking advantage of those things the health care system has to offer that can help one to enjoy an improved quality of life and positively impact the disease process. The stage of the illness, one's personal values and goals, family situation, and other factors will all be significant influences in treatment decisions. It is very important early in the relationship with the physician to be clear about how decisions will be made, who will be making them, and what factors (medical, social, financial, religious, etc.) will influence these decisions. If you think that the doctor you are working with is not able or willing to take your values and goals into account in a way that you feel comfortable with, you should discuss this with the doctor. This may not be easy to do, as many people worry that if they challenge their doctor's advice or judgment, they may be rejected or may not enjoy the same kind of relationship with him that they had before the discussion. However, raising the issue in the context of reviewing treatment decisions with the doctor to clarify one's position can be a way of initiating the discussion. If a resolution cannot be reached, discussing the problem with a patient advocate (such as an ombudsman) or ethics consultant may be of benefit. If this does not resolve the situation, you may want to seek care from another physician.

Discussing Values and Decision Making

The most effective way to be sure that your physician understands the values that are important to you is to have a clear and frank discussion with him or her. Interestingly, data from a study done at the Mayo Clinic (1) show that only about one of eight patients with ALS discussed the issue of life-sustaining care with their physician, despite the fact that 81 percent said that they thought their physician wanted to know their preferences on this issue. In this same study, about half the patients with ALS indicated that they would like to discuss life-sustaining care with someone on their health care team. Many wanted the physician to raise the subject.

On the other hand, physicians are often reluctant to bring up end-of-life decision-making issues because they are concerned that this may frighten the patient or may take away a patient's hope. Some doctors may think that they already know what would be best for their patients and choose not to bring up the issue. However, problems can occur when an acute situation arises. Under these circumstances, decisions must be made rapidly and are often made in the direction of very aggressive care (such as intubation or performing cardiopulmonary resuscitation) when that may not have been what the patient wanted. When this happens, the health care team often turns to family members to make decisions when the patient is too ill to participate. If the family members have not been included in discussions, they will not know how to proceed. One of the greatest gifts a person can give to relatives or other people with whom they have a significant relationship is to reduce the burden of such onerous decision making by indicating how they would want his or her medical care to proceed. Families are much more comfortable carrying out the patient's wishes than trying to make a decision on behalf of another without knowing his or her values (2). Family members may makes choices based on what they think they would want if they were under the same circumstances. They may make decisions to provide aggressive care based on feelings that their ill family member would "want every chance to survive" or even out of feelings of guilt.

A useful vehicle for making preferences known and providing a good mechanism for initiating a discussion about end-of-life decisions is the advance directive. This is discussed more fully later in this chapter.

Optimizing Your Life with ALS

How is it possible to talk about optimizing one's life in the face of a chronic, progressive illness such as ALS? Every one of us must face our mortality, and there are a number of encouraging examples and stories associated with people who have ALS. Consider the lives of Lou Gehrig, Steven W. Hawking (Lucasian Professor of Mathematics at the University of Cambridge, England), Morrie Schwartz (Sociology Professor at Brandeis University and subject of the book *Tuesdays with Morrie*), Justice Sam N. Filer (Canadian lawyer and Judge, Ontario Court of Justice) (3), and many others. It obviously is not expected that everyone will be as inspirational to society as they are, but it is true that each of us in facing death can recognize and celebrate the value of life. In the words of Morrie Schwartz, "Learn how to live and you'll know how to die; learn how to die, and you'll know how to live."

How can a person with ALS feel hopeful about the future? At each stage in our lives, we are all hopeful about different things. As children, we are hopeful about whether we will get what we asked for as a birthday gift or that we will get good grades at school. As young adults, we are hopeful that we will find a meaningful relationship with another person with whom we can share our life, perhaps have children, and enjoy our work. In middle age, our focus turns more toward whether our lives have been meaningful and how we can leave a legacy for those who will follow us. As we approach the end of our lives, whenever that comes, hope centers on the meaningful connections with people we love, a sense of spiritual serenity, and hope that our death will come peacefully and without pain and that we will not be alone. In adjusting to an illness such as ALS, hope may initially lie in science finding a cure or perhaps in thinking that the doctor's diagnosis was wrong. However, as one begins to accept the diagnosis and adapt to the illness, hope shifts to maintaining as much independence as possible, being able to communicate with those around us, spending meaningful time with those we love, and taking pleasure from our surroundings and things we enjoy. At the end of illness, most hope that their care will not be too burdensome to those doing the caregiving and that death will come peacefully and painlessly. As Robert Frost once said, "Hope does not lie in a way out, but in a way through."

An important study (4) examined the role of psychological functioning and survival in ALS. A total of 144 people with ALS in varying stages and severity of illness agreed to participate in a project that included both physical and psychological assessments done at three-month intervals over the course of a year and a half. The psychological assessments included a variety of standardized instruments that measure mood, stress, loneliness, anger expression, social supports, coping, and sense of purpose in life. This battery of instruments included some tests that had been used with people who had other serious illnesses and have been shown to be related to survival. The findings from this study demonstrate that people who have lower levels of psychological distress live longer—and not just a little longer! The median survival time for people who had low levels of distress was more than 1,200 days, for those in the mid-range group it was 609 days, and for people who high levels of psychological distress it was 333 days. The likelihood of this kind of outcome occurring by chance is less than 1 in 1,000. The risk of dying associated with psychological distress was even greater than the risk associated with older age and about equal to that of disease severity. You may think that the reason for these findings is because people with higher levels of distress are those who were the sickest or closest to dying, but this was not the case. There was no major (statistical) difference in the three groups as far as length of illness or severity of illness was concerned. The authors of this paper caution that although psychological status appears to be a strong predictive factor of survival, it should not be used as a "psychological barometer" to predict survival time for a single individual.

Living *longer* does not always equate with living *well*. What is important for most is living as well as you can for as long as you can, taking advantage of the times when you are feeling well. Making the most of the good times includes feeling useful and involved in things; staying connected to people who are important, reconnecting with old friends or making new ones, attaining a sense of spiritual peace, and accepting death as a part of life. Medical care that is focused on optimizing physical and emotional functioning, relieving distressing symptoms, and knowing that the type and direction of the medical care will be consistent with one's own values and life goals is very important to psychological well-being.

Dealing with a progressive, debilitating illness is extremely stressful. It is quite common for people facing this type of situation to develop emotional symptoms, including depression and anxiety. Although everyone is likely to experience these feelings from time to time, for some people they can persist or become pervasive and interfere with quality of life. In these situations, it is helpful to bring these symptoms to the attention of your doctor or seek the help of a mental health professional. Medications and behavioral treatments such as cognitive therapy, biofeedback, and psychotherapy can all be beneficial in helping cope with the stress and symptoms that result from it. One study (5) indicates that the frequency of depression in people with ALS is approximately 25 percent, which is the same as it is in patients with cancer. This suggests that approximately one in every four people with ALS could benefit from medications or other treatment modalities to alleviate a clinical syndrome that adversely effects quality of life.

Another important factor that influences a person's satisfaction with life is that of spirituality. This does not necessarily mean involvement in an organized religion, but rather a sense of connection to a power greater than ourselves. For some people, this may be an appreciation and enjoyment of nature or whatever we understand a "Higher Power" or God to be. Prayer, meditation, personal reflection, and self-examination can all be helpful in coming to a feeling of inner peace. This spiritual aspect of life can provide a significant source of assurance, a sense of peace and hope for what lies beyond our physical existence.

Legal Issues

Advance Directives

Advance directives are legal documents that allow input into medical decisions at times when you are unable to participate in the decision making. All U.S. states and the District of Columbia have enacted statutes that allow people to draft documents indicating their health care choices in the event that they become too ill to talk to their health care providers, or become unconscious. These are frequently called living wills (or medical directives) and health care proxies (or durable power of attorney for health care). Each state has its own guidelines about these documents, but the basic elements of each are similar.

Living Wills and Medical Directives

A living will is like a letter to your doctor telling him or her how you would like your health care handled in the event that you become terminally ill or permanently unconscious (also known as persistent vegetative state). For most people, this document indicates a choice to limit medical interventions that are intended to prolong life such as ventilators, artificial feeding, or kidney dialysis.

You may wish to have either your living will or a separate document spell out what you would want done under specific medical circumstances that differ from terminal illness or persistent vegetative state. Examples might include such circumstances as advanced dementia, being extremely ill with no hope for recovery but not imminently dying, or being in kidney failure and requiring dialysis. Two situations are especially important for people with ALS to consider because of the nature of the disease process: being unable to swallow food and/or fluids (deciding about artificial nutrition and hydration) and being unable to breathe (deciding about forms of assisted or mechanical ventilation). These issues are discussed in further detail later in this chapter. In addition, if you have made a decision that you do not want medical personnel to attempt resuscitation in the event your heart stops beating or you are unable to breathe, this information should be included in the document.

It should be kept in mind that, even though you may have indicated that you would want to have a treatment provided, there may be times when it may be medically inappropriate to offer the treatment. Therefore, it is essential to discuss with your physician various medical scenarios that you might encounter to get input about his or her opinion of the value of the treatment under particular circumstances, as well as whether the interventions in question will be in your best interest.

It is also important to understand that you can always change your mind about what you have written in these documents. As you adjust over time to an illness such as ALS, you may be more or less interested in prolonging your life with medical interventions. For example, people who are healthy may reject the idea of any type of medical intervention that would limit their independence. As people age or learn to adjust to a chronic illness, however, they begin to discover that there are many things about their lives that make continuing to be alive worthwhile in spite of the illness. Conversely, a person may opt for an intervention such as home mechanical ventilation but find after trying it out that it does not work for him. Stopping the ventilator is an acceptable choice in this situation.

Health Care Proxies or Durable Power of Attorney for Health Care

There are many types of "powers of attorney" for various legal circumstances. For example, many people sign a power of attorney so that their spouse can obtain their car license plates for them in their absence. Another common example is a financial power of attorney in which a relative or other agent is named to manage a person's financial affairs. It is important to note that a proxy or power of attorney for medical decisions is a special situation specific only to health care decisions. Even if another person has been named as "power of attorney" for financial o r other reasons, this does not apply to health care decisions. The advantage in executing a durable power of attorney for health care is that you are able to name another person you trust to make health care decisions for you if you are unable, for any reason, to make those decisions yourself. The person named, however, cannot be the doctor who is treating you or any of the health care staff who are involved in your care. This person is known, in legal terms, as your "attorney in fact." A proxy decision maker is not restricted only to situations in which you are terminally ill or permanently unconscious, but it could apply, for example, if you were temporarily unconscious or too ill to participate in the decision making but not considered terminally ill.

The importance of naming an alternative decision maker is having someone who will make the decision you would have made if you had been able to do so. In order for that to happen, you need to have a conversation with the person you name as your attorney about how you want these decisions made and what factors should influence them. Only this way can the person named as your proxy decision maker make the best, most appropriate decisions. In addition, a discussion with your doctor about what kinds of treatments are appropriate under particular circumstances can help to inform your decisions and the way you instruct the person you name as your proxy decision maker.

Palliative Medicine and Hospice

Palliative medicine and hospice programs are described in more detail in Chapter 28. However, it is worthwhile to mention these modalities of treatment because they provide medically and ethically appropriate options for the person with ALS to consider as a part of overall treatment and management.

Palliative medicine is defined as "the active total care of patients whose disease is not responsive to curative treatment. Control of pain, of other symptoms, and of psychological, social, and spiritual problems, is paramount. The goal of palliative care is achievement of the best quality of life for patients and their families" (6). This holistic approach embraces the notion that suffering goes beyond simply the physical aspects of a disease or illness and strives to address the multidimensional aspects of a disease when cure is no longer the goal of treatment.

Hospice is the realization of the goals of palliative medicine in the form of an interdisciplinary team including a nurse, physician, social worker, chaplain, and volunteers. Some programs also involve a physical therapist, art therapist, music therapist, and mental health professional. Most hospice care takes place in the home of the patient, but it can also be delivered in a hospice facility or a nursing home that has dedicated hospice beds or allows hospice involvement.

Not everyone wishes to avail himself or herself of hospice. However, excellent symptom management is still available through palliative medicine, home care, and treatment with a physician specializing in palliative medicine.

Symptom Management

When a person who has a symptom such as pain that may be difficult to control or occurs in a terminal phase of his or her illness, doses of medication, such as narcotics or opioids (a class of drugs related to morphine), may be required in amounts that exceed the doses commonly used in general medical care. Concern has been raised that using large doses of these medications may lead to addiction. However, addiction is not a realistic concern in the situation of advanced disease. Even though a person may develop tolerance to a medication (meaning that increases in the dose may be required to achieve the same therapeutic effect), this is not the same as addiction. It is an expected and predictable physiologic result of prolonged narcotic administration. Studies in the area of cancer treatment have clearly demonstrated that addiction virtually never occurs unless the person had a prior history of chemical dependency (7). Even in the setting of past or current chemical dependency, narcotics can still be used effectively and judiciously, as every person deserves to have pain adequately treated.

Another concern is the possible side effect of respiratory depression that can occur with the administration of high doses of opioids. For physicians, nurses, patients, and family members, the fear that the medication being used to relieve suffering may also be the cause of death is an ethical concern. A principle in bioethics known as the "rule of double effect" applies to this situation. This rule pertains to circumstances in which a treatment may have a good effect (in the case of use of opioid medications, relief of pain, shortness of breath, or other symptoms) as well as an undesirable effect (i.e., decrease in respiratory drive, which may hasten death). When the intent of the clinician is clearly to provide relief of symptoms, even though there is a knowable possible adverse effect, it is ethically appropriate to proceed with the treatment in an effort to alleviate suffering. Frankly, it is extremely rare that the dose of medication used for appropriate alleviation of pain actually results in a person's death.

Ethical Issues Regarding End-of-Life Decisions

Discussing Resuscitation Status

One important decision that everyone needs to consider is whether you wish to undergo cardiopulmonary resuscitation (CPR) in the event that your heart fails or you are unable to breathe. If no decision has been made about this issue, you may be resuscitated against your wishes.

Cardiopulmonary resuscitation is a medical procedure that is initiated on an emergent basis in the hospital, in a long-term health care facility, or in the field (usually by emergency medical technicians, or EMTs, who respond to emergency or 911 calls). Respiratory arrest can occur from a lung disorder or infection or from a neurologic disorder such as ALS, which causes weakness of the muscles of respiration. In this situation, CPR may involve artificial respiration or intubation (putting a tube into a person's trachea, or windpipe) so that the person can be mechanically ventilated. For cardiac arrest (when the heart stops beating or beats so erratically that it cannot effectively pump the blood, known as a cardiac arrhythmia), attempts are made to restore the heart's function with chest compressions, medications, and/or electric shock (defibrillation). Most people's knowledge of CPR comes either from what they see on television or what they read in the media (8). Those settings usually portray CPR as a heroic event that miraculously restores the person to full functioning. This, unfortunately, is not an accurate portrayal.

Cardiopulmonary resuscitation was first used in the early 1960s. It was intended for use in situations in which an otherwise relatively young and healthy person had an unexpected heart attack or cardiac arrhythmia, drowned, or overdosed on medications or toxic substances (9). It was never meant for people who were seriously ill or in whom death was expected. Over time, however, CPR has become a commonly used procedure in hospitals and is now a "default" procedure unless it has clearly been specified by a written order from a physician not to do CPR. This order is usually known as "Do Not Resuscitate" (DNR).

Statistics of the success rate of CPR, taking into account all hospitalized adult patients, show that it is successful (meaning that the patient survives the CPR effort) in about 10 percent to 15 percent of cases (10). For those who are elderly, chronically ill, or physically debilitated, the rate falls substantially below 10 percent, depending on the nature and severity of the illness. It also must be kept in mind that even if a person survives the CPR effort, he or she is not always restored to his or her previous level of function. In fact, it is likely that a person will suffer increased disability or may require increased reliance on technology such as mechanical ventilation after being resuscitated.

It is increasingly recognized that when a person has made the choice against CPR, this choice should carry over to other settings such as rehabilitation or nursing facilities or the person's home. Some states either have enacted or are considering legislation to allow portability of this health care choice. These laws are often referred to as "nonhospital DNR" laws. This would mean that a person who has decided against resuscitation would not have to worry about having this procedure performed on him by EMTs or other health care personnel.

Withholding or Withdrawing Treatments

There are times when the burden of having a treatment outweighs its benefits. Both the legal and the ethical communities are in agreement that it is appropriate not to start a treatment that offers little hope for either cure or return of the patient to a functional state or to withdraw a treatment when its goals are no longer achievable. When a person is actually in a situation such as being on mechanical ventilation, this clear distinction for withholding or withdrawing may be more difficult psychologically, especially when the result of the action or inaction is likely to lead to death. Although it may seem as though the person who withdraws the treatment (or the person making the choice to withdraw) is causing the death of the patient, this is not the case. It is the illness, allowed to run its natural course, that results in the patient's death. One useful way to evaluate whether a treatment should be continued or should not be started is to consider the concept of proportionality—burdens versus benefits. The treatment should be carefully scrutinized as to whether it has the potential to meet the patient's goals and, if so, what burdens are attendant to the treatment. If the burdens or side effects are more oppressive than the patient wishes to bear or it is unlikely that he will survive the treatment long enough to realize any benefit from it, the treatment does not need to be started or may be stopped.

There are many situations in which it will not be clear whether the treatment will be of short- or long-term benefit, and in those situations a "trial" of the treatment is reasonable. It should be clearly understood at the outset that the treatment trial is time-limited and that it will not be continued if improvement or stabilization is not seen in a medically reasonable period of time. This strategy is ethically acceptable and often allows the medical team as well as patient and family to feel that they have exhausted all of the reasonable options and have given the treatment a chance. When treatments no longer can help patients achieve their goals, it is not necessary to continue them. It is extremely important to emphasize that making a choice to discontinue a medical treatment is not physician-assisted suicide or euthanasia. It is simply the exercising of a person's right not to have things done to them that they do not desire, that are too burdensome, or that do not fit with their personal values and medical goals.

Two specific situations that people with ALS will need to carefully consider—mechanical ventilation and artificial nutrition and/or hydration—are discussed in more detail.

Mechanical Ventilation

In Chapter 12, Dr. Schilz explains the problem of respiratory failure resulting from the progressive weakness of the muscles of respiration. It is important to think about and understand the options available to avoid respiratory failure well before the intervention would need to be put into place because respiratory distress may arise rapidly and unexpectedly. In situations in which a clear decision has not been made, medical professionals are likely to use mechanical ventilation to restore respiration and prolong life, and this may not be what many people with ALS would want. A study by Cazzoli and Oppenheimer (11), although this study was simply observational, demonstrated that, among patients with the nonbulbar form of ALS who opt for mechanical ventilation, there is a high rate of satisfaction with the use of noninvasive intermittent positive-pressure ventilation (IPPV), also known as BiPAP, as opposed to ventilation that requires a tracheostomy. Aboussouan and colleagues (12) found that noninvasive IPPV also can be effectively used in some patients with moderate to severe bulbar symptoms. Advantages of the noninvasive IPPV method are that it does not require the same level of nursing care, such as tracheal suctioning and round-the-clock caregivers. Invasive ventilators that require tracheostomy usually involve higher cost and use of resources, including the expectation that family members will serve as caregivers. Nursing home placement may be required for some patients (11). However, studies also demonstrate that people who choose tracheostomy-IPPV tend to live longer (13).

It is important for people who choose mechanical ventilation to indicate to both their family and their physician whether there are circumstances in which discontinuing the ventilator would be desired. Because use of mechanical ventilation may substantially prolong the life of the person with ALS, it may result in a "locked-in" syndrome in which alertness is maintained but the ability to communicate or make wishes known becomes impossible. Reasons given by people with ALS for discontinuing mechanical ventilation include permanent unconsciousness, inability to communicate, becoming a burden to family, not having a caregiver available, insufficient funds, or loss of insurance (14). In another study in which people with ALS were interviewed before the time of a decision about ventilatory support (15), similar reasons were given for those who did not want to use any type of mechanical ventilation. Reasons given for not wanting to start mechanical ventilation were the concern that it would significantly compromise quality of life by causing dependence on others, a feeling of helplessness, and reduced mobility. Those who did consider mechanical ventilation as an option believed that the ventilatory support could improve their quality of life and allow them to live longer. Factors that were also important in their decision were the facts that mechanical ventilation could be provided by nasal mask (noninvasive IPPV) rather than needing a tracheostomy, and that the ventilator could be stopped if they chose.

If a person makes a choice not to include any type of mechanical ventilation in his treatment plan, it is important to know what to do when respiratory distress begins. Some people have clearly made a decision that they would not want to use mechanical ventilation for a variety of reasons, but they may decide to use a ventilator because of discomfort and distress when severe shortness of breath actually occurs. Even more unfortunate is the situation in which a decision to start mechanical ventilation is made in an emergency situation when this is not the person's choice. Having hospice care already established when a decision has been made not to use mechanical ventilation is very advantageous because of the skill and knowledge possessed by hospice nurses about management of these situations. Hospice will support the person in their decision regarding limitation of aggressive treatment options and can administer medication that will ease the discomfort of shortness of breath as well as relieve anxiety, allowing the person to die peacefully and comfortably.

Artificial Nutrition and Hydration

The term *artificial nutrition and hydration* (ANH) encompasses a variety of ways in which nutrition and fluids can be provided to a person in situations in which he is unable to swallow or when problems exist anywhere within the gastrointestinal system (from the mouth and esophagus to the stomach and intestines) that do not allow the intake of adequate food or fluids to sustain life. ANH can be provided by intravenous preparations (know as total parenteral nutrition, or TPN), by passing a tube through the nose into the stomach (nasogastric tube, or NG tube), by opening a small hole in the abdomen and stomach and placing a tube for feeding directly into the stomach (gastrostomy), or by placing a tube directly into the small intestine (jejunostomy). For people with ALS, progressive muscle weakness may begin to affect the muscles of the mouth and throat that are responsible for swallowing and preventing food or fluids from going into the lungs. If a person is unable to keep food or fluids out of the airway, aspiration pneumonia—an infection caused by the introduction of foreign substances in the lungs—often occurs. This is a particular problem for people with ALS because their muscles of respiration typically are compromised as well. This can result in a respiratory crisis that may require hospitalization, mechanical ventilation, and antibiotics. Therefore, some people with ALS who experience difficulty swallowing may opt for ANH.

As you are making decisions, it is important to recognize that ANH is regarded as a medical treatment or intervention, like mechanical ventilation or any other. Therefore, you can choose not to have this treatment or you can choose to stop using ANH if you find that using this form of nutritional support is associated with too many problems or side effects. This can be an emotional issue for some people because we tend to equate the provision of food and drink as an act of caring. However, ANH is quite different from the ordinary act of eating or drinking because it is delivered by "medical" means, and it cannot provide the same source of enjoyment or pleasure as ordinary eating and drinking because the food or drink cannot be tasted or savored.

Every state allows a person to make decisions about ANH, which can be directed through a living will or durable power of attorney for health care. Because some treatment facilities, such as nursing homes that have a religious affiliation, may have policies that do not allow ANH to be withdrawn, and because some health care professionals have strong negative feelings about stopping ANH, it is especially important to indicate to family and physicians in *writing* (through an advance directive) if this is a treatment you would not want or if there are circumstances in which you would want this treatment stopped. Again, it is important to know that it is not suicide, physician-assisted suicide, or euthanasia to withhold or withdraw ANH.

Assisted Suicide and Euthanasia

Despite the success of palliative medicine in relieving symptoms of advanced disease or terminal illness, there remain a small minority of patients whose severe and unremitting symptoms cannot be well controlled despite the most sophisticated and adeptly applied palliative care. In these situations, when patients request aid in dying, it raises the question of whether providing assistance with suicide or euthanasia could ever be ethically justifiable. This is a matter of significant controversy in the fields of bioethics, medicine, and law.

Physician-assisted suicide is defined as the circumstance in which a physician provides the means (such as a prescription) and/or the knowledge of how to use the means, but the person himself or herself carries out the act that results in death by suicide. Arguments for physician-assisted suicide have been championed in the medical community by Dr. Timothy Quill (16). Although Dr. Quill often provides palliative care for terminally ill patients, the patients for whom suffering persists even in the face of compassionate and appropriately delivered treatment trouble him. Quill and some of his colleagues (17) have outlined clinical criteria for physician-assisted suicide. These criteria involve careful assessment of the patient's condition, confirming that it must be "incurable and associated with severe, unrelenting, intolerable suffering"; assessment of the patient's decisional capacity; the voluntariness of the patient's request; and that adequate comfort care has been provided. Additionally, these doctors believe that physician-assisted suicide should only be carried out in the context of a meaningful doctor–patient relationship. Arguments favoring the role of physicians in assisting a patient's suicide include that doctors could humanely oversee this process because of their knowledge of effective methods, their preexisting relationship with the patient, and ability to assess diagnosis and prognosis (16).

Dr. Jack Kevorkian has become a name that is synonymous with physician-assisted suicide. Some laud him as a saint, while others condemn him as a criminal. Major criticisms about Dr. Kevorkian's approach to this very sensitive ethical and personal issue is that he does not have the appropriate training or expertise to evaluate the patient's mental status (i.e., decisional capacity), medical situation, or the thoroughness of attempts to alleviate the person's suffering by use of palliative methods. Furthermore, he clearly has not had a long-term therapeutic relationship with the person who consults for his services. Some published testimonials suggest that this may have been the correct choice for a given individual (18). However, for a practice like this to proceed without appropriate guidelines or review, as some consider the practice as done in the Netherlands, is dangerous and risks considerable abuse.

Positions opposing physician-assisted suicide assert that allowing physicians to actively participate in a patient's death would erode the public's trust in the medical field and would lead to the "slippery slope" of providing physician-assisted suicide or euthanasia for patient's who are not able to request assistance with dying but for whom it is perceived that the patient's quality of life is so compromised that it is assumed they would prefer to be dead. Furthermore, in a society such as the United States, in which not all citizens have equal access to palliative care, some patients may believe that they are too burdensome to their family or community and may be unduly persuaded to choose death as an option.

A study conducted in Washington and Oregon (19) demonstrates that people who suffer with ALS think seriously about physician-assisted suicide. This study included 100 patients who had been diagnosed with ALS, 56 percent of whom indicated that "under some circumstances, I would consider taking a prescription for a medicine whose sole purpose was to end my life." Those who endorsed this statement were more likely to be men, had more years of education, were less likely to be religious, and rated their quality of life as lower than those who disagreed with the statement. Hopelessness, as measured by a standardized scale, was a significant predictor of those for whom assisted suicide was a serious consideration. Interestingly, the presence of depression (as a clinical psychiatric diagnosis) was not associated with the desire for physician-assisted suicide. Of the 56 patients who indicated that they would take a prescription medication to end their life, 44 (79%) also agreed with the statement, "If physician-assisted suicide were available now, I would request a lethal prescription today with the intention of taking it to cause my death within the next month." Most patients, however, indicated that they would reserve the prescription for future use.

Family caregivers were also surveyed in this study. The results demonstrated a significant social, economic, and psychological impact of the caregiving. In the majority of instances (73%), the caregivers and patients had similar attitudes toward physician-assisted suicide, and 62 percent said they would support the patient's decision to take a lethal dose of medication.

Only 24 percent of patients in this study were receiving hospice care. The study did not comment specifically on whether patients who are in hospice were more or less likely to consider physician-assisted suicide. However, this is an area that deserves further consideration from a number of perspectives. First is the concern that in order for a doctor to refer a patient to hospice, he must indicate that the expected life prognosis is six months or less. Predicting life course and signing on to a program with this kind of restrictions is onerous for physician, patient, and family. Palliative care and hospice must be made available for appropriate individuals, such as patients with ALS, without these financial and regulatory constraints (20). If appropriate comfort care and symptom management were available to people with ALS, along with the knowledge that refusing or withdrawing treatments that are no longer able to achieve the goals for which they were originally chosen is an option, it may well be that choosing suicide would not be such a strong consideration.

One of the most celebrated legal cases involving a patient with ALS is *Rodriguez vs. British Columbia* (21). Sue Rodriguez was a 42-year-old woman with ALS who anticipated the day when her illness would be so debilitating that although she might no longer want to live, the extent of the disability at that time would make her physically unable to carry out the act of suicide. This case challenged Canada's assisted suicide ban, alleging that it violated the Canadian Charter of Rights and Freedom (22), which provides that "everyone has the right to life, liberty and security of the person," "everyone has the right not to be subjected to any cruel and unusual treatment or punishment," and "everyone has the right to equal protection and equal benefit of the law without discrimination and, in particular, without discrimination based on race, national or ethnic origin, colour, religion, sex, age or mental or physical disability." In brief, the argument raised by the Rodriguez case involved the view that Sue Rodriguez, as an autonomous individual, has the right to die by suicide if she so chooses, but because she would likely become physically unable to carry out the act, she should be allowed to have assistance from the medical profession to do so. It was further argued that she should not be required to suffer in an "undignified, lingering or painful" fashion but should be entitled to choose a manner and time of death that entails more dignity.

Similar issues have also been considered in the U.S. Supreme Court in *Washington vs. Glucksberg* (23) and *Vacco vs. Quill* (24). Although not specific to ALS, the same issues were debated regarding a person's right to suicide and assistance with suicide in situations in which physical disability prevented the person from carrying out suicide or patients were experiencing unrelenting suffering as the result of a terminal illness. Both the U.S. and the Canadian Supreme Courts have arrived at similar conclusions: that is, there is no constitutionally protected right to suicide or hastening of death. However, the U.S. Supreme Court, in its consideration of *Washington vs. Glucksberg* and *Vacco vs. Quill,* strongly endorsed and encouraged aggressive palliative care and left the door open for further consideration, implying that it would allow decisions about the legality of physician-assisted suicide to be considered at the state level. In fact, the Oregon Death with Dignity Act went into effect in October 1997 (see subsequent section) following this Supreme Court decision.

In contrast to assisted suicide, euthanasia is the intentional taking of life by medical personnel, albeit for reasons of "mercy" or compassion, As defined by Goldblatt and Greenlaw (25), euthanasia "describes a physician's *unilateral decision, inconsistent with acceptable medical standards,* to refrain from offering or to discontinue something that is medically appropriate," or "taking affirmative steps to cause a patient's death, such as administering a lethal injection" (emphasis mine). This is an important distinction because it underscores the difference between the appropriate withholding or withdrawal of treatment when it is no longer medically useful or desired by the patient compared with the situation in which the intent is to cause the patient's death by withdrawing or withholding treatments that could have the potential for patient benefit and of which the patient may choose to avail him or herself.

Laws That Legalize or Allow Physician-Assisted Death

Physician-assisted suicide and euthanasia were legalized in the Northern Territory of Australia under the Rights for the Terminally Ill Act, which became effective in 1995. The Australian Senate disallowed the Northern Province's law on March 25, 1997, primarily because of religious pressures. Two patients availed themselves of physician-assisted suicide under this law before its revocation. This Act allowed for persons who are 18 or older who have decisional capacity and who are suffering from a terminal illness to request a physician's assistance in dying. A second medical practitioner who "holds a diploma of psychological medicine or its equivalent" was also required to examine the patient. The physician must have informed the patient of options including palliative care, counseling, and psychiatric support as well as available medical options that could prolong the person's life. At least seven days had to have elapsed between the time of the initial request and the signing of a formal "certificate of request." An additional 48-hour "cooling off" period was required after the certificate of request was signed before the act of either physician-assisted suicide or euthanasia could take place. It was also required that the medical practitioner who provides the assistance remain present with the patient while the assistance was given and until the time of death. Reporting requirements, including documentation of the patient's illness, prognosis, and oral and written requests, were to be filed with the coroner's office; the coroner would then file a yearly report of assisted deaths with the Attorney General.

Both euthanasia and physician-assisted suicide have been accepted in the Netherlands for more than 20 years. Although not legalized, they are allowed under certain conditions. The guidelines for the practice of euthanasia in the Netherlands include: (1) the patient must be a mentally competent adult; (2) the patient must request euthanasia voluntarily, consistently, and repeatedly over a reasonable time, and the request must be documented; (3) the patient must be suffering intolerably, with no prospect of relief, although the disease need not be terminal; and (4) the doctor must consult with another physician who is not involved in the case (26). It is estimated that in 1991 approximately 1.8 percent of deaths in the Netherlands were the result of euthanasia and another 0.3 percent were the result of assisted suicides. These numbers have remained fairly stable over the last several years according to a follow-up study done through 1995 (27). Of concern is the fact that an additional 1,000 deaths (0.8% of all deaths in the Netherlands) were attributed to euthanasia but in situations in which the patient was not competent when euthanasia was performed. Of these patients, more than half had expressed an interest in euthanasia while they were competent, and most were very near death when euthanasia was performed. It is interesting to note that Dutch physicians see no ethical distinction between assisted suicide and euthanasia, unlike the attitudes of physicians in the United States and other countries.

Although Oregonians passed the Death with Dignity Act in 1994, it did not go into effect until October 1997 because of concerns about its constitutionality. The Act allows for physician-assisted suicide, but not euthanasia, for competent patients who are 18 years or older. Safeguards to the Act include that the patient has been informed of his or her medical diagnosis, prognosis, risks associated with taking the medication to be prescribed, probable result of taking the medication, and feasible alternatives including hospice, palliative care, and other methods of pain control. A consulting physician is also required, as is the request that the patient notify his or her next of kin. A written, witnessed request must be submitted to the physician; this can be done at the same time as the initial oral request. A 15-day waiting period is required from the time of the initial oral and written request until the time a prescription can be written for the patient. At the time of the writing of the prescription, the patient must make a second oral request and must be informed that he or she has the opportunity to rescind the request. Patients must be legal residents of the state of Oregon. If a physician believes that he cannot in good conscience carry out the requested assistance, the patient and their records must be transferred to another health care provider.

Your Rights in the Health Care System

It is hoped that the information presented so far has assured the reader that a person with ALS has the right to make decisions about how his or her health care will proceed, can make decisions to accept or reject medical treatments or interventions that are offered, and can choose to discontinue treatments after they have been started if they are too burdensome or do not meet his goals. Despite the legal and ethical support for these choices, some people have encountered difficulty trying to exercise these rights. What can you do if you believe your rights are being violated or that a health care facility, physician, or other medical personnel are overriding choices you have made?

The first step should always be an attempt to facilitate open and clear communication with your health care team. Asking to have a conference with the doctor or entire team often can serve to have everyone's perspective stated and clarified. It often is difficult for health care personnel to feel comfortable stopping or not providing life-sustaining treatment because they see their role to be one of preserving life. If the doctor thinks you are being coerced to make a decision or that your decision is being influenced by pain, depression, anxiety, or other factors, he or she may request consultants such as a psychiatrist, ethicist, pain management specialist, or others to see you to be sure that you are not making an irreversible decision when options are available to improve your quality of life. It is in your best interest to cooperate fully with these consultants to facilitate the process. This also allows you to be fully informed of any options you may want to consider.

If this is unsuccessful, you may wish to discuss your concerns with the office or person designated at the health care facility as the ombudsman or patient advocate. Another alternative is to ask to meet with the facility's ethics consultant or committee. Every health care facility that is accredited by the Joint Commission for Accreditation of Health Care Organizations (JCAHO) is required to have a mechanism available for the resolution of ethical problems or disputes. Ethics consultants or patient advocates can meet with you and the physician or health care team to mediate and attempt to resolve the conflict. As a last resort, you may choose to seek your health care from another provider or in another facility in a setting in which your choices will be respected.

References

1. Silverstein MD, Stocking CB, Antel JP, et al. Amyotrophic lateral sclerosis and life-sustaining therapy: Patients' desires for information, participation in decision making, and life-sustaining therapy. *Mayo Clin Proc* 1991; 66:906–913.
2. Bascom PB, Tolle SW. Care of the family when the patient is dying. *West J Med* 1995; 163:292–296.
3. Goldblatt D. A life-enhancing condition: The Honourable Mr. Justice Sam N. Filer. *Semin Neurol* 1993; 13:375–379.
4. McDonald ER, Wiedenfeld SA, Hillel A, Carpenter CL, Walter PA. Survival in amyotrophic lateral sclerosis: The role of psychological factors. *Arch Neurol* 1994; 51:17–23.
5. Sauders C, Walsh TD, Smith M. Hospice care in motor neuron disease. In: Sauders C, Summers DH, Teller N (eds). *Hospice: The living idea*. London: Edward Arnold Ltd., 1981:126–147.
6. *Cancer pain relief and palliative care*. Technical Report Series 804. Geneva: World Health Organization, 1990.
7. Kanner RM, Foley KM. Patterns of narcotic use in a cancer pain clinic. *Ann NY Acad Sci* 1981; 362:161–172.
8. Diem SJ, Lantos MPH, Tulsky JA. Cardiopulmonary resuscitation on television: Miracles and misinformation. *N Engl J Med* 1996; 334:1578–1582.
9. Kouwenhoven WB, Jude JR, Knickerbocker GG. Closed chest cardiac massage. *JAMA* 1960; 173:1064–1067.
10. Miller DL, Jahnigen DW, Gorbien MJ, Simbartl L. Cardiopulmonary resuscitation: How useful? *Arch Intern Med* 1992; 152:578–582.
11. Cazzoli PA, Oppenheimer EA. Home mechanical ventilation for amyotrophic lateral sclerosis: Nasal compared to tracheostomy-intermittent positive pressure ventilation. *J Neurol Sci* 1996; 139(Suppl):123–128.
12. Aboussouan LS, Khan SU, Meeker DP, Stelmach K, Mitsumoto H. Effect of noninvasive positive-pressure ventilation on survival in amyotrophic lateral sclerosis. *Ann Intern Med* 1997; 127:450–453.
13. Cazzoli PA, Oppenheimer EA. Use of nasal tracheostomy positive pressure ventilation in patients with amyotrophic lateral sclerosis: Changing patterns and outcomes. *Neurology* 1998; 50:A417–A418.

14. Moss AH, Oppenheimer EA, Casey P, et al. Patients with amyotrophic lateral sclerosis receiving long-term mechanical ventilation: Advance care planning and outcomes. *Chest* 1996; 110:249–255.

15. Young JM, Marshall CL, Anderson EJ. Amyotrophic lateral sclerosis patients' perspectives on use of mechanical ventilation. *Health Social Work* 1994; 19:253–260.

16. Quill TE. *Death and dignity: Making choices and taking charge.* New York: WW Norton, 1993.

17. Quill TE, Cassel CK, Meier DE. Care of the hopelessly ill: Proposed criteria for physician assisted suicide. *N Engl J Med* 1992; 327:1380–1384.

18. Poenisch C. Merian Frederick's story. *N Engl J Med* 1998; 339:996–998.

19. Ganzini L, Johnston WS, McFarland BH, Tolle SW, Lee MA. Attitudes of patients with amyotrophic lateral sclerosis and their care givers toward assisted suicide. *N Engl J Med* 1998; 339:967–973.

20. Walsh TD. The Medicare hospice benefit: A critique from palliative medicine. *J Palliative Med* 1998; 1:147–149.

21. 107 D.L.R. 4th 342 (Can. 1993).

22. Can. Const. (Constitution Act, 1982) pt. 1 (Canadian Charter of Rights and Freedoms), Sections 7, 12, 15(1).

23. 117 S Ct 2258 (1997).

24. 117 S Ct 2293 (1997).

25. Goldblatt D, Greenlaw J. Starting and stopping the ventilator for patients with amyotrophic lateral sclerosis. *Neurol Clin North Am* 1989; 7:789–806.

26. Angell M. Euthanasia in the Netherlands—good news or bad? *N Engl J Med* 1996; 335:1676–1678.

27. Van der Maas PJ, van der Wal G, Haverkate I, et al. Euthanasia, physician-assisted suicide, and other medical practices involving end of life in the Netherlands, 1990–1995. *N Engl J Med* 1996; 335:1699–1705.

Suggested Reading

Schwartz, M. *Letting go: Morrie's reflections on living while dying.* New York: Dell Publishing, 1996

This inspirational handbook offers advice about living with physical limitations, grieving your losses, dealing with your mind and emotions, developing a spiritual connection, and reviewing the past. It is written by Morrie Schwartz, who was the subject of three "Nightline" special television programs and the focus of the book *Tuesdays with Morrie* (Albom M. *Tuesdays with Morrie.* New York: Doubleday, 1997).

Choice in Dying, Inc. publishes a number of pamphlets related to end-of-life choices such as advance directives, cardiopulmonary resuscitation, dying at home, artificial nutrition and hydration, and other life-sustaining treatments (such as mechanical ventilation, dialysis, etc.). These are excellent resources presented in a question-and-answer format. They can be obtained through Choice in Dying, Inc., 200 Varick Street, New York, NY 10014; telephone: 1-800-989-WILL.

26

Financial Realities

Linda Boynton De Sepulveda, R.N., D.N.Sc., and Michael C. Graves, M.D.

There is no predictability to life's experience, including that of ALS, as the disease varies considerably from individual to individual. The changes in health status over time must be met with flexibility. ALS affects every aspect of one's being—physical, emotional, social, financial, and spiritual. However, one can acquire hope and strength through the acquisition of knowledge. This chapter will assist you to identify resources and liabilities.

Providing satisfactory medical care to everyone at a cost they can afford is a compelling issue. Many people do not receive medical care that is adequate in either quantity or quality, and the cost of that care is inequitably distributed (1). The economic impact of ALS may begin long before the actual diagnosis is made. (2) Patients with ALS do not begin the journey with the diagnosis; it comes after a long process of evaluations and referrals. The length and extent of these evaluations are governed by four types of payment systems. There is the indemnity insurance payment system (IP), the managed care payment system (HMO, PPO, EPO), the governmental payment systems called Medicare (FMC) and Medicaid (SML), and the self-payment system (Pay), also known as the noninsured.

Financial Realities:
There Is Health Care and There Is ALS

Alphabet Soup: IP, HMO, PPO, EPO, FMC, SML, Pay

Indemnity Insurance Payment Systems (IP)

The indemnity insurance payment system pays physicians' bills on the basis of billed charges, after the deductible and coinsurance are met. The deductible and coinsurance are the patient's responsibility. The indemnity insurance approach is rapidly declining as more insurance companies are paying only up to the "usual and customary level." This change in reimbursement has inflated the out-of-pocket expenses for most people.

Managed Health Care (HMO, PPO, EPO)

Managed care is defined as a prepayment system. The care providers are paid in advance a preset amount for all the services the client may or may not need in a given period. This form of health care service is intended to provide high-quality, cost-effective care. The most common forms of managed care are health maintenance organizations (HMOs) and preferred provider organizations (PPOs). The exclusive provider organization (EPO) is a group of fee-for-service providers operating in much the same way as a PPO but granting the beneficiary no coverage outside the network. Managed care groups work from the belief that the primary care doctor plays a key role in the management of patient care. Patients are assigned a primary care doctor, who determines the need for referrals and arranges the consultation if he or she deems it appropriate. These referrals are normally made with specialists who are salaried or have contracted with the specific managed care group. Referral to a specialist not in the group is rarely done and usually requires a petition to a medical review board.

Disability, Medicare, Medicaid, and COBRA

Disability under Social Security is based on an individual's inability to work. The person with ALS must be unable to perform any work for which he is trained or suited for, and the disability must last longer than one year or lead to death. To qualify for Social Security Disability benefits, the person needs to have worked. Qualification for benefits is dependent on the number of years worked and the number of credits earned in that period. To apply for Social Security disability, you need to file a claim with the Social Security office either by phone, by mail, or in person. Certain information is necessary to process your claim: (1) social security number; (2) names, addresses, and phone numbers of doctors, clinics, and institutions that treated you and dates of treatment; (3) a summary of where you worked in the past 15 years and what kind of work you did; (4) a copy of your W-2 form or, if self-employed, your federal tax return for the past year; (5) date of marriage if your spouse is also applying. Once the person with ALS has been approved for disability benefits, he will receive his first Social Security check dating back to the sixth full month from the date the social security office decides the disability began. For more information, call the Social Security's 24-hour toll-free number: 1-800-772-1213.

In 1965 President Johnson signed the Medicare program into law. Medicare provides health benefits to people over age 65 years or those who have been receiving Social Security disability payments for two years. The program has two complementary but distinct parts: hospital insurance (known as Part A) and supplemental medical insurance (known as Part B). After the deductible and coinsurance payment are met, Part A will pay for (1) inpatient hospitalization, (2) nursing care at a skilled nursing facility following acute hospitalization, (3) some in-home health care, and (4) hospice. All services have specific time limitations, and reimbursement is based on a specific set of criteria. In Part B recipients pay a monthly premium and must meet a yearly deductible. Part B will help pay for (1) physician services, (2) diagnostic tests, (3) durable medical equipment (limited to specific equipment), and (4) ambulance services and other health services and supplies not covered in Part A (details of the extent and type of coverage are presented throughout this chapter) (3).

If the patient with ALS disagrees with what Medicare has paid on a claim (e.g., services, DME, deductibles, payments) he or she can appeal. The claimant has six months from the date of denial to file an appeal. In requesting an appeal, the claimant must be sure to include his Medicare number, address, and phone number and describe what portion of the denial he is appealing. Or, complete the "Request for Review of a Part B Medicare Claim" form, which is available at your local Social Security office. There is no charge for the appeal process or review. The appeal process takes 45 days. You will receive a letter detailing the decision, outlining the reason for the decision, and providing information on the next appeal decision level. If the amount is greater than $100 and your initial appeal was denied, you have six months to appeal for a carrier hearing. If the amount is greater than $500 and the second appeal is denied, you may request a hearing with an Administrative Law Judge. If this appeal is denied, you can ask for the Appeals Council to review the decision within 60 days. To request an Appeals Council review, you must make your request in writing. If the amount is greater than $1,000 and the decision is not in your favor, you can bring suit in Federal District Court. You should have legal counsel at this stage.

Until 1965 there was no federal participation in medical care for poor people; the state provided whatever care was necessary. This changed in 1965, when Medicaid, Title XIX of the Social Security Act, was implemented. Medicaid is a joint federal and state program that provides health benefits for poor people. Eligibility for Medicaid is determined by each state and level of income. In the early years of Medicaid, families had to "spend down" all their assets so that a family member could be cared for. Under the new guidelines, assets are divided and only those of the patient need to be spent down, thus preventing the impoverishing of the surviving spouse. There are specific legal issues and timing of the spend down that are important to know. It is important to know that the rules about what can be spent or kept vary between states. Second, the interpretation of the rules can vary between welfare offices. Third, a negotiation process is possible when the division of assets is not considered equitable. We advise anyone wishing to go through this process to seek legal assistance from a lawyer who is experienced in Medicaid laws. Otherwise, a person with ALS may unnecessarily incur losses.

While people with ALS are still employed, it is important for them to determine how they can maintain insurance coverage while they go through the disability process. The Consolidated Omnibus Budget Reconciliation Act of 1985 (COBRA) is an employer group health plan that people with ALS can pay for if they must stop working because of their disability. If they worked for a company that had fewer than 20 employees and are not eligible for COBRA, they can seek legal council to determine their recourse under state laws.

No Insurance

More than 37 million Americans, including many people with ALS, do not have health insurance. Some say it is because insurance is not provided where they work, others say it is too costly, and others believed they would never get this sick. Whatever the reason, they need to apply for disability benefits as quickly as possible. There are guidelines for working while disabled; you should check with your local Social Security office.

Financial security is something we can all relate to. Making the right choices, knowing the limitations of our insurance coverage, and knowing alternative resources can instill well-being (Table 26-1). Everyone at one time or another has been overwhelmed by insurance forms, deductibles, authorizations, justifications, and appeal processes. But knowing the system can greatly increase the chance for success in acquiring what may be necessary for survival. If people with ALS find that their insurance is inadequate, they need to know what alternatives exist.

Medical Evaluation

This section addresses the process of diagnosing ALS, how to pay for it, and how your insurance can affect the process. The first part applies to everyone and deals with the various steps people go through in arriving at a diagnosis. The second part discusses the challenges presented to patients by the health care industry. This part should assist the patient and family in navigating through the obstacles that these systems all too often place in the way of obtaining proper medical consultation.

Steps in the medical evaluation of the ALS patient:
- Initial evaluation by the primary care physician

Table 26-1. Know Your Insurance Policy

General Information	Insurance card	Know: 1. Name of subscriber, 2. Insurance phone number, 3. Group number of insurance plan, 4. Policy holder. Who is the subscriber (date of birth, Social Security number)?
	Policy	1. Is there an annual deductible? 2. What are your annual out-of-pocket expense? 3. Are there claim forms? 4. Is there a capitation in services provided (expense limit or maximum)? 5. Can I have access to case management services? 6. What is the appeal process?
	Doctor visits	1. Is there a fee for service or is it prepaid? 2. Is there a deductible? And how much? 3. What is the referral process in order to see a specialist?
	Pharmacy plan	1. Do you have one? 2. Is there a spending limit (capitation)? 3. Does it include nutritional supplementation?
	Durable medical equipment (DME)	1. Do you have DME coverage? Deductible? 2. What equipment is covered under your policy? 3. Is there a preferred provider? 4. Forms? Preauthorization? Review process?
	Long-Term Care	1. Do you have long term, in-home health and/or Hospice care coverage?
	In-Home Care	2. What are the limitations of these benefits (number of days, justification, preferred agency)?
	Hospice	

- Referral for a second opinion
- Referral to a neuromuscular specialist
- Application of the "El Escorial Criteria"
- Tests: blood tests, electromyography (EMG), and magnetic resonance imaging (MRI) scans or X-rays

Initial Evaluation

It is important for a person with the possible diagnosis of ALS to begin by consulting a general internist or family practitioner. A routine evaluation of your general health is important whether you eventually turn out to have ALS or not.

Referral for a Second Opinion

A neurologist should be seen to diagnose ALS and to rule out the alternative neuromuscular conditions that can resemble it. What is a neurologist? Historically, the recognition of the existence of ALS and the development of the neurologist as a modern medical specialist occurred together in the mid to late nineteenth century (see Chapter 3). Today's neurologist will have completed about 12 to 13 years of higher (post–high school) education before taking his board examinations in the specialty. After that he may choose to become a "neuromuscular specialist" by taking a one- or two-year neuromuscular fellowship, in which he concentrates on the skills of examination, EMG, and muscle biopsy needed for ALS and other neuromuscular diseases. Everyone suspected of having ALS should see a neurologist for careful examination, especially one who specializes in neuromuscular diseases including ALS (see "third opinion, the neuromuscular ALS specialist neurologist").

Cost and Benefit of the Neurologist

The cost of the first evaluation by a neurologist averages $350. This office consultation is of more value than the expensive diagnostic tests that are frequently done. The neurologic examination depends on a knowledge of the structure and function of the brain, spinal cord, nerves, and muscles. The cost of seeing a competent neurologist is money well spent because no brain scan, X-ray, or other test can replace this expertise. If the correct diagnosis is not made, patients may have surgical operations for such conditions as carpal tunnel syndrome, tarsal tunnel syndrome, ulnar nerve compression, and spinal conditions. An opinion from a neurologist specializing in neuromuscular disorders is also a good idea.

Sometimes the Diagnosis Is Difficult

For some people with ALS who have typical symptoms and are seen by a knowledgeable physician, the correct diagnosis is clear very early. When a neurologist examines these patients, the typical signs of ALS are present, and alternative diagnoses are unlikely. For other patients, the diagnosis can be difficult, even by experienced physicians. Failure to establish the correct diagnosis can lead to anxiety and unnecessary medical testing, potentially harmful medical treatments, and fruitless surgery. Delays in diagnosis usually are due to one or more of the following:

1. Delay by the primary care physician in referral to a neurologist.

2. Referral for a second opinion directly to a neurosurgeon or to an orthopedic surgeon, with the assumption that the problem is one that needs surgical treatment.

3. Failure of referral to a neurologist who specializes in neuromuscular diseases and ALS.

4. Denial (the psychological kind, not the HMO kind). There is an old attitude that early diagnosis of a disease such as ALS is of no benefit to the patient because there are so few effective treatments to offer. This leads to denial by both physicians and patients and their families.

Early diagnosis will benefit the patient and also will ultimately cost less than delayed diagnosis, for both the patient and his insurance company (4). The anxiety produced by the fear of the unknown may be higher than that of facing a known and defined enemy. Other benefits of early diagnosis allow patients to:

- Choose new drugs that may slow down the disease.

- Find specialty centers to volunteer for clinical trial and to contribute to research that may help others in the future.

- Avoid unnecessary and expensive medical testing.

- Avoid expensive, fruitless, and potentially harmful treatments and surgeries.

Even when examined by an expert, some people with ALS may not have enough signs and symptoms to meet the criteria for the diagnosis of ALS. These criteria are known as the "El Escorial" criteria (see Chapter 2). Patients may need MRI scans, muscle biopsies, and various blood tests. If even these tests are not helpful, more time is needed. These patients need to have appointments every three to six months for careful reexamination.

Application of the "El Escorial Criteria"

Chapter 2 covers the details of the system developed by the World Federation of Neurology to confirm the diagnosis of ALS. These criteria are now available for neurologists to use to diagnose ALS.

Tests and More Tests: Blood Tests, EMG, MRI Scans or X-rays, and Muscle Biopsy

Blood Tests

Most patients with ALS seen in our clinic have had many blood tests in the hope of finding some disease that might be curable. However, no blood test can be used to rule in or rule out ALS. Diagnosis of this disease depends completely on the skills of a neurologist. If, based on his examination, the neurologist believes that another diagnosis is possible, appropriate blood tests are needed.

Electromyography

The details of EMG and other tests that the neurologist may order are found in Chapter 3. The EMG alone cannot diagnose ALS. Only a physician who has done a complete neurologic history and examination can do this. EMG testing can also demonstrate a number of diseases of nerves and of muscles that can sometimes mimic ALS. All patients with suspected ALS need to have EMG testing done by a physician who is familiar with ALS and related conditions.

MRI Scans and X-rays

Just as they have had many blood tests, many patients seen in our clinic have large packets of scans and X-rays. These are only needed in specific situations. If a patient does not meet the "El Escorial criteria" when the neurologist first examines him, these tests are needed to rule out other conditions.

Muscle Biopsy

Muscle biopsy is only necessary in a few ALS patients. These biopsies should be sent to a major neuromuscular research center. Otherwise the test may not be helpful and may need to be repeated.

The Influence of Type of Insurance on the Diagnostic Process

As outlined earlier, every patient needs to take a series of steps in the diagnostic journey, including the primary doctor, the neurologist, the ALS specialist neurologist, and appropriate testing. Changes in how medical care is financed have begun to affect the ease of taking each of the preceding steps. However, any shortcuts that eliminate the steps outlined may lead to a wrong or delayed diagnosis. The type of insurance you have can effect the process of evaluating a diagnosis of ALS. As you compare the different kinds of insurance available, it may seem that private insurance is the best and HMOs are the worst in getting access to the experts needed to diagnose ALS. This is true if we only consider diagnosis and ignore treatment. Obviously, you need to consider more than just diagnosis in planning your budget, and that is when the various managed care plans may show their real value.

The Conflict Between Managed Care and Specialists

Before 1950 there were very few medical specialists and only rarely would general practitioners send a patient with ALS to a specialist. Beginning in the 1960s many physicians became specialists and even provided the primary source of care for the diseases within their specialty. For example, neurologists gradually developed experience in the day-to-day care of conditions such as Parkinson's disease and epilepsy. Additionally, patients could go directly to the specialist without any special permission. Insurance would pay the costs. However, the costs of medical care increased rapidly from 1970 through 1990. Part of this was attributed to this easy accessibility of patients to specialists.

Managed care was devised to save money, in part by limiting access to specialists. However, this approach failed to recognize that a great deal of primary care was already being provided by the specialists. The general practitioner, or a committee, was given the responsibility to decide which patient could or could not go to a specialist or have a certain laboratory test or even a surgical operation. This is inappropriate for neurologic conditions such as ALS. At times the primary care doctor loses personal income for every patient sent to a specialist or for diagnostic tests ordered. For a number of reasons, it may be hard to get the attention of the proper specialist physician to help determine exactly what is wrong and what is needed. On the positive side, the low monthly premiums of the managed care options are appealing for the healthy young person with limited income. For patients who do have a disease such as ALS, managed care plans may offer better coverage for drugs and in many cases lowered or eliminated copayments.

People with ALS frequently have little choice about what kind of insurance they have. Patients and families must take the responsibility for receiving services. This is known as "requesting an authorization." If conscientious and ethical, the managed care plans should still approve all requests that are medically necessary. However, the patient with ALS may need to be persistent in requesting an authorization.

Private "Fee for Service" Insurance

In the IP system, the primary care doctor, usually an internist or a family practitioner, can more easily make a referral to a neurologist. The average cost for the consultation is approximately $350. The neurologist may decide that testing is needed. EMG and nerve conduction velocity (NCV) testing (see Chapter 3) are almost always needed and cost upward of $500. Blood tests and MRI scans are sometimes needed, adding several thousand dollars more. If you add muscle biopsies and spinal taps, the bill can come to tens of thousands of dollars. Inappropriate treatments and surgery can increase the bill to hundreds of thousands of dollars. Because the patient must pay the 20 percent to 25 percent copayment, it is in his financial interest to make sure that the requested tests are really necessary. Unless one is a medical professional, it is difficult to decide what testing to get. The best guide is to seek the advice of a good neurologist before all testing and to get the advice of a neuromuscular specialist at a neuromuscular center if there is any question about what is necessary.

Medicare

As discussed previously, private insurance generally converts to Medicare when you reach age 65. Medicare has most of the same rules as private insurance, but it may pay less. Most neurologists accept Medicare. There generally is a copayment.

State Medical Assistance

In California the state program for low income people is called Medi-Cal. This program pays very little to the doctor. Occasionally, depending on the locality, neurologists will see a limited number of such patients as a charitable act. Patients facing this type of situation should always try to go to an ALS–Neuromuscular Research Center. Although Medi-Cal pays very little to doctors, it is one of the best programs in paying for drugs and durable medical equipment such as wheelchairs.

Managed Care: HMO, PPO, EPO

These are now the most popular types of insurance. In the large HMO, there generally is little or no out-of-pocket expenses to the patient. In one large California HMO, patients can get a second opinion or even a third opinion from neurologists within the HMO. You usually can find out which neurologist in the large HMO has completed a fellowship in neuromuscular diseases or otherwise is especially interested in ALS. The large HMO will sometimes give authorization to go to a specialist outside the HMO when it is really necessary to get the correct diagnosis. In the PPO care plan, the insurance company gives you a book that lists all the doctors you are allowed to see. There usually is a wide selection of neurologists, including those at the ALS and Neuromuscular Research Centers nearest you. Smaller managed care programs (e.g., PPOs or EPOs) often have only a few neurologists in their system. These neurologists usually are general neurologists who can take care of problems such as strokes, Parkinson's disease, Alzheimer's disease, and all the more common conditions that require neurologic care. A referral to a neurologist who specializes in neuromuscular disease should be firmly requested for every patient who is in one of these smaller HMOs.

Role of Charitable Foundations

The Muscular Dystrophy Association (MDA) and the ALS Association (ALSA) both support a number of ALS Neuromuscular Research Clinics around the country. The MDA clinics allow patients who have little or no ability to pay to see the experts. The MDA is able to pay for expenses that health insurance plans or HMOs should cover. These clinics frequently serve the valuable role of identifying needs. They then help the patient articulate their need in the form of a request for authorization to the HMO or other insurance company. You can find a list of these clinics on the World Federation of Neurology ALS Web Page (www.wfnals.org) or by calling your local MDA or ALSA office (see Chapter 32).

Medical Care

Drug Management

Cost-Controlling Issues

Prescription medications have been another area of great concern to the person with ALS. In addition to the rapidly escalating cost of drugs, there has been an explosion in the number of agents used to treat various associated medical problems, as discussed in other chapters. In an attempt to control costs, many states have passed legislation that allows pharmacies to fill prescriptions with a generic equivalent. Another attempt by insurance companies, HMOs, and federal programs to curtail costs is the development of formularies. A formulary is a restrictive list of available medications from which physicians can choose. In the outpatient setting, HMOs, PPOs, state Medicaid, and IPs are beginning to restrict physician prescribing practices by the use of a drug formulary. The patient with ALS can still receive drugs that are not on the approved formulary, but they probably will have to pay for them.

Pharmacy Plans: What Are They, What Do They Offer, and How Do I Get One?

A few IP insurance programs have pharmacy plans. Medicare does not cover the cost of prescriptions, but Medigap plans (Medicare supplement insurance) have 10 standard plans that can be purchased. Three of those plans (H, I, and J) cover a portion of prescription costs. The H and I plans have a $250 deductible and a maximum benefit of $1,250 per year. The J plan also has a $250 deductible with a maximum benefit of $3,000. Access to prescription coverage may or may not be included under managed care. Typically, the cost for prescriptions under these plans can vary from $2 to $10 per prescription and the amount of drug dispensed per prescription may be limited to a one-month supply unless there is a mail-order plan.

It is important to know if the person with ALS has a prescription plan. If he does, you need to determine the amount and type of coverage. Generic drugs are less expensive than brand-name drugs, but injectable prescriptions may or may not be covered. In addition, some prescription programs may limit access to drugs. Some HMOs have a drug formulary. Drugs are dispensed from that list either free or at reduced rate. The variety of drugs at the patient's disposal for treatment also will be limited. At present, only one drug has been approved by the U.S. Food and Drug Administration (FDA) for the treatment of the underlying disease process in ALS (see Chapter 4), but numerous medications may be needed for the management of conditions associated with the disease.

Symptom Management

Medications used to treat such problems as excessive saliva, spasticity, cramps, insomnia, depression, emotional lability, or difficulty breathing may or may not be listed on a drug formulary; there may not be a generic equivalent; or the drug may be in limited supply. Therefore, choices to treat a specific medical problem may be limited, restricted, or constrained by financial resources (see Chapter 4).

Treatment of ALS (Riluzole, Vitamins, Homeopathic)

The only FDA-approved treatment for ALS at this time is Rilutek (riluzole). Over-the-counter vitamins and herbs usually are not covered by pharmacy plans. Multi-vitamin pills can cost as little as $5 per 100 tablets, but the annual cost could be considerably more when you add vitamin C, vitamin E, vitamin B complex, ginkgo biloba, superoxide dismutase (SOD), and enzymes. This figure does not include all the other drugs that may be tried during the course of the disease. One of the most difficult decisions a person with ALS has to make is whether to pay for drugs that are only modestly effective in treating the disease, especially if they do not have a pharmacy plan. Most HMOs have approved riluzole for the treatment of ALS and pay the full cost of the medication ($650–$800 per month), but pharmacy plans such as Medigap may cover the cost of the drug only for the first few months of the year.

Recourse: Alternative Funding Sources

Are there any? If the person with ALS does not have a pharmacy plan or if his plan has a capitation, he needs to explore other options and develop strategies to save money. Generic drugs generally cost 30 percent to 50 percent less than brand-name medications. Prescriptions that are filled by mail tend to cost less, but you may need to shop for the best price. People with ALS should not forget to ask about the cost to fill the prescription, shipping, and any other fees (membership) that may be required. A few pharmacy programs are AARP Pharmacy Service, APP (American Preferred Prescription, Inc.), Action Mail Order, Health Care Services, and Medi-mail order. Some national and state pharmaceutical programs may assist patients in the purchase of medications. One such program is sponsored by the National Organization for Rare Disorders (NORD). Financially needy individuals can obtain prescribed medications through the NORD medication assistance program. The amount of financial compensation is determined by the applicant's financial need. NORD currently dispenses Rilutek (riluzole) tablets through the Patient Assistance Program, which provides free drugs to patients who are not eligible for public or private reimbursement. For more information, call 1-800-999-NORD. The Prescription Drug Patient Assistance Program is another national program that provides drugs at no cost to those who qualify. The physician applies to the pharmaceutical company for a 90-day supply of medication. He needs to reapply each time the drug is reordered. The Veterans Affairs office can also help individuals who were veterans. It may provide some drugs at a reduced rate, depending on the facility's formulary. The patient needs to contact his local Veterans office, hospital, or outpatient facility

Table 26-2. Prescription Services Resource List

	Agency	Notes	
Prescriptions	AARP Pharmacy Service	Don't need to be AARP member	1-800-456-2226
	APP (American Preferred Prescription, Inc.)	No membership	1-800-952-7779
	Action Mail Order	No membership required	1-800-452-1976
	Health Care Services	Membership $12 if you are member of National Council of Senior Citizens. You don't have to be a senior citizen to join.	1-800-758-0555
	Medi-mail order	No membership required	1-800-331-1458
	NORD	Dependent upon financial need	1-800-999-NORD
	Prescription Drug Patient Assistance Programs	The doctor coordinates a 90-day supply of medication with the pharmaceutical company. Restrictions are given in booklet.	1-800-548-9034
	Veterans Administration	Veterans can receive drugs at a reduced rate or sometimes for free	Local VA facility

for information. Table 26-2 provides a summary of prescription services resource list.

Durable Medical Equipment (DME)

The term *durable medical equipment* refers to items that can withstand repeated use. The item must be prescribed by a physician, must be medically necessary

(Certificate of Medical Necessity is required), must be appropriate for home use, must fill a medical need, must be something that can be used repeatedly, and must be something that would not be useful if the patient were not sick. Medicare Part B helps pay for DME and other supplies used in the home, including oxygen equipment, canes, walkers, commode chairs, patient lifts, wheelchairs, braces, hospital beds, and seat lift mechanisms. Medicare approves some DME items for purchase, while others must be rented. Some items, such as scooters and seat lift mechanisms, require prior authorization. A prior authorization request can be submitted by the patient, doctor, or supplier. It is also important to note the order in which equipment is requested (e.g., walker or cane before wheelchair); otherwise a denial can be expected.

Under Medicaid guidelines, the definition of DME is similar to that of Medicare. Based on the estimated time of medical need, Medicaid will determine the need to rent or purchase DME. The physician needs to complete a medical necessity form, and the provider needs to complete a claim form. DME that has been purchased or rented by the state may be reclaimed for the use of other individuals when the original recipient no longer needs it.

Insurance companies and managed care organizations often do not cover DME or offer only limited coverage. The cost of DME can add to the overwhelming financial burden of ALS. In addition to problems with financial support, there may be delays in receiving the needed equipment or service. Various patient advocate groups have expressed concern that there is no incentive to create laws or policies to protect the consumer. "Managed care organizations and private insurers have nothing to lose and everything to gain by automatically denying or delaying coverage for DME" (5).

Adaptive devices such as grab bars, stair glides or elevators, emergency call devices, or built-up utensils are not considered DME. Therefore, these items are considered an out-of-pocket expense.

Implication for Treatment Decisions

The person with ALS should know what his policy covers. He should know what equipment is covered and the limitations in either type or price. An example of limitations in coverage is a portable suction machine. Medicare covers the rental of a high-volume aspirator that weighs approximately 8 pounds and needs an electrical outlet. Unfortunately, Medicare does not currently cover the rental of a more useful portable aspirator, which weighs less than 3 pounds and is wired for both AC and DC. Both devices cost approximately the same amount. One device can be used anywhere, thus not limiting the patient to one room. Health care professionals, patients, and family members can become frustrated at times when attempting to get the most appropriate equipment for patient use and then finding that the equipment is not part of the approved list! Table 26-3 outlines DME equipment costs and coverage.

The person with ALS also needs to know what is required to process a claim. Always ask questions, and if the supplier does not know, you should call your

Table 26-3. DME Equipment Costs and Coverage

DME	Cost (US$)	Coverage based on insurance carrier:				
Type of equipment	range	FMC	SML	HMO	EPO/PPO/IP	
Wheelchair: standard manual	400–3,500	cap on rental	Yes	Yes	%	
Wheelchair: standard electric	3,500–12,000	4,500 purchase	Yes	Yes	%	
Wheelchair: full electric (tilt and recline, leg elevation, seat elevation, special trunk/head support)	12,000–25,000	No	Yes	Usually No	%	
Cane	9–50	Yes with Cap	Yes	Yes	%	
Walker: standard	70–150	Yes	No	Yes	%	
Walker: heavy duty, large wheels, special attachments	275–400	Yes	Yes	Yes	%	
Commode	90–1,200	Yes with Cap	Yes	Yes	%	
Shower chair or shower bench	50–120	No	Yes	Yes	%	

Yes = full coverage, with justification (HMO may have limited selection)
No = no coverage, patient responsible for full cost
% = percentage of cost covered by insurance, balance patient's responsibility after deductible met
Cap = capitation on rental or purchase price

insurance carrier. If the claim is denied, you should know the appeal process. If all else fails, you should know where to turn for assistance. ALSA and the MDA both have local loan equipment pools. You can contact the local service representative and ask about borrowing the needed equipment. MDA will assist with the purchase of a wheelchair or orthotic device in some circumstances. Contact your local representative for more information. Another potential source for assistance is community programs, such as church groups or aid groups.

Augmentative and Alternative Communication Devices

Augmentative and alternative communication (AAC) devices include but are not limited to portable computer-generated messages, either verbal or nonverbal (see Chapter 10). Medicaid funding has been established in most states, and many insurance providers offer AAC devices. However, Medicare usually does not support funding for these devices. The patient can appeal a denial. First he must determine that the device meets one of the DME criteria, such as AAC devices are durable, they are a treatment for severe expressive communication disabilities, they are not needed by persons without this disability, and/or they are portable. He then must follow the appeal process previously described.

Implication for Treatment Decisions

When all appeals have been exhausted, the person with ALS should seek additional support. Contact the ALS Association and the Muscular Dystrophy Association, both of which have local loan equipment pools. Contact your local service representative and ask about borrowing the equipment you need. The ALS Association in some areas has set aside funds to assist in the purchase of AAC devices.

Ventilation (Tracheostomy and Ventilator and/or Bi-PAP or CPAP)

At some point the person with ALS may experience difficulty breathing. The decision to use mechanical ventilation can be difficult. Factors that affect that decision are not limited to the availability of insurance coverage but also include whether there are caregivers in the home or other funds to support private duty nursing to assist the patient with ALS in the management of these devices.

What Are Invasive Ventilation and Noninvasive Ventilation? Does the Policy Cover the Patient's Needs?

Invasive ventilation refers to the placement of an endotracheal tube in the nose or mouth or a tracheostomy (tube in the neck) and attachment to a mechanical breathing device. Invasive ventilation is considered a permanent method of support (see Chapter 12). A noninvasive device refers to positive pressure air delivered through a nasal mask, nasal pillows, or face mask. These methods of ventilation assist the person with ALS to breathe. Some insurance companies consider these modes of ventilation as DME rather than life support equipment. The result may be that they will not cover the cost or rental of the equipment. The person with ALS will need to examine not only the cost of the machine but all the ancillary equipment that is necessary, especially if the device is invasive (i.e., tubing, suctioning catheters, trach replacement, dressings). The financial impact could be significant.

Implication on Treatment Decisions

We encourage the person with ALS to seek medical and financial counseling before making a decision about the use of any respiratory device. Noninvasive ventilation is simpler, less expensive, and nonsurgical; it often is used only at night. Invasive ventilatory support requires surgery (tracheostomy), hospital admission, and nurse or family training. The cost of noninvasive equipment rental is not less than $6,000 per year, and invasive equipment can cost as much as $20,000 per month if the cost of 16 hours of nursing care per day is included. Typically, insurance companies may pay for the rental of the equipment and some supplies, but the cost of nursing care may be limited to the first month to six weeks and then becomes the financial responsibility of the patient and family.

Nutrition

What does one do to maintain proper nutrition and hydration? Dietary supplements can be used if the person with ALS has no difficulty swallowing or has some difficulty but is not aspirating (choking) foods and fluids. However, if he does have significant difficulty with swallowing, a surgical procedure to insert a tube (percutaneous gastrostomy tube, or PEG) into the stomach can be performed (see Chapter 11). Feeding tubes are not a life-sustaining measure, but they do improve quality of life. Malnutrition and dehydration have been shown to increase (1) the rate of disease progression; (2) feelings of fatigue; and (3) the risk of further complications, such as aspiration pneumonia, malnutrition, and dehydration.

Insertion of a feeding gastrostomy tube is usually done as an outpatient procedure, although some ALS patients may require a one- to two-day hospital stay. The cost of the procedure normally is covered by most insurances. However, Medicare requires that the patient have a modified barium swallow test and that the test indicate that aspiration of food and liquids is present. Otherwise, Medicare will not pay for the surgical procedure. Managed care health programs require referral to a specialist within their provider group. Other insurance programs require payment of a deductible (if applicable) and coinsurance. The cost of the procedure may be as little as $1,500 (same-day stay). Additional charges depend on overnight stay and physical condition at the time of the procedure.

Feedings consist of special formulas or prepared products. The average cost of feedings per month is $250. Feeding tubes and syringes normally cost $30 per month. However, if bolus feedings are not tolerated, slow drip feedings are recommended. The cost for the rental of a drip pump is approximately $220 per month. Medicare will cover the cost of feedings when nutrition is through a feeding tube. Other insurance programs vary in the amount that is reimbursed. The patient with ALS needs to review the specific coverage with his or her insurance company.

We are not aware of any programs that assist with the cost of surgery, supplies, or nutritional supplement.

Nursing Care

Skilled nursing care refers to patient services that are necessary to meet specific care objectives. Registered nurses, physical therapists, occupational therapists, and speech pathologists all provide short-term skilled care. The terms *custodial care* and *in-home care* refer to those services used to maintain or support the care of an individual but not to rehabilitate him or her. Nursing homes can serve several functions, either as a skilled nursing facility, an extended care facility, or a hospice. Nursing homes at one time were the mainstay of long-term care. Over the years, however, more and more individuals have decided to remain at home through the disease and dying process. Skilled nursing facilities are used as short-term stays for the management of a specific health care problem. Extended care facilities attempt to meet the patient's long-term care needs. Hospices or hospice services are designed to provide palliative care to individuals with a terminal disease who choose not to seek curative or life-sustaining care (i.e., invasive ventilation) (see Chapter 12).

Table 26-4. National Patient Service Resources

National Organizations	Amyotrophic Lateral Sclerosis Association (ALSA)	National nonprofit health organization. They provide several patient support services.	1-800-782-4747 http://www.alsa.org
	Muscular Dystrophy Association (MDA)	National nonprofit health organization. They provide several patient support services, including MDA/ALS clinics throughout the USA	1-800-572-1717 http://www.mda.org
	National Respite Locator Service	This is a national directory for Respite services	1-800-773-5433 http://www.chtop.com
	National Hospice Organization (NHO)	This is a national directory for Hospice services	1-800-658-8898 http://www.nho.org

Out-of-Pocket Expense Based on Health Care Program

Most insurance companies cover the cost for skilled nursing services when a planned program has been developed and a letter of justification and a prescription has been provided by the attending physician. Custodial care or extended care services generally are not covered by insurance companies unless the patient has specifically selected a policy with an in-home program feature. Medicaid, on the other hand, may provide for a home health aide to assist with activities of daily living, and Medicare covers the cost of extended care service if the patient was discharged from an acute care facility; that coverage is limited to the first 100 days. Extended care facilities normally are not covered by insurance companies unless the patient is on a ventilator. The cost for care in any of these facilities can be quite high, and personal resources can be spent at an alarming rate. Hospice is covered under Part A of the Medicare benefits and by most HMO and private insurance plans.

Implication for Treatment Decisions

Whatever choice is made for assistance—short-term, long-term, or palliative—the person with ALS needs to identify what coverage he has, what he needs to do to get that coverage, and what his out-of-pocket expense will be. For some individuals there is no help available unless they pay for it. If this is their only option, they need to talk to their case manager, local hospital social worker, ALSA or MDA Patient Services Coordinators, and ALS Clinic coordinators about alternative resources in their community.

Recourse: Alternative Funding Sources

The Spousal Impoverishment Program allows for the division of a patient's assets, enabling the healthy spouse to retain resources. To apply for this program, you should seek the assistance of an attorney experienced in this field.

Voluntary Not-for-Profit Agencies and Health Care Alternatives

Non-Profit Agencies

Amyotrophic Lateral Sclerosis Association (ALSA). ALSA is a nonprofit organization dedicated to the ALS patient, family, caregivers, and health care professionals. Its purpose is to provide funding for research, education, community-based support groups, and identification of local resources as well as to serve as an advocate at the local and national levels (see Table 26-4).

Muscular Dystrophy Association (MDA). MDA is a nonprofit organization dedicated to over 40 neuromuscular diseases including ALS. It supports more than 200 hospital-affiliated clinics that specialize in neuromuscular diseases and several ALS subspecialty clinics. MDA also provides educational material, funding for research, and community-based support groups for ALS patients (Table 26-4).

United Way. United Way is a national nonprofit organization that provides support to various other charitable or nonprofit organizations. Through various interface programs it can assist individuals in locating rent subsidy, utility subsidy, child care subsidy, and food programs in their area.

The Amyotrophic Lateral Sclerosis (ALS) Patient and Caregiver Resource Guide was developed by Rhone-Poulenc Rorer Pharmaceuticals Inc. (currently Aventis) in 1996 (6). It provides an extensive list of organizations and description of their services.

Health Care Alternatives

Both MDA and ALSA support clinics across the country that specialize in the care of the ALS patient. Information about these clinics can be found on the web page (wfnals.org) (see also Chapter 32). The types of services and treatment costs are variable. The patient with ALS should contact the local clinic to determine what resources are available and what cost is entailed. The typical clinic supports the cost of the physical examination, limited testing procedures, access to rehabilitation services (PT, OT, speech pathology), and some may have a social worker and nurse.

References

1. Levvy G. The role of the amyotrophic lateral sclerosis and motor neurone disease community in health-care resourcing. *International Journal of Clinical Practice* 1998; 94:4(Suppl):14–17.
2. Klein LM, Forshew, DA. The economic impact of ALS. *Neurology* 1996; 47 (Suppl 2):S126–S129.
3. Mitsumoto H, Norris FH. *Amyotrophic lateral sclerosis. A comprehensive guide to management.* New York, Demos, 1994.
4. Munsat T, et al. Economic Burden of Amyotrophic Lateral Sclerosis in the United States. Poster presentation at the 9th International Symposium on ALS/MND, 1998.
5. Pennell, Frances. Talking Points. Barriers to Accessing at Through Private Insurance. Http://wata.org/meeting/t-pennell-attach.htm. March 4, 1998.
6. Rhone-Poulenc Rorer Pharmaceuticals Inc. "Amyotrophic Lateral Sclerosis (ALS) Patient and Caregiver Resource Guide," 1996.

Suggested Reading

1. Appleby C. Values. *Hospitals & Health Networks.* July 5, 1996:20–26.

2. Baldor, R. *Managed care made simple.* Malden, Mass.: Blackwell Science, 1996.

3. Corrigan JM, Ginsburg PB. Association leaders speak out on health system change. *Health Affairs* 1997; 16(1):150–157.

4. Edwards JC, Donati RM. *Medical practice in the current health care environment.* Baltimore: Johns Hopkins University Press, 1995.

5. Meslin EM. An ethics framework for assisting clinician-managers in resource
allocation decision making. *Hospital & Health Services Administration* 1997; 42(1):33–48.

6. Orchard DW. Health policy and the quality of life. *Journal of Palliative Care* 1992; 8(3):31–33.

7. Roberts CC. Keeping managed care in balance. *Health & Social Work* 1996; 2(3):163–166.

8. Shortell SM, et al. *Remaking health care in America.* San Francisco: Jossey-Bass, 1996.

9. Stroud Jackson. Financing ALS (unpublished manuscript).

10. Sultz HA, Young KM. *Health care USA. Understanding its organization and delivery.* Gaithersburg, MD: Aspen, 1997.

27

Home Care Agencies

Dallas A. Forshew, R.N., B.S.N.

Supportive care is the term used for care that supports the person but does not take away or change the course of the disease. Good supportive care in amyotrophic lateral sclerosis (ALS) means that the people helping you have experience with ALS, have an awareness of your future needs, can anticipate and help plan for those needs, and can help take care of problems when they arise. Let me give you an example. Many people with ALS develop weakness of leg muscles. If you begin to have a little leg weakness, your health care professionals can look ahead and tell you that you may eventually need a walker. As more weakness appears, it may be time for you to talk with your physician, nurse, or therapist about the different types of walkers that are available and what the best choice for you might be. It may be appropriate to go shopping at this time. It is important to check with your insurance company before buying. Finally, when it is time for a walker, you will have already checked out the possibilities and can easily purchase one. The walker will help prevent falls and prolong independence, allowing participation in previous activities without the help of other people. It is hoped that the walker will enhance quality of life better than if it were not used.

Let us explore what can be done to treat your symptoms, improve your quality of life, and help your family cope with the disease through home care services.

What Is Home Care?

Home care refers to the care given to a patient by outside people who are paid

349

to come into the home. Home care can include many kinds of help, from professional therapists to aids who help with bathing and dressing. Home care agencies are available to provide this care, but *your physician must order the care.* Your physician or nurse probably will want to guide you in the choice of an agency and then will work with the agency to arrange the services that you need. The agency should report regularly to your physician and nurse to tell them of further needs.

Home care is designed for people who have trouble leaving the home. Your insurance company may require that you be "homebound." The definition of "homebound" may vary from one insurance company to another, but it usually means that you need special equipment to leave the home, such as a walker or a wheelchair, and that you leave the home infrequently. Your physician will certify whether you are homebound, but he must follow insurance guidelines.

The Need for Home Care

Many people ask, "How do I know when I should have home care?" The answer is different for different people. Many people with ALS never need home care but need care in the home from a hospice agency later on (see Chapter 29). However, many people with ALS will need some help in the home. You will have a good idea of what home care services are after you read this chapter. As you look at your personal needs, do not forget the needs of your caregivers, the family members who help you with your daily activities. A caregiver who is becoming overly tired is a clear signal that some help is needed in the home. If you think you could benefit from home care, talk with your physician, nurse, or therapist.

Large ALS specialty clinics, such as those certified by the ALS Association or the Muscular Dystrophy Association (MDA), include a health care team. The team may include a physician, nurse, therapists, and others who provide much of the clinical care. However, any physician or clinic can use the team model and call in or refer you to other professionals. The challenge of the professionals who provide home care is to bring a team approach to care of ALS patients in their home.

Services Offered by Home Care Agencies

The services offered by home care agencies vary among agencies and regions of the country. An experienced nurse manages the evaluation and overall care provided by home care agencies. She will oversee day-to-day care provided by aids such as bathing and dressing, as well as services provided by professionals such as physical, occupational, speech, and respiratory therapists, and social workers who are available to address specific care needs. Many agencies also offer ancillary services such as volunteers for respite care, running errands, or light housekeeping.

Services

Skilled Nursing Care	Home Health Aids
Physical Therapy	Occupational Therapy
Speech Therapy	Social Work Services
Nutritional Therapy	Homemakers
Respite Care	Ventilator Care
Respiratory Care	Emergency Response

Skilled Care and Basic Care in the Home

You will soon become familiar with the terms *basic care* and *skilled care* because your insurance company will limit services based on how your needs fit into these two categories. Many insurance companies pay for skilled care but not for basic care. The insurance company may also have a limit on the number of yearly visits.

Skilled care can be described as care that needs to be provided by someone who is *professionally trained.* This might be a registered nurse, a physical therapist, or a speech therapist.

Basic care can be described as care that anyone could provide and does not require special training or skills. Basic care includes things that your family may help you with, such as bathing and dressing.

It is important to talk with a representative from your insurance company to find out what your particular policy offers. An excellent method of working with your insurance company is to have a case manager, who usually is a nurse. If a case manager has not already been assigned by the insurance company, call and ask to have one assigned to you. Use your case manager as your contact person whenever you need to consult the insurance company. She will become familiar with you, your disease, and your needs. Case managers can sometimes "cut red tape" because they are aware of ALS and your whole situation.

What If Your Insurance Does Not Cover Home Care?

This is one of the most difficult problems in ALS. If your breathing test is good and you do not qualify for hospice, you will look to home care if you need help. But what do you do if your insurance does not have an adequate home care benefit?

A social worker or nurse can help you to investigate resources in your community. People at your place of worship may be able to give assistance. Your friends and family may have been asking "What can I do?" Now is the time to tell them to come over to your home for a few hours each week so your caregiver can go to the store or, even better, so your caregiver can visit friends or see a movie. Family and friends have a very real need to "do something" for you. Allowing them to help is therapeutic for them, so do not hesitate to ask.

You may need to "private pay" for home health aid help. You can contact an agency, ask for a home health aid, and be billed for the service. This is relatively expensive, but it gives you a trained person with an agency behind them. If the aid does not show up on a day, you can call the agency and they should send another. In addition, the performance of the aid will be covered by the agency's liability insurance if there is ever any serious problem. You may choose to find an aid on your own, someone who is not working under the auspices of an agency. This will be much less expensive, but it does carry some risk if there are ever any problems.

Some volunteer agencies may provide services in your home. Some ALSA chapters employ nurses who will perform home visits to give support and advise. Contact ALSA or MDA for information.

How to Choose a Home Care Agency

The home care agency must receive orders from your physician that specify what services you need. Most communities have many home care agencies. The most important thing to remember is that your physician and nurse know the agencies in your community and will choose the best one for you. Your physician will have listened to the comments of other patients and families about the agencies. Trends in these comments over time provide valuable information about agencies. Your physician should welcome suggestions and ideas from you and the agency about your services.

Agencies should be accredited through JCAHO or CHAP and certified by Medicare. They also should be licensed by your state. They should offer experience in a full range of services. Furthermore, a home care agency that is also a hospice agency is of great benefit. Most people with ALS will need hospice services late in the course of the disease; if your home care agency is also a hospice agency, you will not have to change agencies when you eventually need hospice.

It may be difficult to choose between agencies when advertised services appear to be comparable at many different home care agencies within a community. Many ALS centers have found it helpful to develop a relationship with a few reputable agencies and to foster their knowledge of ALS care through lectures and referrals. The more experience an agency has with ALS patients, the more likely it is that the patient's care will be good and comprehensive.

The Initial Home Visit and
What to Expect from a Home Care Agency

As a "customer," you have the right to receive quality service from the agency. You also have the responsibility to be a wise consumer.

There is a lot to do at the initial home visit. The nurse must learn about you, your medical condition, and your social situation (family, friends, other supports you may have in the community such as religious affiliation). You also need to get to know the nurse at this visit and learn about what the agency can offer. Remember to speak up and be a partner in making the plan for your care.

There are a number of other "pieces of business" that usually occur at the initial home visit. The agency should provide you with a copy of the Patient's Bill of Rights and Responsibilities and discuss these with you. You should be given a full description of the agency's available services. In addition, the agency should give you information about services that are available through other means such as community support and resource services. The agency should research your insurance benefits and explain what is covered and what is not. It should describe its billing procedure and how it will notify you of noncovered services. The agency is required to fully inform you before services are started.

Skilled Nursing Care

A registered nurse (RN) will oversee your care and coordinate the activities of other people who come into your home to provide services.

The first duty of the registered nurse is to meet in your home with you and your family, assess your needs, and develop a plan of care. This is called the *intake visit.* You also have some responsibilities during the intake visit. You and your family should advocate for yourselves and speak up. Let the nurse know what you need and work with her to develop your plan of care.

In addition to the intake assessment, the nurse is responsible for ongoing assessment of your situation as it changes. Other things the nurse can do include patient and family education, basic counseling, and performing any medical procedures.

Home Health Aid Care

Home health aids (HHAs) take care of basic needs such as bathing, dressing, and feeding. Depending on the agency and the level of the aid's training, the aid may also help with range of motion or other exercises. They may do some light housekeeping.

After a time, your caregiver and other family members may need some help. ALS is a difficult disease for both family and patients. Your family will need both emotional energy and physical energy to give you support over the months and years. We want to keep your family caregiver(s) in good shape so they do not become overtired or burned out. We want to take care of the caregiver(s). One way to do this is to have a home health aid from a home nursing agency. The insurance company might pay for the services of a home health aid if a skilled service is being provided at the same time.

Social Workers and Psychological Care

Amyotrophic lateral sclerosis changes the lives of everyone it touches. This includes patients, their families, and their friends. Some people say that ALS is harder on the family than it is on the patient. It also is a progressive disease, and it seems that every time the patient and family become accustomed to a situation and begin to manage, the situation changes and everyone has to adjust again. This is a difficult process for everyone.

Social workers are specially trained to help patients and family members cope with physical and emotional changes in their lives. Although most people affected by ALS can cope on their own, it is hard! It is much easier to have some guidance from someone who is trained in this area. Just as a home health aid can help to conserve your and your caregiver's physical energy, a social worker can help to conserve your emotional energy. A social worker can help to guide your feelings and help your family as everyone adjusts. Social workers are an important part of the home care team and should be used by all ALS patients.

The social worker does not help only the patient. The emotional well-being of each of us is a compilation of our life experiences, expectations, and fears. Issues of the past, the present, and loss of the future need to be talked about openly. Family members have concerns very similar to yours, not only with respect to themselves but also related to their relationship with you. Family relationships are complex. The social worker can give guidance toward resolution of both old and new concerns.

Death and dying issues are in the forefront of the minds of all people with ALS and their families as soon as the diagnosis is made. These issues remain of concern throughout the illness, whether you and your family are talking about them or not. Concerns will be easier to deal with if a social worker helps.

It is common to have difficulty coping when you are first told about ALS entering your life. Some depression is not unusual but it deserves full attention. If you feel "blue" or depressed, talk with your social worker or nurse, who can refer you or your family member for ongoing counseling. Also, tell your physician because sometimes medication can be helpful.

In addition to helping with feelings, social workers are often knowledge-able about insurance matters and social agencies. Most communities have a wide range of social agencies. Some are federal or state funded and some are locally sponsored. Community service clubs, "good works" agencies, and church groups are some of the resources available. Others include Centers for Independent Living, equipment loan closets, support groups, and Meals on Wheels. Social workers can sort through the maze of agencies and make appropriate referrals.

Physical Therapy

Physical therapists provide help with mobility issues. Their services are considered "skilled." Although it would be nice to have a physical therapist come to your home regularly to do exercises, this is not practical in the long run. There are specific times when a physical therapist will be of most use to you. These include the home safety evaluation, teaching exercises for stiff or painful joints and muscles, teaching transferring techniques, and equipment selection.

A home safety evaluation is a good idea if you are weak and falls are a concern. The physical therapist can come to your home and make suggestions for such things as the rearrangement of furniture, the placement of handrails, and the selection of equipment for the bathroom.

The physical therapist can decide which exercises would be most useful to you. He or she can do the exercises and then teach them to you and your family. Exercises are necessary to keep joints and ligaments limber. Range-of-motion exercises are needed if you are no longer stretching your joints in your day-to-day activities. For example, if arm weakness prevents you from reaching for items that are on the second shelf in the cupboard, you will need exercises to keep the shoulder free from stiffness and pain and prevent the development of a frozen shoulder. This is an area of your care where you can really make a difference in how you feel. You often can prevent pain by starting exercises when needed and keeping up with the exercises on a daily basis.

Your insurance company may allow physical therapy only as long as you are showing some improvement. This assumes that your family will take over once your stiffness has been stabilized and you have regained the "range" in which you can move your joint and the pain is gone or diminished.

A physical therapist can help with transfers. Transferring from a wheelchair to a car can be tricky, as can many other transfers in the home. It is important to learn how to move someone properly to prevent injury to the patient and caregiver. A physical therapist can teach techniques that keep both you and your helper safe. This teaching should be done at the home using your bathroom, your bed, your favorite chair, and your car. The physical therapist may need to come for several teaching sessions until you and your caregiver have practiced and feel comfortable showing the therapist your new techniques.

Equipment selection, such as deciding which type of walker or wheelchair is best, can be confusing. The physical therapist can suggest appropriate equipment for your situation and teach its use. It is a good idea to get some advice before you spend a lot of money. A physical therapist can be especially useful in measuring you for and helping select a wheelchair.

Occupational Therapy

People are often confused about the difference between an occupational therapist and a physical therapist. An occupational therapist usually works with the arms and with activities of daily living. A physical therapist usually works with the legs and with mobility issues. Either can perform a home safety evaluation. They both work with exercises and suggest equipment.

An occupational therapist provides expertise with issues related to activities of daily living, such as bathing, dressing, and feeding. He can teach you "tricks" that will help you remain independent for as long as possible. An occupational therapist often suggests helpful equipment or exercises. He may be the person to perform a home safety evaluation for you.

Many insurance companies (including Medicare) do not consider occupational therapists as giving "skilled" care. Medicare will allow occupational therapy visits only if a "skilled" health care provider (such as a registered nurse, physical therapist, or speech therapist) is also coming into your home.

Speech Therapy

Speech therapists, sometimes called speech pathologists, are trained to work with both speech and swallowing problems. Swallowing problems usually are evaluated by a speech therapist in a clinic or hospital. Communication is the main concern of a home speech therapist.

The speech therapist can help you maximize your current ability to speak and swallow by teaching you useful tricks. Examples for swallowing might include tucking your chin slightly as you swallow, taking smaller bites of food, and chewing more slowly and carefully. Examples for communication might include speaking more slowly, facing the person to whom you are speaking, and writing out words if you become frustrated.

An important role of the speech therapist is to teach you many ways to communicate if your voice cannot be understood. These methods may range from handwriting to the use of a sophisticated computer system. Substitutions for vocal communication are sometimes called "augmentative communication." Home speech therapists should be able to teach the basics of augmentative communication, but a specialist in augmentative communication is needed for "high-tech" equipment such as computers. Specialists in augmentative communication often work in larger hospitals or clinics.

Some patients become neglectful of their communication needs and do not pursue alternatives to speaking. However, the ability to communicate is one of the most important human activities. If you are not able to speak, that does not mean that you cannot communicate. You might have to learn a new way to make your needs and feelings understood. Communication should remain free-flowing. You must not only be able to make your physical needs known ("I'm hungry") but also be able to express your thoughts ("I've thought a lot about Sam and want to explain to him why . . .").

Nutrition Counseling

Dietitians assess your nutritional status and help both you and your family to adjust your diet as your needs and swallowing abilities change. Dietitians may suggest avoiding certain foods, offer suggestions for foods or liquids that will be easier to handle, and suggest appropriate nutritional supplements if you are losing weight.

Some people with ALS eventually have trouble swallowing and cannot maintain their weight. The main purpose of the mouth and throat is to get food and fluids down the esophagus and into the stomach. The mouth, throat, and esophagus make up a "tube." If your own tube does not work well, you can replace it with a tube that does work well—a feeding tube. A feeding tube is a good idea if you take a very long time to eat, if food or fluids are "going down the windpipe" and you are coughing or choking, if you get tired eating, if food no longer appeals to you, or if you are losing too much weight. A feeding tube is often called a PEG tube, which stands for percutaneous endoscopic gastrostomy. It will be much easier for you physically if you have a feeding tube placed earlier rather than later, especially if you wait until you have lost a lot of weight or your breathing is not good. A dietitian is best able to suggest the formula used for tube feedings and to keep your bowels functioning properly.

Respiratory Therapy

Respiratory therapists can help you with breathing problems. The therapist can perform tests in your home to measure your ability to breathe. These tests are called pulmonary function tests (PFTs) and might include forced vital capacity (FVC), maximum inspiratory flow (MIF), and pulse oximetry. Pulse oximetry measures the amount of oxygen in your blood by using a clip on a finger. Respiratory therapists install, monitor, and teach the use of equipment such as noninvasive bilevel positive air pressure (BiPAP) machines.

Respiratory therapists often are available not through standard home care agencies but through agencies that specialize in home respiratory needs. Some larger medical equipment companies employ respiratory therapists to serve patients who use their equipment. A home care agency may contract with another agency for respiratory therapy services, but frequently these services must be arranged separately from the patient's regular home care. This is easily arranged through your physician.

Invasive ventilation for the ALS patient in the home is a complex issue and is not addressed here. However, you should know that tracheostomy and invasive ventilation (a life-support breathing machine) is an option and can be handled in your home with the help of a respiratory therapist.

Resources

Amyotrophic Lateral Sclerosis Association 800-782-4747 www.alsa.org

Muscular Dystrophy Association 800-572-1717 www.mdausa.com

National Association for Home Care 202-547-77424 www.nahc.org

National Hospice Organization 800-658-8898 www.nho.org

National Council on the Aging 800-424-4096 www.ncoa.org

National Association of Area Agencies on the Aging 800-677-1116

National Family Caregivers Association 800-896-3650 www.nfccacares.org

Well Spouse Foundation 800-838-1338 www.wellspouse.org

National Respite Locator Service 800-773-5433 www.chtop.com

National Rehabilitation Information Center 800-346-2742 www.naric.com

AbleData Database 800-227-0216

A.C.C.E.S.S. Program (Advocating for Chronic Conditions, Entitlements, and Social Services) 888-700-7070 This is a toll free number and a free service to help with insurance and disability qualifications.

Your Medicare Handbook is a comprehensive guide from the Department of Health and Human Services. You can receive a copy by calling the Medicare Hotline at 1-800-638-6833.

Hints: A Helpful Guide to Understanding Medicare: Simple step-by-step directions to help beneficiaries with their hospital and medical bills. A booklet from Medicare Part B, Blue Cross and Blue Shield of Utah.

Summary

Home care services are used by many people with ALS, some for relatively brief periods of time and some for longer periods. All people with ALS and their care-givers eventually will benefit from hospice services.

The goal of home care is to provide services in your home that are similar to those you would receive in your clinic—a team approach with a nurse overseeing the services in your home. Remember that you are a partner in your care, so you need to let your wishes be known to the home care team and to your physician's team.

28

Palliative Care: The Management of Advanced Disease

Mark J. Stillman, M.D.

Recent initiatives by lay organizations to pass physician-assisted suicide laws in Oregon, Washington State, and New York have served to highlight the glaring deficiencies in end-of-life care in the American medical system. A recent study highlighted the need for open discussion of end-of-life issues in the amyotrophic lateral sclerosis (ALS) patient population. In this 1998 survey, 56 percent of patients with ALS said they would consider assisted suicide, nearly 90 percent would consider it if it were legalized, and three quarters of all caregivers concurred.

Until recently the United States had no training programs dedicated to the study and care of patients with advanced incurable diseases such as ALS and cancer. Educators in medical and nursing schools are now finally recognizing the role of palliative care—the management of advanced disease—as a new field of medicine devoted to these patients and their families, and medical training is slowly changing.

What Is Palliative Care?

The World Health Organization defines palliative care as the care offered by a multidisciplinary team of doctors, nurses, social workers, therapists, clergy, and volunteers and describes it as: "The active total care of patients whose disease is not responsive to curative treatment. Control of pain, of other symptoms, and of psychological, social, and spiritual problems is paramount. The goal of palliative care is the achievement of the best quality of life for patients and their families. . . . Palliative care . . . affirms life and regards dying as a normal process, . . . neither hastens nor postpones death, . . . provides relief from distressing symptoms, . . . integrates the psychological and the spiritual aspects of care, . . . offers a support system to help the family cope during the patient's illness and in their own bereavement."

The components of a typical palliative care service are listed in Table 28-1. (Hospice care, as it relates to ALS, is discussed in more detail in Chapter 29.) In the United States, it is predominantly a home-based system of care, and its development and refinement have been fostered by the Medicare Hospice Benefit, written into law by Congress in 1982. Regardless of which component of palliative care establishes first contact with a patient with ALS or some other disease, the goals and principles of care are the same: to treat the patient and his family, using a multidisciplinary approach, for the purpose of comfort and symptom relief and to improve quality of life for as long as feasible.

Many medical practitioners and lay people equate hospice care with palliative care, failing to realize that it is only one component of it. At least in the United-States, hospice care is a form of home-based palliative care that a patient and family elect when life expectancy is limited to six months or less. On a broder basis, as it applies to cancer care, palliative care is the management of anticipated and unanticipated complications of a disease during the disease's natural trajectory.

Palliative Approaches to Patient Care

Little has been written about palliative care of the ALS population in comparison to a larger literature devoted to the diagnosis of ALS, its pathophysiology, and attempted cures. What has been written is derived from small studies, but the work is thoughtful and applicable to the whole. Certain principles of care—universal principles of care for any patient population—should be followed:

Table 28-1. Components of a Palliative Care Service

1. Hospice (a) Home-based (b) Inpatient or residential
2. Inpatient acute care facility for the management of acute medical or symptom control issues that cannot be managed as an outpatient
3. Inpatient palliative care consultation service for consultation of patients with palliative care issues on surgical and medical services
4. Outpatient consultation services

- Open communication between health care practitioners with patient and family
- Good nursing care, with particular attention paid to body positioning to prevent skin breakdown in the bedbound patient
- Awareness that patients have a normal mental status even when they are mute
- Special attention to facilitation of communication, swallowing, and breathing
- Anticipation of consequences of immobility: constipation, pain, anxiety and depression, insomnia, fatigue, bedsores, and urinary retention

It cannot be overemphasized that the recipients of care include not only the person with ALS but also his family and primary caregivers. Considering that the progression of ALS implies an inevitable dependence in toileting, eating, and such seemingly routine tasks as changing position in bed, failure to recognize the physical and psychological stresses on the caregiver is a grievous oversight. The inclusion of psychiatric social workers, specially trained nurses, home health aids, volunteers, and respite time (brief hospital admissions to allow a family under stress a period of rest) in the benefit package of hospice under the Medicare Hospice Benefit is an indicator that the hospice–palliative care approach anticipates such problems.

Communicating with the Patient and Family

Like any seriously ill patient, the person with ALS is in danger of sudden fatal deterioration resulting from respiratory failure or intercurrent medical complications. The family needs to be informed of this from the outset in order to make an informed decision about the level of care in such a circumstance. Involved in this decision is a consideration of cardiopulmonary resuscitation and placement of an endotracheal tube for ventilation, as well as the eventual surgical insertion of a breathing tube (tracheostomy) for long-term respiratory support. As discussed subsequently, some people with ALS choose to have a tracheostomy to help them breathe when diaphragmatic and chest wall muscles weaken to the point that independent breathing is no longer possible. Failure to anticipate such emergencies or to be informed of their possibility can lead to the imposition of unwanted treatment by emergency medical staff.

Symptom Control

Table 28-2 lists the symptoms that most commonly plague the person with ALS and that present a challenge to the palliative care or hospice team.

Pain

Although classic neurology textbooks regard pain as an uncommon symptom of ALS, the fact is that as many as two-thirds of all patients may experience pain. The pain is described as aching, cramping, or burning, and it may be attributed to either loss of innervation (muscle cramps), abnormal stress on the musculoskeletal system from immobility (e.g., bedsores, stiff joints), or spasticity (increased muscle tone) from involvement of the upper motor neuron tracts.

Clearly, good nursing care is important, with frequent positioning and passive mobilization of joints. That is all that is needed for some patients, but pain medications are necessary for others. The pharmacologic treatment of spasticity and stiffness is limited. Baclofen and tizanidine both work in the spinal cord to inhibit spasticity and muscle stiffness around a joint, but they do so at the expense of sedation and weakness. For those patients who rely on their spasticity to walk, the drug-induced weakness can be a problem. The dose of baclofen is between 10 and 80 mg a day in three or four divided doses, with a maximum dose of 200 mg per day. The recommended dose of tizanidine is between 6 and 24 mg per day in divided doses. Other medications such as dantrolene sodium have been used for ALS-related muscle spasms and spasticity, but they are used less frequently because of side effects.

When specific attempts to treat the pain fail, the use of pain medications should follow the guidelines established by the World Health Organization for cancer pain and acute pain. The "stepladder" approach, as it has come to be known, starts with the recognition of pain and the initiation of treatment with a drug suited to the type of pain the patient describes. Mild pain is treated with low doses of an opioid medication (narcotic) or a non-opioid analgesic. As the pain increases, either a stronger opioid replaces the initial weaker analgesic or larger doses of the opioid are added (Figure 28-1).

The successful management of pain depends on the clinician's familiarity and understanding of the mechanism of pain and the appropriate use of analgesics.

Table 28-2. Symptoms Common to Patients with ALS

- Pain
- Dysphagia (difficulty swallowing)
- Drooling
- Dyspnea (shortness of breath)
- Weakness
- Bedsores
- Inability to sleep
- Anxiety and depression
- Constipation

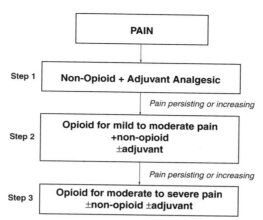

Figure 28-1. The WHO stepladder approach to the management of cancer pain.

The use of opioids requires the experience and skill to balance beneficial effects with side effects. A brief description of the most commonly used agents follows.

The opioid analgesics are the cornerstone of therapy for cancer pain and are the most useful class of analgesics for the management of any pain that is resistant to non-narcotic medications. The drugs belonging to the morphine (or mu opioid) family are the most frequently used group of opioid analgesics and the ones most familiar to physicians. Weak analgesics such as hydrocodone or oxycodone are prescribed for mild or intermittent pain. Hydrocodone and oxycodone both come as combination tablets attached to either aspirin or acetaminophen. This combination is convenient, but it tends to limit the number of tablets taken in a day because of concerns about toxicity from either aspirin or acetaminophen. Fortunately, oxycodone comes in a pure preparation and is available as a liquid concentrate; it also is available in a delayed-release tablet preparation, which is ideal for patients with prolonged pain. In the delayed-release form it may be taken by mouth on a 12-hourly basis instead of every four hours, which is the recommended interval for the immediate-release liquid or tablet formulations. The dose depends on the severity of the pain—hence the importance of careful assessment by the clinician—and the patient's tolerance to the medication. Doses start at 5 to 10 mg oxycodone every four to six hours and increase as needed to control the pain, either as pure oxycodone or combined with 325 mg acetaminophen or aspirin per tablet. Delayed-release oxycodone tablets come in 10 mg, 20 mg, 40 mg, and 80 mg.

Of all the mu opioid drugs, morphine sulfate remains the most versatile because it is available in short-acting liquid and tablet, long-acting tablet, and injectable formulations. It can be prescribed by mouth, under the tongue, by feeding tube, by rectum, or by injection (subcutaneously, intravenously, or intramuscularly), and charts are available that outline dosage and routes of administration. In turn, the route and dosage of morphine depends on the severity and persistence of the pain, while the route of administration is determined by the patient. One of the pill formulations can be prescribed if the patient is able to swallow. If a percutaneous endoscopic gastrostomy (PEG) is available and the patient cannot swallow, liquid immediate-release morphine can be prescribed via tube on a four-hourly basis. For the patient who is unable to swallow and without a PEG, immediate release morphine can be provided under the tongue as either a solid tablet or liquid formulation (10-, 15-, or 30-mg tablet, or liquid concentrate 20 mg/ml), and the dose can be repeated as needed in two to four hours. Rectal preparations of morphine come as immediate-release 15-mg suppositories or delayed-release oral tablets, which dissolve slowly and are absorbed. The delayed-release tablets are available in 15, 30, 60, 100, and 200 mg doses.

When absorption through oral or rectal mucosa is inadvisable or impossible, morphine can be infused by the intravenous or subcutaneous route. Portable pumps that infuse concentrated solutions of morphine have been in use for a number of years and have remedied many previously intractable pain management problems. A "rescue" button can be installed in the pump's program to permit the delivery of small doses of morphine in situations in which pain breaks through (patient-controlled analgesia).

The dose of morphine depends on the severity and duration of the pain, and careful evaluation and reassessment are necessary to adjust the dose. Oral doses as small as 5 mg every four to six hours, as needed, may be adequate for a patient with mild or intermittent pain, whereas other patients may require high subcutaneous infusion rates of morphine for comfort.

The recent introduction of a narcotic patch, the fentanyl transdermal system, has promised to replace expensive opioid infusions. Available in 25-, 50-, and 100-microgram patches, they can be placed on the skin every 72 hours in situations in which the patient is unable or unwilling to take medications by mouth. The 25-microgram patch provides approximately the same analgesia as 15 mg of oral morphine every four hours, but exact doses must be individualized. A sublingual preparation of fentanyl will soon be available for the management of cancer pain, and it should be useful for any opioid-tolerant patient with severe breakthrough pain.

Side effects of opioids, including respiratory depression, constipation, nausea and vomiting, and concerns for addiction, are widely recognized. As in the cancer population, addiction or psychological dependence is virtually unheard of; nausea and vomiting can occur with any opioid agent, and constipation is assured. Use of antiemetics and laxatives is advised. Avoiding respiratory depression requires a skilled hand and the knowledge that tolerance to the depressant effects of opioid analgesics develops rapidly; it should be remembered that any patient who is awake and comfortably breathing on a stable dose of a short-acting opioid probably is not in danger of respiratory depression, no matter how high the dose.

Dysphagia

Dysphagia, or difficulty in swallowing, is a common symptom of ALS and occasionally is the presenting symptom. The problem extends not only to foods but also to a patient's own secretions, resulting in the embarrassment of drooling. It is not difficult to understand how dysphagia occurs if one keeps in mind that ALS is a disease of motor function. Weakness of the striated muscle—the tongue, pharyngeal muscles, and the upper esophagus—makes chewing and propulsion of food to the back of the throat and the esophagus increasingly difficult, leading to pooling of secretions and foodstuffs. Liquids, in particular, follow the quickest and most direct route directed by gravity, leading to aspiration down the trachea, and followed by reflexive coughing ("choking"). As a consequence, oral intake decreases and weight loss ensues out of fear of choking or exhaustion from coughing spells. Few things are as disconcerting to the sympathetic caregiver or friend than to see a patient suffering in this manner—wasting away from starvation despite a strong desire to eat.

There are several approaches to this problem. The first and simplest approach is to alter the texture of the food. If necessary, the advice of a dietitian who is familiar with swallowing disorders should be sought. Under the Medicare Hospice Benefit, a speech pathologist trained to evaluate swallowing disorders should be available on an as-needed basis. Blenderized food or food thickened with starch will enable many people to get the liquid and calories needed to maintain weight.

Other options are available for those patients in whom swallowing is impaired. In the past, a procedure known as a cricopharyngotomy (the surgical sectioning of the pharyngeal muscles) was reserved for patients with "spastic" swallowing disorders, but technical advancements in feeding tubes have made this procedure obsolete. Until recently, the procedure of choice was a nasogastric (NG) feeding tube, a small rubber tube placed through the nose into the stomach. Pliable, latex NG catheters are much more comfortable than the rubber nasal tubes, but they have a small diameter and tend to clog. Several procedures to deal with the problem of feeding people who cannot swallow have been developed in the last 10 years, including percutaneous endoscopic gastrostomy (PEG) and, less commonly, percutaneous endoscopic jejunostomy (PEJ). Feedings with clear liquids can safely commence within 24 to 48 hours of endoscopic (fiberoptic) tube placement through the abdominal wall, gradually building up to 100 percent supplementation of caloric needs through the use of commercial liquid diets.

The widespread use of the PEG tube feeding has led to symptomatic improvement in the ALS population—less "choking" to be certain—but has not led to prolongation of survival when compared with NG feeding. Moreover, the procedure of inserting the tube is not without complications, and there may be abdominal wall pain severe enough to warrant opioid therapy for the first 24 to 48 hours. Even in the most experienced hands, there is a 1 percent to 4 percent 24-hour postoperative mortality as a result of pulmonary complications; post-procedural pain leads to abdominal splinting and places patients at great risk for developing pneumonia, pulmonary embolus, and respiratory failure. As a result, it is recommended that patients be considered candidates for PEG tube placement earlier rather than later—when weight loss approaches 5 percent and bulbar symptoms (dysphagia , dysarthria, or aspiration of oral secretions) first develop. Patients should have preoperative pulmonary function tests to document enough reserve lung function to mount an adequate cough.

The patient's and family's reluctance to submit to a surgical procedure in favor of more natural attempts at feeding frequently delays this procedure. When the patient finally agrees, it often is too late to reverse the weight loss or forestall the operative complications. Every effort should be made to perform placement of a PEG relatively early.

Drooling

Drooling is an embarrassing and distressing symptom that results from a patient's inability to swallow saliva often enough to prevent overflow. Beyond the obvious use of a handkerchief, control of drooling requires drying out or suppressing the salivary glands. Surgical and radiotherapeutic control of salivation has been attempted, but medicinal manipulation is usually just as effective. A number of drugs may be useful.

Anticholinergic agents such as scopolamine hydrochloride and medications with anticholinergic side effects are frequently used to control drooling. A scopolamine patch used to treat motion sickness provides a convenient way to dry the mouth without the need to ingest yet another pill. This 1-mg patch is placed on the skin, usually behind the ear, and can be left in place for three days. Anticholinergic antidepressants such as amitriptyline, nortriptyline, or desipramine predictably cause dry mouth as a side effect, even in doses as low as 10 mg per day. These agents have additional benefits such as pain relief, appetite stimulation, and the treatment of depression. Another medication whose side effects are use-ful in drying salivary secretions is the antihistamine cyproheptadine. This medication stimulates the appetite and usually is effective in a dose of 4 to 8 mg at bedtime, although higher doses sometimes are needed. A related antihistamine, diphenhydramine, in a dose of 25 to 50 mg every 6 to 8 hours, can have the same effect.

Other anticholinergic drugs that have been used to dry up saliva include benztropine (1–6 mg/day by mouth or tube in divided doses), trihexyphenidyl (6–10 mg/day by tube or mouth in divided doses), and glycopyrrolate (3–8 mg/day by mouth or tube in divided doses). The shortcoming of all these drugs, with the exception of glycopyrrolate (Rubinol), is the tendency to cause confusion and sedation. Most of them have been used to treat Parkinson's disease for the very reason that they penetrate the brain's natural barrier to chemicals.

Two other useful agents are propranolol and lithium. Beta blockers, of which propranolol is the standard, have been used to control mucus-rich secretions when anticholinergics have failed (propranolol 10–20 mg twice a day or metoprolol 12.5–25 mg twice a day.) Lithium carbonate, the medication for bipolar (manic-depressive) disorder, has mucosal dryness as one of its side effects and has been used for this purpose in ALS patients. The dose is 600 to 1200 mg per day in divided doses.

Caregivers should be aware that saliva is essential not only for food ingestion but also for dental maintenance and health. The loss of the protective effect of salivary antibodies against bacteria increases the risk of tooth decay; good dental hygiene is essential.

Shortness of Breath (Dyspnea)

The sensation of shortness of breath is a serious symptom in ALS. In general medical practice, there are numerous causes of dyspnea, including pneumonia, chronic lung disease (e.g., emphysema, chronic bronchitis), congestive heart failure, venous thromboembolism, and asthma. Although a person with ALS can have any of these, the progressive muscle weakness that accompanies the disease causes ALS patients to develop restricted ability to breath. Simply stated, they do not have the chest wall strength and mobility to take deep breaths. Portions of the lung may therefore collapse and pneumonia may develop. Patients describe a force or a weight restricting their ability to take a deep breath or to fully empty their lungs. The great fear is "choking" or "suffocating" to death.

Initial Treatment

Initial medical management should be directed at correcting any potentially treatable cause. This should include (1) controlling secretions and preventing regurgitation of tube feedings; (2) optimizing the patient's position in bed to minimize any chance of aspiration and maximize the ability of the diaphragm to function properly; (3) providing oxygen when needed; and (4) treating lung infections, bronchitis, or asthma. When these options fail or do not exist, the only therapeutic choices are to provide mechanical ventilation for the patient or to suppress the symptoms of breathlessness medicinally.

The ultimate consequence of respiratory failure is death as a result of elevated carbon dioxide level (hypercapnea) and decreased oxygen level (hypoxia). If the symptoms accompanying dyspnea—agitation, anxiety, and air hunger—can be controlled, death can be peaceful, with the patient quietly entering a coma. Any agitation can be suppressed with sedative hypnotics. The alternative—the prolongation of life on mechanical ventilation after tracheostomy or intubation (insertion of a plastic breathing tube into the trachea)—is viewed as heroic therapy by many patients, families, and clinicians.

It is therefore essential that families and caregivers of patients with ALS be aware of the natural history of the disease from its onset. Symptoms indicating that some form of ventilatory support is needed include disrupted sleep, orthopnea (the inability to breathe while lying flat), daytime sleepiness, dyspnea with exercise, ineffective cough, and less than 50 percent of the predicted ability to exhale (forced vital capacity). All too often patients and families confront impending respiratory failure without prior knowledge of treatment options. In particular, they may not be aware that the patient can receive breathing support from either a closely fitting mask, a tube placed in the trachea (endotracheal tube), or a surgically inserted hole in the trachea (tracheostomy). A patient who is mechanically ventilated for more than two weeks eventually will need a tracheostomy because an endotracheal tube cannot be tolerated for a longer period. One recent study found that 92 percent of patients who were on mechanical ventilator machines after tracheostomy had not decided in advance that this was what they would have wanted. Almost one-third were not satisfied with their quality of life as respirator-dependent patients. Sadly, many patients would have not have opted for mechanical ventilation if they had known of the financial and social burdens placed on their families or if they had known they would have to go to a skilled nursing unit. The role of advance directives and living wills is apparent in such a situation, as discussed in Chapter 25.

The alternative to tracheostomy and ventilation is noninvasive ventilation (NIV) using a tight-fitting nasal mask or face mask. This is an adequate option if the patient can tolerate the mask, has no problems managing secretions, and does not aspirate. *Patients who have poor airway protection are at risk of aspiration with this ventilation technique.*

Nasal NIV is therefore indicated for willing patients who do not have brain stem dysfunction (i.e., altered swallowing mechanisms) and who do not need suction. It is covered under the Medicare Hospice Benefit, costs less, and is associated with less complex care than mechanical ventilation and tracheostomy. More than 90 percent of patients are able to stay at home on NIV. Success with NIV can be predicted by the following:

- Absence of excess secretions

- Properly fitting face or nasal mask

- Willingness to wear mask

- A desire to live

- A good caregiver

Symptomatic Treatment

There are well-described techniques for the relief of dyspnea, borrowed from intensive care medicine, where they are routinely used for people with cardiac or pulmonary ailments. The benefits of opioid analgesics have been amply demonstrated for the treatment of air hunger related to dyspnea caused by cardiac pulmonary edema (severe heart failure). When given in small intravenous injections, morphine reduces shortness of breath and the inflated filling pressures of a flooded heart in heart failure. Oral preparations of morphine sulfate and morphine-related narcotics have been used in a similar manner and given on a round-the-clock basis for constant shortness of breath. The few studies that confirm the utility of opioids have demonstrated improved exercise tolerance for patients suffering from chronic obstructive lung disease.

Recent interest in inhaled or nebulized opioids has led to their increased use for patients with end-stage disease and associated breathlessness. No data have been published for nebulized drug therapy in ALS. The only exception has been the treatment of pooled saliva with nebulized lidocaine. The benefit of nebulized or aerosolized drug is its direct delivery to the sites (and presumably the receptors) where it is needed. Systemic absorption and side effects are limited. Despite few data in ALS, morphine sulfate and other drugs are being used in handheld bedside nebulizers with seemingly good results. Starting doses of morphine are 5 mg of injectable solution nebulized in normal saline every four to six hours as needed. The dose can be increased to 10 to 20 mg per treatment, as indicated. If the patient cannot tolerate morphine, a suitable alternative is fentanyl, 25 to 100 mcg nebulized in normal saline every four to six hours as needed.

Even with nebulized drugs, there are concerns about side effects, especially respiratory depression in patients with impaired ventilatory function. This fear has not been borne out in chronic obstructive lung disease, although there have been anecdotal reports of respiratory depression with nebulized morphine. Although nebulized morphine has rarely been associated with wheezing, fentanyl has been used safely.

Other medications have been useful in treating dyspnea and associated anxiety. Sedative hypnotics have been used for years in the intensive care unit to treat agitated ventilated patients when the agitation interferes with ventilation. Benzodiazepines (diazepam, lorazepam, midazolam) and barbiturates have all been used in this situation. There has been recent interest in the phenothiazines, a class of drugs designed for the treatment of agitated psychoses. Their use has now been extended to the agitation caused by dyspnea. Chlorpromazine and methotrimeprazine have been extensively used on palliative medicine services in both the United States and Europe.

Bedsores

Bedsores, or decubitus, are a common complication of immobility, although they are rare in patients with ALS. Frequent turning and positioning in bed is needed to prevent them from developing. Special beds using airflow or continuously moving pellets have been designed for patients with ALS, spinal cord injury, and Guillain Barré syndrome. Once a decubitus develops, however, meticulous attention must be paid to keeping pressure off the wound so that blood flow and airflow are maximized. Dead tissue must be removed and infection treated with dressing changes and wound cleaning; only in this way can new skin grow in and surgical grafting be avoided. There are a variety of ways to debride decubitus in the home, including wet to dry saline dressings, wet to dry iodophor dressings, specially developed adhesives, and spray granules. Severe wounds with superinfection and exposure of bone and deep tissues require surgical consultation and debridement (regular removal of damaged tissue) with or without skin grafting. It is best to prevent the development of skin breakdown by keeping the patient dry and well positioned.

Constipation

Constipation is common in ALS, even though the disease does not affect the smooth (automatic) muscle function in the bowel wall. Immobility and drugs such as opioids induce constipation. When this problem is combined with the patient's inability to self-toilet, it can create an unpleasant situation. As for patients without ALS, the treatment of constipation should follow a stepped approach starting with the maintenance of bowel hydration through the use of food fiber and adequate liquids as well as the institution of a set pattern of bowel elimination. A daily rectal suppository or a phosphosoda enema may help regulate the bowels, and stool softeners such as docusate should be used daily. For more severe constipation, cathartics such as magnesium compounds (milk of magnesia or magnesium citrate) or senna pills (maximum 6 pills twice daily) may be started on a regular basis. If persistent constipation is anticipated, especially with the use of opioid analgesics, the addition of other agents may be necessary. Osmotic agents that induce bowel motions, such as lactulose (30–60 ml one to three times a day) or 70 percent sorbitol (30–60 ml one to three times a day) can be very effective for the most resistant cases of drug-induced constipation.

Insomnia

Many people with ALS complain of an inability to fall asleep. Table 28-3 outlines the possible causes of insomnia. The first task is to correct any reversible causes such as pain and dyspnea. Many agents are now available for the treatment of depression and anxiety. Once again, the tricyclic antidepressants are effective agents for depression, and their side effects of sedation, dry mouth, and appetite stimulation can be useful. Newer nonsedating antidepressants have been introduced in the last few years, including the selective serotonin and norepinephrine reuptake inhibitors, such as fluoxetine, sertraline, paroxetine, and venlafaxine. Table 28-4 lists the medications for the treatment of depression and their range of doses. The antipsychotic chlorpromazine remains an excellent medication for inducing sleep and at the same time is effective for treating anxiety, agitation, nausea, and vomiting. The dose is 12.5 to 100 mg per mouth at nighttime, given by g-tube, intramuscularly, or intravenously.

Special Considerations

In a large medical center, the practitioner in hospice or palliative care eventually will help you deal with the decision to withdraw a ventilator or feeding tube. Tested bioethical principles underlie the decision by hospital personnel to support the with-

Table 28-3. Causes of Insomnia in the ALS Population

- Depression/ anxiety
- Inability to adjust posture
- Cramps/pain
- Dyspnea
- Reversal of sleep/wake cycle

drawal of life support when efforts to reverse medical and personal deterioration are futile and to help you deal with the personal tragedy of this decision. The practice guidelines used in intensive care units for withdrawing ventilatory support for brain-dead patients can be applied to ALS. Obviously, it is easier to withdraw ventilatory support in a comatose patient, as is frequently the case in intensive care units dealing with trauma and out-of-hospital cardiac arrests, but medications are available to sedate patients so that there is no perceptible respiratory distress when the ventilator is disconnected from the tracheotomy tube. It is important that the managing team be absolutely sure that your entire family agrees with the decision and to document this in your medical record. This family decision often is based on an advance directive or a living will. If the person with ALS does not have such a document, careful discussions should precede any action, and ethics consultants or social workers may enormously facilitate this difficult decision for your family.

The procedure basically involves sedating the patient before disconnecting the ventilator. This can be done with an opioid analgesic, a sedative hypnotic (e.g., pentobarbital), a sedating phenothiazine (e.g., chlorpromazine), or a combination of these medications; extra medication should be on hand should respiratory

Table 28-4. Antidepressant Medications

Tricyclic Antidepressants	Dose (mg)	Comment
Amitriptyline	10–250	Given at night preferably
Nortriptyline	10–250	" "
Doxepine	10–250	" "
Imipramine	10–250	" "
Quartenary Antidepressants		
Trazadone	25–150	Given at night to enhance sleep
Selective Serotonin Reuptake Inhibitors		
Fluoxetine (Prozac)	10–60	Tend to energize; give in A.M.
Sertraline (Zoloft)	25–200	" "
Paroxetine (Paxil)	10–40	" "

distress develop. Depending on your family's desires, family members can be present in the room, or the withdrawal can be done in their absence.

Conclusion

The symptomatic or palliative management of the person with ALS is a challenging problem for clinicians and caregivers alike. In addition to the emotional turmoil that accompanies this degenerative neurologic disease, progressive weakness and immobility create unique clinical problems. As with cancer, incorporation of palliative techniques early in the course of the disease, including the enlistment of hospice services if necessary, is not only advisable but also warranted.

Suggested Reading

1. Borasio G, Voltz R. Palliative care in amyotrophic lateral sclerosis. *J Neurol* 1997; 244(Suppl 4):S11–S17.

2. Cazzolli P, Oppenheimer E. Home mechanical ventilation for amyotrophic lateral sclerosis: Nasal compared to tracheostomy intermittent-positive pressure ventilation. *J Neurol Sci* 1996; 139(Suppl):123–128.

3. Ganzini L, Johnston W, et al. Attitudes of patients with amyotrophic lateral sclerosis and their care givers toward assisted suicide. *N Engl J Med* 1998; 339:967–973.

4. Mathus-Vliegen L, Louwerse L, et al. Percutaneous endoscopic gastrostomy in patients with amyotrophic lateral sclerosis and impaired pulmonary function. *Gastrointest Endosc* 1994; 40:463–469.

5. McDonald E, Wiedenfeld S, et al. Survival in amyotrophic lateral sclerosis: The role of psychological factors. *Arch Neurol* 1994; 5:17–23.

6. Moss A, Casey P, et al. Home ventilation for amyotrophic lateral sclerosis patients: Outcome, costs, and patient, family, and physician attitudes. *Neurology* 1993;43:438–443

7. Newrick P, Langton-Hewer R. Pain in motor neuron disease. *J Neurol Neurosurg Psychiatry* 1985; 48:838–840.

8. Newall A, Orser R, Hunt M. The control of oral secretions in bulbar ALS/MND. *J Neuro Sci* 1996; 139(Suppl):43–44.

9. Norris F, Smith R, Denys E. Motor neurone disease: Towards better care. *Br Med J* 1985; 291:259–262.

10. O'Brien T, Kelly M, Saunders C. Motor neurone disease: A hospice persective. *Br Med J* 1992; 304:471–473.

11. Rose F. The management of motor neurone disease. *Adv Exp Med Bio* 1987; 209:167–174.

29

Hospice Care

Barbara Thompson, OTR/L, CSW, and N. Michael Murphy, M.D.

Amyotrophic lateral sclerosis (ALS) can create pain, unrest, and mourning in everyone it touches. Hospice is dedicated to providing care and comfort to everyone involved with far-advanced illness when the pursuit of a cure is contributing little or nothing to the quality of life. Because these issues are major concerns of hospices and curative treatment is not available for ALS, it is appropriate that the hospice become involved as early as possible to temper the stresses and strains in your family and so improve your quality of life.

The modern hospice evolved within the last half century mainly as a response to the rampant technology that engulfed medicine, paid little attention to the feelings of all involved, and usually promoted treatment of one sort or another right up to the bitter end. It was becoming difficult to die in peace and rare to die in the comfortable and familiar surroundings of home. The hospice is still considered by some as a death sentence and a place of doom and gloom, and some fear that if a patient becomes involved then she will give up or lose hope. Our experience has been much more optimistic; with enhanced communication among family members and the necessary support, the ever-present tension related to the fear of dying lessens, and it becomes more possible to focus on the possibilities of each day, and for eventual death to be peaceful.

The first part of this chapter is concerned with a short history of the hospice movement together with organizational details. There is then some consideration of ALS as it affects the whole family and an outline of the family meeting, which we consider to be a necessary and powerful catalyst to a more satisfying last weeks

373

and months of life. The chapter ends with a review of how hospice can assist with the management of the more common symptoms of ALS, and considerations for caregivers.

The History and Philosophy of Hospice

Records of ancient hospices date to the fourth century A.D. As way stations for travelers and pilgrims, hospices proliferated in the Middle Ages. Often based in monasteries, these early hospices provided refuge for those in need. Hospices subsequently disappeared and did not reappear until the seventeenth century, when the Sisters of Charity in Paris opened several houses to care for people who were ill, indigent, or dying. In the nineteenth and twentieth centuries, the Irish Sisters of Charity began to use the word *hospice* to refer to homes for dying patients (1)

The hospice movement of the twentieth century developed in response to unmet needs of patients dying in traditional medical environments. Dame Cicely Saunders recognized the necessity for an alternative program of care for persons with advanced illness for whom there was no hope of a cure. In 1967 she founded St. Christopher's Hospice in London, which subsequently became the model for hospice programs in the Western world (2).

The Connecticut Hospice in New Haven was the first hospice in the United States, opening a home care program in 1974 and an inpatient facility in 1980. Hospice programs then spread throughout the United States through grassroot community efforts (3).

By the late 1970s there were more than 200 hospice programs in the United States, with much variation in the scope of services and organizational models. Explosive growth in the type and number of hospices led concerned providers to recognize the need for principles of hospice care and standards for developing programs. The National Hospice Organization (NHO) identified the basic tenets and characteristics of a hospice program, and the National Hospice Organization Standards (1979) provided the following statement on the philosophy of hospice:

> *Dying is a normal process, whether or not resulting from disease. Hospice exists neither to hasten nor to postpone death. Rather, hospice exists to affirm life by providing support and care for those in the last phases of incurable disease so that they can live as fully and comfortably as possible. Hospice promotes the formation of caring communities that are sensitive to the needs of patients and families at this time in their lives so that they may be free to obtain the degree of mental and spiritual preparation for death that is satisfactory to them (4).*

With the surge in the hospice movement during the 1970s, Congress mandated the Health Care Financing Administration (HCFA) to study hospice and its potential impact on the Medicare and Medicaid programs. This study showed that hospice was a cost-effective means of caring for people with terminal illnesses, and 1982 legislation provided hospice benefits to Medicare beneficiaries. These regulations established beneficiary requirements, reimbursement standards and procedures, the required scope of services, and the conditions for a program to become Medicare-certified. Additional legislation, approved in 1986, allocated federal funds for an optional state Medicaid hospice benefit. Individual states could thereby choose to amend their Medicaid plans to provide beneficiaries with coverage for hospice care. In 1990 Congress passed legislation extending coverage to eligible beneficiaries. As a result, residents in nursing homes are now eligible for Medicare hospice benefits when their stay is reimbursed through Medicaid or private pay (5).

The Hospice Medicare Benefit

Under the Medicare hospice benefit, care must be provided by a Medicare-certified hospice program. In 1997 there were 3,000 Medicare hospice programs in the United States, 80 percent of which were Medicare-certified (NHO, personal communication, July 15, 1998). The National Health Organization maintains a list of Medicare-certified hospice programs throughout the Unites States. Their telephone number is 1-800-658-8898. Referral to a hospice program can be initiated by an individual with ALS, a family member or friend speaking on behalf of someone with ALS, the attending physician, or other health care provider familiar with the needs of the individual. There usually is an identified staff person at hospice, often referred to as the intake or admissions coordinator, who screens referrals, answers questions about eligibility for hospice, or redirects the referral if hospice is not an option. If a referral is appropriate, a hospice nurse will visit with the individual and make arrangements for admission to the program. The following information describes general eligibility criteria and entitlements under the Medicare hospice benefit.

To receive hospice care under Medicare, an individual must be entitled to Part A of Medicare and have a physician certify a prognosis of approximately six months or less. Eligible beneficiaries then transfer their coverage from traditional Medicare to the Medicare hospice benefit, which is divided into time segments called election periods. In electing the hospice benefit, which is more comprehensive than regular Medicare, the individual waives the right to regular Medicare benefits except for payment to the attending physician and treatment for medical conditions unrelated to the terminal illness. The individual may revoke the hospice benefit at any time and resume regular Medicare benefits. If revoked in the middle of an election period, the remaining days in that election period are forfeited.

Medicare hospice beneficiaries are entitled to receive hospice care for two election periods of 90 days each, and an unlimited number of 60-day election periods thereafter, as long as there is evidence of disease progression. Following each benefit period, the hospice medical director and the attending physician must certify that the person remains terminally ill, and the individual must choose to continue receiving services under the Medicare hospice benefit (6). Private health insurance coverage usually includes hospice care. The specifics of coverage vary from one policy to the next, and some policies have deductibles and copayments that will apply. Hospice will discuss insurance issues at the time of referral and will do the billing and paperwork necessary for reimbursement of hospice services.

Along with the eligibility requirements defined by the Medicare hospice benefit, participating hospices usually develop additional criteria for admission to their programs. These are discussed at the time of referral and are reviewed in more depth during the admission process. Some hospices require that there be an identified person, referred to as a primary careperson, present in the home who is able to provide or arrange for the necessary caregiving. Other hospices serve people who live alone if they can develop an alternative caregiver system through a network of friends and/or privately paid help. Hospice will discuss care and safety issues at the time of admission and throughout the course of the illness to ensure that the needs of both patient and family are considered. Certain types of care such as intravenous antibiotic or fluid replacement therapy may not be available through the hospice. Most hospices do not admit people who are ventilator-dependent.

Regardless of whether a hospice is an offspring of a hospital, freestanding, or community-based, it must meet the criteria established by HCFA in order to be Medicare-certified and eligible for reimbursement through Medicare and Medicaid. The hospice must provide a full complement of services in both home and inpatient settings. An individualized plan of care is developed and continuously updated based on the needs of the patient and family.

Services of a Medicare-Certified Hospice

Certain core services must be provided by a Medicare-certified hospice, including:

- *Nursing care by or under the supervision of a registered nurse.* A registered nurse, who usually visits at least weekly, serves as the coordinator of services and contact person for the family.

- *24-hour on-call availability of nursing services.* If there are problems or concerns during the nighttime hours, family can use the on-call system to receive immediate consultation with a hospice nurse, who will contact other people or make a home visit as needed.

- *Physician services.* The hospice medical director assumes overall responsibility for the medical component of the hospice program. He or she does not, however, replace the primary care physician who has been caring for the individual with ALS. The hospice medical director works in tandem with the primary care physician and ALS experts in addressing medical needs.

- *Social work services.* As a hospice team member, the social worker is available for emotional support to family members and friends as well as the person with ALS. She can assist with location and coordination of community services and resources, such as transportation, supplemental personal care assistance, and support groups. Considerable attention is given later in this chapter to the role that a social worker may have in helping to orchestrate family meetings.

- *Chaplaincy services.* Each hospice has a chaplain who can provide pastoral care to family members on request or can assist with location of services within the individual or family's community.

- *Volunteer services.* Hospice trains and supervises volunteers who are available to families as needed in home, hospital, and nursing home settings. They can be a source of companionship, emotional support, and practical assistance. Typical activities for volunteers include running errands, providing transportation, visiting in the home or assisting people with community outings, providing respite for the caregiver, and helping with household chores.

- *Bereavement follow-up.* Hospices provide support for family members and significant friends for approximately a year following the death of a patient. Typically, a variety of support groups are available along with some intermittent contact on an individual basis. If there are special needs, such as those of young children who have experienced the death of a parent, hospice can provide or help families obtain assistance with the grieving process (2).

The following services can be provided directly by hospice staff or indirectly by the hospice program through contractual arrangements with other agencies or individuals:

- *Home health aide and homemaker services.* Hospice provides intermittent coverage for home health aid and homemaker services. Hospice will provide home health aid or licensed professional nurse (LPN) services in the home if necessary for the physical care of the patient. The days and times for this service are determined on the basis of availability and individual care needs. Typically, hospice provides a maximum of 10 to 20 hours per week of home health aid coverage. Families often choose to supplement this care with privately paid help. Some families have health insurance that covers private help over and above hospice. Hospice may provide continuous care (24-hour) in the home if needed as a short-term alternative to hospitalization during the dying process.

- *Occupational, physical, respiratory, and speech therapy.* These services are available as needed for symptom control. Indications for use are discussed in a later section.

- *Medical supplies and appliances, including drugs and biologicals deemed necessary by the interdisciplinary team for symptom management, such as medications to control excess secretions or spasticity.* Hospices will review the issue of Riluzole use and payment on a case-by-case basis. Now that Riluzole is approved by the U.S. Food and Drug Administration (FDA) for ALS and is no longer considered "experimental," people with ALS can continue taking Riluzole while on hospice. Hospice will pay for medications related to ALS when such medications are considered to be of benefit in managing the disease (G. Davis, personal communication, January 11, 1999). ALS clinic physicians, knowledgeable regarding Riluzole, can be helpful in recommending its continued use when it is in the person's best interests and consistent with their wishes regarding treatment

- *Durable medical equipment.* Items such as manual wheelchairs, commodes, walkers, electric beds, and electric recliners are typically available. Some hospices may be more generous or restrictive in the types of medical equipment that they will provide. Hospice will arrange for the delivery of covered equipment (2).

Although the primary thrust of hospice care is in the home setting, inpatient care must be available as needed for symptom control, respite care, or terminal care in the last days of life if it becomes impossible at home. Some hospices operate freestanding facilities or hospice units within hospitals; others use designated hospice beds within affiliated hospitals or nursing homes when inpatient care is needed. If hospitalization is needed, the hospice home care nurse will arrange for admission to a designated hospice bed or specialized hospice unit in the hospital. Home care is resumed after the crisis is stabilized through hospitalization. In many cases, hospitalization is prevented by using the hospice's 24-hour on-call nursing system to handle a crisis at home. The goal of hospice is to assist people in staying in their home environments through the remainder of their lives.

Hospice and ALS

The philosophy and structure of hospice are ideally suited to assist people with ALS and their families in living as fully and comfortably as possible in the final stage of illness. Meticulous attention to symptom control, experience in providing care to people who are approaching death, and resources to support families through this process can ease the anxiety, fear, and worry that invariably accompany the progression of ALS. Increasingly, people with advanced ALS are benefiting from support available through hospice programs.

Hospice programs in the United Kingdom have the longest history of caring for people with ALS. In particular, St. Christopher's Hospice (1967) opened with at least 10 percent of its ward beds for people with advanced neurologic illnesses (7).

In the United States, the relationship between people with ALS and hospice is younger and less developed than in the United Kingdom. This is due in part to the relative newness of hospice in the United States and as to structural differences between hospices in the United States and the United Kingdom. Additionally, hospice programs in the United States have traditionally served people with end-stage cancer. Some hospices are unfamiliar with management of other terminal illnesses and hesitate to admit patients because of concerns regarding prognosis and length of stay. To facilitate increased referral of non-cancer patients to hospice programs, the NHO published *Medical Guidelines for Determining Prognosis in Selected Non-Cancer Diseases,* 2nd. ed. in 1996 [8]. This document includes a section on ALS and seeks to identify which patients are likely to have a significantly shorter prognosis if the disease runs its normal course. The guidelines provide criteria for determining when someone is likely to have a prognosis of six months or less, which is an eligibility requirement under the Medicare-Medicaid benefit. Hospices with more experience in caring for people with ALS are able to interpret the guidelines more flexibly, allowing their clinical experience to guide judgments regarding admission.

Collaboration between hospices and health care professionals or ALS clinics experienced in the care of people with ALS can enhance the willingness of hospices to become more involved and effective in caring for people with the disease. This collaboration among health care providers not only improves the quality and continuity of care from diagnosis to death but also can help to sustain the caregiving abilities of involved health care professionals through pooling of resources, experience, and support (9).

Hospice is not synonymous with "giving up." We have seen people on hospice take trips abroad that they had always hoped to take; attend a jazz festival, rock concert, or symphony performance when they thought it was impossible; do advocacy work on behalf of other people with ALS; teach a daughter how to make a favorite pie; go to an important wedding, bar mitzvah, or graduation; create a book of photos and writings as a legacy for a newborn grandchild; reconcile with an estranged family member; read, write, or publish poetry for the first time; learn how to use a computer or how to meditate; continue to perform important functions in their roles as parents, spouses, and volunteers, to name a few; delight in the company of friends and family; and joyously celebrate the return of the light at the beginning of the new year.

Hospice Referral Considerations

It is essential that the needs of people with ALS and family members be addressed from the earliest stages of the disease. Hospice programs can provide a comprehensive range of services that are well-coordinated and accessible once they are admitted to the program. Although it would be ideal if people with ALS and their families could utilize the full range of hospice services throughout the course of

ALS, there are constraints on hospice programs. It also is necessary to determine whether hospice is the best fit for the needs of the person with ALS.

The following criteria can be used to determine eligibility for admission to a Medicare-certified hospice:

1. *Approximate prognosis of six months or less,* bearing in mind that the longer the family is on the program, the more closely developed will be the interpersonal relationships that improve the effectiveness of hospice care.

2. A *"Do Not Resuscitate" (DNR) order is not required.* A DNR order is a legal document advising health care providers of an individual's wish not to be resuscitated in the event of respiratory or cardiac failure. People with ALS who have decided not to use long-term mechanical ventilation through tracheostomy will find it helpful to formalize and communicate this decision through the use of documents such as a DNR order. Hospices previously required a DNR order before someone could be admitted, but this is no longer the case. At the time of admission to hospice, people with ALS may be undecided regarding whether they want to use any form of assisted ventilation. It is helpful to meet with people who are familiar with the pros and cons of assisted ventilation, in an atmosphere that is conducive to open and ongoing exploration of this issue, and within the family context. Under these circumstances, ambivalence usually clears over time, rendering a well-considered decision. Knowledgeable hospice personnel can be helpful in discussing this choice. No decision is irrevocable; if someone decides to use mechanical ventilation through tracheostomy after being admitted to hospice, they can do so by transitioning off of hospice and onto a program that can provide the necessary care. Noninvasive forms of assisted ventilation such as BiPAP are usually considered to be palliative care, which is treatment aimed at promoting comfort. Providing excellent palliative care is a prime objective of hospice (see Chapter 29).

3. *Progressive swallowing problems* that prevent intake of nutrients and fluids by mouth needed to sustain life. Indications of nutritional impairment would include progressive weight loss and dehydration. Dehydration is an excessive loss of fluid. It is recognizable when the urine becomes a darker yellow, has a more noticeable odor, is less frequent or in smaller amounts, and is accompanied by a constant dry mouth. If nutritional impairment is apparent and the person with ALS elects not to have a feeding tube, a hospice referral can be considered. People with supplemental feeding support (e.g., feeding tube) may be appropriate for hospice care if they are experiencing a progressive decline in breathing capacity.

4. *Progressive breathing difficulty* can be monitored through regular pulmonary function testing (PFT) throughout the course of ALS. A referral to hospice can be considered if the forced vital capacity (FVC) is less than 50% of predicted and is deteriorating. Respiratory fatigue is generally experienced when the vital capacity (VC) is less than 1.5 liters (10). Other symptoms of advanced breathing difficulty that would support a hospice referral include: (1) visible use of muscles in the neck and upper chest for breathing, and shallow breaths; (2) abnormal arterial blood gas measurements; (3) underventilation during sleep— symptoms include morning headache, lethargy, daytime sleepiness, poor appetite, shortness of breath, restlessness during the night, and interrupted sleep; or, (4) confusion or hallucinations resulting from too little oxygen or too much carbon dioxide in the blood.

5. *Life-threatening complications in combination with rapid progression of ALS.* One example of a life-threatening complication is aspiration pneumonia. Aspiration occurs when food or liquids, including saliva, slips into the airways and lungs. This can occur if there are swallowing problems, difficulty clearing secretions, or an ineffective cough. When coughing is ineffective or secretions increase, aspiration can cause parts of the lung to fill up, resulting in pneumonia. Pneumonia also can be caused by bacteria or viruses and may be a complication of a flu or bronchitis. A hospice referral may be indicated if there are recurrent pneumonias or if the pneumonia is unresponsive to antibiotic treatment.

These criteria are used routinely by the ALS Regional Center in Albany, New York, as a guide for timing a referral to hospice. We reviewed 23 people with ALS who were referred to Community Hospice in upstate New York by the ALS Center during a three-year period. All 23 patients had pulmonary function tests within one month of admission to hospice, and the average vital capacity was 44% of expected. The average length of stay on hospice was 144 days—well within the hospice guidelines.

The 1996 NHO guidelines suggest more stringent criteria for *critically impaired ventilatory capacity,* which is one category cited as an indicator for a prognosis of six months or less. *Critically impaired ventilatory capacity* is defined as follows:

> The patient should have, within the past 12 months, developed extremely severe breathing disability. Examples include: I. VC less than 30% of predicted. 2. Significant dyspnea [shortness of breath] at rest. 3. Requiring supplemental oxygen at rest. 4. Patient declines intubation or tracheostomy and mechanical ventilation (8).

If hospice programs or other health care providers interpret the NHO guidelines too narrowly, they can prevent timely admission of people with ALS to hospice programs and limit patient and family access to valuable and necessary services.

Other criteria cited in the NHO guidelines are in accord with the parameters previously described in this chapter.

Contraindications for Hospice

Hospice is not the best option in some circumstances:

- Hospice programs usually provide intermittent care in the home and typically limit home health aid coverage to 10 to 20 hours per week. Some people have private insurance that provides for more extensive nursing and home health aid services under non–hospice home care policies. Therefore, it is important to compare regular home care and hospice home care benefits before choosing hospice.

- Hospice is not appropriate if someone is firmly decided on a course of long-term mechanical ventilation.

The Family and ALS

At Community Hospice, we invite every family to meet with us soon after admission to the program, whether the admission has occurred in the short-term inpatient unit, at home, or at another place of residence such as a nursing home. We believe that life-threatening illness affects everyone in the family and that coming together to share experiences, concerns, and worries can lessen the additional stress of hiding fears. Giving voice to feelings and thoughts that arise in response to ALS can help each involved person feel less isolated and more informed regarding the likely course of the disease and more hopeful regarding the possibilities for mutual support and a peaceful death.

For most families, often despite loud protestations of their closeness, the idea of coming together as a group is terrifying. Strong feelings, with their attendant images and ideas, usually have not been openly expressed, especially in front of strangers, even when they are keenly felt. If the family has had little experience in sharing powerful everyday experiences, they will be terrified at the thought of sharing the avalanche of emotions and thoughts that can be set off by loss: fear, rage, grief, confusion, helplessness, sorrow, or a sense of unreality, to name but a few.

At a time when death is near, people are often skeptical about the usefulness of talking and fear that it will only make the situation more painful. Most of us have had little practice in finding ways to be with our own suffering and the suffering of others, even those with whom we share the most intimate ties. Far too many families remain silent, unable to bridge a sense of separateness in the face of pain that seems unbearable. The everyday complexities of living may temporarily supplant opportunities for thoughts and feelings to simply unfold in the company of others. A sense of urgency or incessant business can further deepen a sense of isolation and contribute to feelings of hopelessness or despair. There may be precious little opportunity for conversation and mutual listening without interruptions or a sense of interfering obligations. Alternatively, when there is the opportunity to be lovingly heard by each other, there is the magic of soul-to-soul connection. This helps us live with the aches and pains of everyday life, even the frightening manifestations of ALS, which seem so much more powerful when we feel alone, unheard, and unwitnessed.

Some hospices do not arrange family meetings routinely but will do so at the request of family or if there is extreme chaos. It is our belief that gatherings for every family are valuable because life-threatening illness always brings with it some degree of chaos, and there is always much to say even though we might be afraid to say it.

In anticipation of a family meeting, there often is a thick atmosphere of tension, distrust, and doubt. Stories of old hurts and disputes may emerge along with descriptions of who is allied with whom and how the family does or does not communicate. Mourning for family members who died earlier can be reawakened by ALS. If parents and children are present, there may be warnings not to upset "Mother" and not to say anything to "Father," because it will "only make matters worse." Skeptical, frightened, or angry family members may ask us what we could possibly hope to accomplish and why we would want to upset people "at this time." Doubt and distrust can derail a meeting before it has begun. If, however, there is someone skillful to guide the family meeting, there is a willingness on the part of participants to suspend judgment for a while and let go of the expectation that the meeting will "provide a fix," there is the possibility for those present to become more fully attentive and available to one another. When this occurs, we begin to notice that once shunned feelings can be shared, hurts relinquished, and old losses mourned. Healing can begin. Although there may be times when it seems that there is hardly any movement, quite often there is a feeling of peace, spaciousness, and lightness after a gathering. What once seemed forbidden or intolerable has lost some of its hold, and it is now possible to breathe more easily.

Most people with ALS in the hospice program live and die at home. We suggest that family meetings be held in the comfort and convenience of the home environment. The gathering may be small or large. Whether there are 30 or more family members and friends or no family present, we gather with the belief that our lives and our connections with the world depend on the telling of tales to anyone who will listen and be witness.

The Story of the Illness

The facilitator usually begins the meeting by asking the patient to tell the story of the illness. The accuracy of dates and facts is of little importance. It is the images and feelings that need expression. If it is the father who has the illness, he may turn to his wife and ask her to tell the story. If she is the designated family storyteller, she may be the one who talks to the doctors, relays news to the family, and comforts them. But it is a family myth that capacity to nurture resides only in the mother and that it is her role to run interference for death. The father may be gently encouraged to speak of "the unspeakable," to acknowledge his own wounds as well as the reality of his impending death. Perhaps this is the first time they have heard the story from him, have seen his vulnerabilities, heard his fears, and been given the opportunity to offer comfort and understanding. As the father reveals his story in the supportive company of others, he is reclaiming and remembering himself.

The Story of His Worries and Fears

"Father" may say that his principle concerns are for his wife and children. The facilitator asks him how he met his wife, what she is like, how he feels about her, and how he views their marriage. These powerful questions usually evoke jokes or nervous laughter, sometimes verging on uproar in the family, but gentle persistence can encourage him to speak. There can be surprise when disappointments, disillusionments, or resentments can be voiced and let go, making room for the expression of vulnerability, tenderness, and love. These words may seldom if ever have been heard from the father, as men so often hide behind their unemotional and strong facades like the Wizard of Oz, encouraged early on to armor themselves and diminish or devalue feelings.

Dark secrets can also be aired. For example, his alcoholism, which may have created immense pain and a volatile emotional environment, leaving all around him in a perennial state of apprehension and distrust. For years, the silence surrounding his alcoholism may have produced torrents of anger and guilt within the family, unexpressed but palpable. Now the father may speak about his alcoholism and acknowledge the pain it has caused himself and others. He may tell the untold story of his own parents' alcoholism and speak of the regret he now feels for having missed out on his children and they on him. Listening without interruption and a minimum of judgment can leave open the possibility for compassion and forgiveness.

When he is asked to talk about each of his children, he usually starts with facts and figures—their grades, degrees, and successes. It is much more difficult for him to express feelings of love and the heartbreaking sadness of having to leave them. He may say that they know he loves them without his having to say so. He is nevertheless encouraged to relate the story of his connections with family, expressing whatever worries and concerns as well as hopes and dreams he has for each of them.

Then the father can be asked about concerns he has for himself. He may dismiss the question initially but when pressed may say that he does not wish to suffer. Then, if he permits himself to voice his concerns, he may say that he is fearful about "choking to death," "suffocating to death," "being completely paralyzed and unable to communicate," or "being a burden." At this point, it is possible for the hospice facilitator to talk about each of these fears, letting him know that they are very commonly experienced by people who have ALS, whether they are expressed or not. In an atmosphere that is open, honest, and supportive, it is possible to talk about the probable way in which his ALS will progress, along with the likely manner of death. He can be told that eventually, perhaps in his sleep, he will simply breathe out—expire—and not have the strength to breathe in again. Simply, quietly, and without emergency, he will let go. This discussion often is followed by a relieved sigh with some variant of "Oh! Is that all it is?"

Death, too, can be brought from out of the shadows, and fear-laden images and ideas can be replaced with those based on more accurate accounts of death from ALS. Death from ALS can be quite peaceful. Most people die at home, and there is help available to address changes that occur over time. Family and caregivers can be prepared for what lies ahead so that there is an atmosphere of greater calm and more opportunity to appreciate the beauty of life.

Remembering the Children

It is most important that young children and grandchildren be involved in family meetings. This may be very difficult for adults who want to shield them, and they may say that the children are too young to understand. Although three-year-olds may not understand the words, they are very much in touch with the feeling tone of those they love. Excluding children can convey a message that death is something to be hidden.

> In the early days of the hospice, there was a family gathering presided over by a gentleman we will call Mr. Ryan. Mr. Ryan, his wife, eight children and their spouses, and several grandchildren were all present for the meeting. Mr. Ryan told stories of a wonderful marriage with many struggles and offered love and encouragement to everyone in the room. In turn, they shared colorful tales of Mr. Ryan, celebrating their years together. There was much laughter and many tears. After some time, all were exhausted and the meeting was winding down. When asked if he had any questions or anything more to say, Mr. Ryan sat up on the couch and said that he wanted to speak to his five youngest grandchildren, who had been wandering in and out of the room but had not been directly addressed. Ranging in age from about six to nine years old, they sat on the floor in a semicircle by his feet, and this is what he said to them: "Children, I am going to die and it is nobody's fault. It just happens. I won't be there to see you grow up, but I want you to know that you have each been a joy in my life, and you will always have my blessing and my love." There was not a dry eye in the room for those who witnessed this most sacred event. Mr. Ryan reminded us of how important it is for grandparents to take leave of their grandchildren face-to-face, if at all possible. So often they are best friends and love each other unconditionally. The loss can be compounded for children when a grandparent leaves without saying goodbye, delegating the heartbreaking task to the parents.

There was a sequel to this family meeting. Six years after Mr. Ryan's death, hospice staff had occasion to meet with one of Mr. Ryan's sons in law. During that visit, he spoke of how powerfully moved he had been by the family meeting with Mr. Ryan. The experience, he said, had given him the courage to become deeply connected with his 22-year-old daughter during her final months of life and eventual death two years after the family meeting. A family meeting can have far-reaching effects, and simply voiced blessings can empower and enrich the lives of others in ways that are quite unanticipated.

Stories of Roots

This can be a chance to speak of connections with one's ancestors. It is surprising how little many people know of parents, grandparents, and beyond. A few facts but not many stories, and it is the stories that provide us with an appreciation for the lives and contributions of those who have come before us. Stories can provide us a sense of continuity, linking generations of people. Many will say that their parents or grandparents came from abroad and that they seldom heard them speak of their past struggles or early lives. This leaves subsequent generations without any tales to tell and pass along, with a history devoid of color, dimension, and feeling. We need to tell and hear the sad stories along with the happier ones; otherwise the picture of our roots is incomplete. Reflections about parents, siblings, and growing up often reveal continuing pain from deaths unmourned and loving words unspoken. Bringing these memories, images, and feelings into the present can allow grieving to take place, lessening the deep pain that can result from holding on to fragments of an incomplete and untold story. Unattached to the rage or grief of preceding losses and deaths, it becomes easier to die in peace.

The Family Tells of Him

The mother may start by telling her story—how they met and her view of the ups and downs of the marriage. She is always asked how the illness has affected her, and this often evokes tears and worries about present and future, together with stories of other losses and disconnections in her life. Her worries may be for the relief of his suffering, her children's grief, or her future.

Some secrets may emerge, such as a history of substance abuse. The following is a typical scenario: the mother or one of the children reveals the father's history of alcoholism. Then mother may say that the 20 years of his drinking were awful for her and the children, and she may describe a repetitive sequence of drunkenness, disregard for others, financial problems, and absence. Family may interject that the father was wonderful when he was sober. The children are invited to say what it was like for them. They may express embarrassment, shame, anger, fear, a sense of never having known their dad, or constant worry for their mother. In talking about this type of painful experience, the object is not to judge or to inflame guilt. Rather, the intent is to acknowledge and speak of history that had been banished into the underworld so that it does not reappear in subsequent generations, often in more disguised form. If the family is able to speak of their collective past with a willingness to listen to one another, individual members may be able to construct a new and more useful understanding of themselves in relation to others, rather than harbor unnecessary feelings of responsibility, resentment, or shame for many years to come.

Some family secrets are harder to let go of than others, so the suffering is likely to be handed on.

> There was a family meeting around the bedside of a middle-aged woman who was dying in the hospice inpatient unit. Her husband was by her side and had been extremely attentive and almost over-solicitous in recent days. Her daughter sat at the end of the bed with her husband. There was an impenetrable stiffness and superficiality at the beginning of the meeting. The mother lay with her eyes closed, said she had no worries, and did not have much to say about husband or daughter. The husband held her hand, rhapsodizing about his wife and their marriage and how heartbreaking her illness had been for him. The daughter was initially quiet and said a few things about her mother, but then she suddenly stood up and delivered a startling and heartrending story. She said that she had been immersed in an incestuous relationship with her father for 10 years and talked of the pain, shame, and nightmares of her childhood, from which she was only now emerging with the help of both a therapist and a loving husband. Her father made a variety of attempts at denial, but her mother listened with eyes open. It was to her mother that she was talking. This dialogue continued off and on for the several days before she died. The daughter forgave her mother's lifelong closed eyes, and they struggled with their new intimacy. Father remained denial-coated and disconnected.

Most children are not plagued by such painful memories, and the family meeting is an opportunity for them to remember, laugh, cry, hug, thank, and take their leave. Even if their father appears to be unconscious, the children are encouraged both in the family meeting and when they have time alone with him to hold his hand and tell him anything they would like to say. Even in the most wanting of relationships, we can express our sadness that we missed out on one another and thank our parent for giving us life. Although the task of sorting things out may seem impossible in such a short time, the power of impending loss can facilitate openings, insights, and new directions, both internally and within the family as a whole.

Variations on the Family Meeting

There are times when, through a series of prior disconnections or deaths, a person with ALS does not have family members who are present and involved in caregiving. When possible in such instances, hospice can assist in building a viable community of alternative caregivers and friend networks that can serve as surrogate family. Family meetings can then be offered as a way to facilitate the interpersonal communication and collaboration necessary to meet the challenges of ALS. Along with this more practical objective, these meetings can provide those involved with an opportunity to revisit their internalized connections with family through the stories that survive and can be told. Inner connections with family remain for all of us and continue to change despite physical absence or the passage of time. Having ALS, or caring for someone with ALS, can constellate feelings from the past and invite a reworking of the stories that we have constructed about our lives and relationships with others. Family or friend meetings can be an invitation to acknowledge our connections with others, the suffering that is shared, as well as the beauty and brevity of life.

Symptom Management in Hospice

Each person with ALS has a nurse, usually called a nurse case manager, who visits at least weekly to review the needs of patient and caregivers. As ALS progresses, symptoms such as constipation, muscle cramps, and pain or discomfort from prolonged immobility can be effectively addressed. The nurse case manager will consult with members of the hospice team, the primary care physician, and available ALS experts to develop and coordinate the plan of care. Medication for management of ALS symptoms such as increased salivation and muscle cramps is discussed elsewhere in this book. Occupational and physical therapists, speech-language pathologists, dietitians, and respiratory therapists can provide valuable help in promoting health, comfort, function, and well-being. Their specific contributions also are discussed elsewhere in this book. In addition to these traditional health care providers, hospices often have affiliations with massage therapists and practitioners of other complementary approaches such as Reiki, Therapeutic Touch, and various forms of meditation.

Management of the following symptoms of advanced ALS is discussed within the context of hospice:

- *Sleep problems are common.* They occur for a variety of reasons, including depression, anxiety, changes in respiratory status, and positioning problems or discomfort associated with immobility. Various management approaches should be considered depending on the contributing causes. Alternative positioning, more frequent position changes, and bed pads that improve weight distribution can help with problems related to immobility. Anxiety can be reduced with medications, relaxation training, and conversations that address fears associated with the progression of the disease and the manner of death. The need for ongoing conversations with people who have ALS and their caregivers was discussed earlier. Some people are afraid they will not be able to call for help during the night when caregivers are sleeping, so having a reliable call system is essential. It is important to rule out clinical depression because sleep difficulty is a related symptom.

Various antidepressants and mild relaxants can be used to aid sleep. Loss of sleep, for whatever reason, can contribute to a depressed mood, lowered level of alertness, poorer functioning, and a reduced capacity for coping with day-to-day concerns. Therefore, sleep deprivation should always be taken quite seriously. When ALS affects the nerves that control the respiratory muscles, breathing becomes weak and sleep can be disturbed. People with ALS who do not have significant impairment of speech and swallowing function can consider using noninvasive devices, such as bilevel positive airway pressure (BiPAP), to assist nighttime ventilation (11) (see Chapter 12). Hospice programs may or may not consider BiPAP a palliative (i.e., comfort) measure, however, and may be concerned about its use because BiPAP can influence one's prognosis. Some people with far-advanced ALS do not want to use devices that assist ventilation, and this wish should be respected.

- *Anxiety* may result from worries and fears related to the progression of the disease or from physiologic changes such as those resulting from impaired ability to breathe. People often do not report that they are feeling "anxious." Rather, the following may be present: physical agitation or restlessness; complaints of general discomfort and frequent requests for repositioning; reports that the mind is racing or that it is difficult to think clearly; fearfulness; and increased requests for companionship, especially at nighttime. Giving attention to fears and worries, using methods to improve physical comfort, and the selective use of medications such as lorazepam (Ativan) can help with the management of anxiety. The literature provides extensive description of the benefits and use of stress management approaches such as guided visualization and various forms of meditation for the management of anxiety [12,13]. Massage and Therapeutic Touch can also be helpful for some people.

- *Depression* is a normal and expected consequence of a life-threatening diagnosis and the multiple losses that occur during the course of a disease such as ALS. It is important for this normal and expected form of depression, which can be viewed as a component of the grief and mourning process, to be distinguished from what is referred to as clinical depression. When present, clinical depression can be debilitating, compromising a person's capacity to respond to the challenges of ALS and find any enjoyment in life. Symptoms of clinical depression are:

  - loss of pleasure and interest in activities, including those still possible for the person to enjoy

  - changes in sleep (too much, too little, trouble falling asleep, or waking up during sleep)

- changes in appetite accompanied by weight loss due to disinterest in eating
- difficulty concentrating during activities
- difficulty thinking clearly and more trouble with problem solving
- hopelessness and ongoing thoughts of suicide
- symptoms of depression are greater in the morning, with lessening of depression as the day goes on
- significant and unexpected withdrawal from social relationships, including family
- a depressed mood most days, for most of the day
- an experience of emotional flatness that is not punctuated by periods of happiness or enjoyment in activities
- severely distorted and negative perceptions of self (e.g., lowered self-esteem, guilt-ridden or self-accusatory ruminations)
- the persistence of symptoms over time with no significant change in spite of favorable environmental circumstances, including the presence of supportive and encouraging people in close relationship with the person who is depressed (14,15).

Clearly, some of the symptoms of clinical depression, such as problems with sleep and appetite, are also symptoms of ALS progression. Treatment with antidepressant medication should be considered when there is a combination of symptoms that are severe and/or of long duration, when the symptoms affect the person's involvement in day-to-day activities, when the level of distress experienced by the individual is high, and when there is a personal or family history of clinical depression. We are in no way suggesting that medications substitute for the types of support and counsel described elsewhere in this chapter. Rather, antidepressant medications can be effectively used to complement other approaches, helping people to access innate coping abilities, creatively respond to problems associated with ALS, enjoy simple day-to-day pleasures, and prepare for death. All too often health professionals dismiss symptoms of clinical depression with the comment "I'd be depressed too," overlooking an opportunity to provide some relief for those who are suffering unnecessarily from clinical depression. It also is not uncommon for people who are clinically depressed to refuse treatment because they do not recognize that they are depressed or believe that their depression is somehow a deficiency of character or will rather than a phenomenon that has a biological component.

- *Dysphagia* (i.e., difficulty swallowing): Various problems and concerns can arise if the muscles of the mouth and throat become weak (see Chapter 10). One study involving the review of 124 people who died of ALS showed that none "choked to death" (16). Nevertheless, people with ALS commonly say that this is a fear, and it is helpful to provide reassurance that, although they may experience "choking episodes," "choking to death" is not the manner of death from ALS. These episodes can be anxiety-producing for everyone, so it is helpful to reassure family members that as long as the person is coughing and there is no evidence of food obstructing the trachea (i.e., windpipe), their best response is to be a calm presence until the coughing ceases. The speech-language pathologist can provide instruction on how to decrease the likelihood of problems associated with dysphagia through training in compensatory swallowing techniques and dietary modifications (see Chapter 10).

The option of using a feeding tube usually has been discussed well in advance of admission to hospice. Although it is possible to have a feeding tube inserted after hospice admission, it is not common. People with ALS, family members, caregivers, and health care professionals may express concerns about "starving to death" as the ability to take food and fluid by mouth becomes more difficult. People with advanced ALS typically do not complain of a gnawing hunger or pain resulting from decreased ability to take food by mouth. The process usually is gradual and not painful. Appetite wanes and fatigue increases, along with visible weight loss. Likewise, dehydration need not be an overshadowing concern. It is important to maintain scrupulous attention to mouth care as fluid intake decreases. Even for those who elect to use a feeding tube, the amount of fluids given often is decreased in the advanced stages of the disease so that the body is not burdened by excess fluids. The zeal of physician and family to promote intravenous fluids at this stage may delay death for a short time, which may in turn create problems rather than relieve discomfort.

A hospice patient occasionally may elect to discontinue use of a feeding tube for nutritional support. It is important for this type of decision to be discussed openly with the family because caregivers can sometimes interpret the decision as a failure on their part to provide adequate support or care.

- *Respiratory problems* are the hallmark of ALS and the usual cause of death. Discussion of respiratory complications and management options, including hospice, should take place within the context of the family system so that there is agreement on how to respond as breathing problems develop. Advance discussion prevents crises later. As mentioned earlier, a DNR is not required for admission to hospice. If hospice admission criteria are met and the person has not decided in favor of long-term mechanical ventilation, a referral is appropriate. Knowledgeable hospice personnel can provide information and support that can assist the decision-making process. Once a person with ALS has been admitted to hospice, various forms of palliative treatment can be used to ameliorate the effects of respiratory compromise. These may include noninvasive ventilatory support, such as BiPAP; nasal oxygen; proper positioning; relaxation training; and medications to reduce anxiety. Respiratory therapy is a covered benefit under hospice when it is deemed necessary for symptom management. More detailed descriptions of ways to manage respiratory problems are provided elsewhere in this book.

A fear of "suffocating to death" commonly produces anxiety for both the person with ALS and family members. Gentle yet open discussion surrounding the likely progression of the disease and manner of death can soften fear. When decline in breathing ability occurs gradually over time, people often can adapt to very low levels of respiratory reserve without evidence of distress. If the decline is more rapid, the person may be more in need of active symptom management. There still is some reluctance to use morphine in far-advanced illnesses, especially when there is any hint of respiratory compromise. Hospices have clearly demonstrated its efficacy in pain control. In ALS, toward the end of life, there may be a mixture of restlessness, agitation, aching discomfort, fear, anxiety, and sleeplessness that can respond extremely well to the use of low-dose morphine and/or lorazepam (Ativan). In no way does this imply physician-assisted suicide but rather appropriate and ethical end-of-life care. Reiterating the 24-hour on-call availability of support through hospice and the option of hospice inpatient admission for terminal care can also be reassuring.

Providing people with ALS and their families with knowledge of what to expect helps to prepare them for death, prevent crises, and enhance their ability to make the most of their remaining time together. Even in the final hours of life, people can connect with loved ones in ways that can later sustain family members during the bereavement process. An essential vehicle for helping people with ALS and families throughout the course of the disease is the family meeting, as discussed earlier.

The Dying Process

Respiratory decline is usually discernible over time; with proper identification, symptoms can be managed so that people die peacefully at home. Making accurate predictions about prognosis is difficult. Some of the symptoms of advanced ALS and indications for a referral to hospice have been presented as general benchmarks. Once on program, the hospice staff monitors changes, discusses options for symptom management, and provides support to the person who has ALS and those involved in caregiving. During the last days or few weeks of life, the following changes may also occur, indicating that death is close:

- *Increased disengagement from the world of the living is common (17)*.
  In the last few days or weeks, people who are dying often seem to withdraw into themselves for increasingly long periods. People may prefer to communicate less, seem preoccupied or "elsewhere," request that visits be limited to members of the immediate family, or withdraw from even their most intimate relations. Some people will clearly communicate their

wish for undisturbed time, while others will communicate this nonverbally by becoming less responsive to others and the environment. While recognizing and respecting the dying person's need for disengagement, it is equally important not to abandon the person. Even though people may not talk about dying, they often know intuitively that death is near. Whether or not there are direct conversations about dying, it is always important to give people gentle reassurances of continued presence and concern. This can be communicated by caregivers through the tone of one's voice, gentle touch, and, depending on individual history and beliefs, various forms of spiritual practice or ritual.

- *Reports of "visitations" from friends or relatives who have predeceased the person who is dying are not uncommon and are described in the death and dying literature.* Less common are reports of angels or religious figures [17]. There may be some reluctance on the part of people to share these experience with family because they are outside the usual range of experience. It is helpful for families to know that this type of experience is not uncommon, lest they become overly concerned and fearful that the their loved one is "going crazy."

- *Decreased interest in taking food and fluids by mouth or feeding tube usually occurs as the appetite wanes and body functions slow.* At this stage, forcing foods can cause uncomfortable symptoms. Adequate mouth care, such as keeping the lips moist with lubricants or a wet compress, can offset the effects of decreased fluid intake.

- *Certain physiologic changes are indicative of impending death:* decreased sphincter control resulting in urinary and rectal incontinence; sluggish circulation resulting in diminished sensation, discoloration, or mottling of the extremities, cold skin (progressing from feet to hands, ears, and nose); sensory impairment resulting in blurred vision or altered taste and smell (hypersensitive or hyposensitive); changes in vital signs such as decreased blood pressure, slow and weak pulse, shallow and irregular respirations; and decreased gastrointestinal activity resulting in nausea, flatus, distention, or constipation (17).

- *Physiologic signs of imminent death include the following:* dilated and fixed pupils; inability to move; loss of reflexes; weaker and more rapid pulse; changes in the appearance of the face such sunken cheeks and a gray pallor to the skin; noisy breathing ("death rattle"); lowered blood pressure; and breathing characterized by increasingly long gaps between inspirations (gaps initially last a few seconds and can lengthen to 45–60 seconds), visible use of the neck muscles on inhalation, mouth-breathing with the jaw relaxed in an open position (17).

- *A period of increased agitation or restlessness, symptomatic of advanced respiratory dysfunction, can precede death by a few days or weeks.* These symptoms are not always present before death, and some people experience little or no apparent distress. More often there is a "transition period" characterized by increased agitation, especially at night. Medications to reduce anxiety can be helpful during this time. Thankfully, this period does pass, and people usually experience a time of calm lasting from a few hours to a few days before death.

- *A period of calm before the death is not uncommon.* Some who work with people who are dying describe this calm or heightened sense of well-being before death as the "shooting star" phenomenon. The transition from restlessness to calm can be quite dramatic at times. One memorable example involved a young man who had experienced a steady and rather rapid progression of ALS. For approximately one week, he had experienced sleeplessness, agitation, general discomfort, and other symptoms of advanced respiratory dysfunction. Then, for 24 hours before his death, there was a dramatic shift. He became not only calm but also by all appearances euphoric. Infused with a sense of well-being and initiative, he spent the day making detailed funeral plans for himself, even composing his own light-hearted obituary. He then communicated his wishes and goodbyes to family and intimate friends with the delight of someone making final preparations before a trip. This gentleman's last day will be long remembered by those who were present, and it was later described by his family as his remarkable and final gift to them.

- *Coma, or a period of unresponsiveness to sensory stimulation, can precede death by less than an hour or for several days.* Although people may not be able to respond in any way that is apparent to the observer, we always tell caregivers to assume some level of awareness on the part of the person who is dying. Hence, family can continue speaking softly to the person who is dying and, if able to do so, may offer reassurances that "it is OK to go."

- *Certain metaphorical themes appearing in conversation may herald that death is near.* For example, it is not uncommon for people to talk about "going home" or, in their own frames of reference, speak of preparations for travel [18]. Days before she died, one woman had a series of dreams about taking care of some important business and getting on a bus with a driver who knew how to take her to her beloved childhood home and early family. These dreams prompted actual discussions with her children around some final legal arrangements she wanted to make, and she was not content until she was assured that her affairs were in order. Then she seemed to relax, having made preparations alluded to in the dream, and she enjoyed her final days with an attitude of relaxed anticipation.

When faced with the relentless decline of ALS, family distress, and a personal feeling of inadequacy or helplessness, we are eager to prescribe something to take it all away. Fight and flight are deeply conditioned responses; we fight disease and then back away when our doings are no longer helpful. We are not taught that we have a vital place in mourning with others. When we are dying of ALS or anything else, we need someone to mourn along with us; we need someone to listen, witness, and be thoroughly present. When we are the caregiver, this type of witnessing can give us clues on how to best help the person who is dying. Just as each person's life is unique, so the experience of death is unique for each person. It has almost become a truism that people will die as they have lived. We each bring our personality, history, sense of meaning, and magic to the process. Ultimately, when we participate in the dying process of another, we are preparing for our own death. Those who are facing death in the immediate future have much to teach us both of dying and of living.

Care for the Caregivers

It seems fitting to close with a few words about caregivers, whose needs can be eclipsed by the day-to-day demands of caring for a loved one with ALS. It may seem that just as one settles into a manageable routine or accommodates to a loss, disease progression presents another loss, necessitating yet another accommodation. At times, the rate of physical change in ALS can seem to outpace your capacity for adaptation and a caring response. This has been referred to as "compassion fatigue." Even the most loving, conscientious, capable, resilient, and physically fit caregiver has limits. Thus, it is imperative that the physical, emotional, and spiritual needs of caregivers assume importance. This can be difficult because the needs of people with ALS are compelling. Yet it is in everyone's best interest for caregivers to remain well and fit. Utilizing sources of support available through hospice and the types of services previously discussed can be of benefit.

It may initially feel intrusive and unsettling when ALS requires that we accept help from others and involve strangers in our lives, homes, and intimate daily routines. It may be difficult for people with ALS, who have come to rely on the loving care of family members, to entrust themselves to the care of someone new. Caregivers may choose to continue providing most of the physical care for loved ones and accept help with other responsibilities such as household chores, transporting children to activities, or planning for holidays. For others, relieved of some responsibilities for providing physical care, caregivers may once again experience themselves as wife, husband, daughter, son, or friend to the person who has ALS. Providing personal care is a time of intimate connection for some people, while for others it is not. When the needs of caregivers conflict with those of the person who has ALS, it may be difficult to talk and tensions may escalate. At times, caregivers may feel that caring for themselves is "selfish," or they may not recognize their own own needs in the midst of caring for another. Hospice staff can help address these issues and help families respond creatively to the difficulties brought about by ALS.

Amyotrophic lateral sclerosis turns lives upside down, challenges the assumptions upon which we base our lives, and alters our customary ways of doing things. Hospice, while not a panacea, can be of help in living and dying with ALS. Hospice also follows the family for approximately a year following the death. Hospice can provide useful information on the grieving process, along with various options for support such as small bereavement groups, intermittent contact with bereavement staff or trained volunteers, and referral to community resources including counselors who can companion and assist those who are mourning.

Ultimately, it is the aim of hospice to bear witness to both individuals with ALS and their companions, while providing tangible support and personal presence. In doing this, it becomes a privilege for us to be invited into the lives of people with ALS. Those who live with ALS, as well as their families and friends, are our most generous teachers.

References

1. Hadlock D. Physician roles in hospice care. In: Corr CA, Corr DM (eds.). *Hospice care: Principles and practice*. New York: Springer, 1983.
2. Thompson B, Wurth MA. The hospice movement. In: Tigges KN, Marcil WM (eds.). *Terminal and life-threatening illness:* An occupational behavior perspective. Thorofare, NJ: Slack, 1988.
3. Corless I. The hospice movement in North America. In: Corr CA, Corr DM (eds.). Hospice care: *Principles and practice*. New York: Springer, 1983.
4. National Hospice Organization. Standards of a hospice program of care. Alexandria, Va.: Author, 1981.
5. Thompson B. Occupational therapy with the terminally ill. In: Kiernat JM (ed). *Occupational therapy and the older adult: A clinical manual*. Gaithersburg, Md.: Aspen, 1991.
6. HCFA. Hospice Care Benefit Periods. Program Memorandum #628. Implementation of the Balanced Budget Act of 1997.
7. Saunders C. Walsh TC, Smith M. Hospice care in motor neuron disease. In: Saunders C. Summers DR, Teller N (eds.). *Hospice: The living idea*. London: Edward Arnold, 1981.
8. NHO. Medical Guidelines for Determining Prognosis in Selected Non-Cancer Diseases, 2nd ed. Alexandria, Va.: Author, 1996.
9. Thompson B. Amyotrophic lateral sclerosis: Integrating care for patients and their families. *Am J Hospice* 1990; 7:27–32.
10. Hillel A, Miller R. Bulbar amyotrophic lateral sclerosis: Patterns of progression and clinical management. *Head Neck* 1989; 11:51–59.
11. Sufit, R. Symptomatic treatment of ALS. *Neurology* 1997; 48(Suppl 4):S15–S22.
12. Carrington P. Modern forms of meditation. In: Lehrer PM, Woolfolk RL (eds.). *Principles and practices of stress management,* 2nd ed. New York: Guilford Press, 1993.
13. Barber TX. Hypnosuggestive approaches to stress reduction: Data, theory, and clinical application. In: Lehrer PM, Woolfolk RL (eds.). *Principles and practices of stress management,* 2nd ed. New York: Guilford Press, 1993.

14. APA. *Diagnostic and statistical manual of mental disorders,* 4th ed. Washington, DC: Author, 1994.
15. Rando TA. *Treatment of complicated mourning.* Champaign, Ill.: Research Press, 1993.
16. O'Brien T, Kelly M. Saunders C. Motor neuron disease: A hospice perspective. *Br Med J* 1992; 304:471–472.
17. Samarel N. The dying process. In: Wass H, Neimeyer RA (eds.). *Dying: Facing the facts.* Washington, DC: Taylor & Francis, 1995.
18. Callanan, M, Kelley P. *Final gifts: Understanding the special awareness, needs, and communications of the dying.* New York: Poseidon Press, 1992.

30

Mourning

N. Michael Murphy, M.D.

With reasonable physical health, or even in the face of considerable sickness, we seldom contemplate or allow into full consciousness the possibility that we can die at any time. Denial of death is everyday fare for most of us, but that inner innocence or naivete which maintains the myth of our physical immortality becomes sorely tried or even shattered by the diagnosis of any life-threatening illness. The implications of ALS are particularly hard to ignore since all the literature speaks of a fatal outcome, and the muscular decline is an ever-present reminder of finitude and death. This loss of health and innocence in ALS evokes the expression of a whole range of feelings that may be frozen by denial or given full exposure, which is the prelude to acceptance of what is happening. These responses, induced to varying degrees in patient, family, and caregivers are the subject of the first part of this chapter. The second part focuses on some aspects of care for those who are suffering or have suffered from loss, be they the ones with ALS, their families, or their caregivers.

Mourning and the Response to Loss

Loss transports us into a journey that ranges back and forth along a path that ends with integration and acceptance. In ALS or any other terminal illness, death may intervene at any time with the trials and tribulations imposed by the loss still unresolved. We will retain some degree of denial, but most of the time will move

399

beyond it. Most will not continue to rage incessantly against the coming of the night, but may become stuck in a state of bereavement and need a kindly nudge in order to leave it behind. Grief is a prelude to letting go or dying and will be shunned as long as death is denied or avoided or while we are consumed by our response to bereavement.

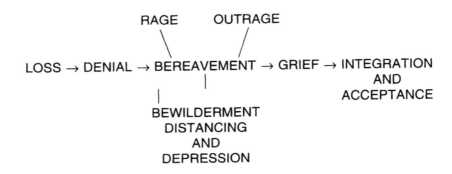

Denial is a natural, self-protective response to any event that disconnects us from that which provides nurture or self-esteem. In the event of sudden death of someone close, or the sudden, unexpected diagnosis of an illness such as ALS, the immediate response is usually some variant of "Oh, no!" Taken literally, this is an exclamation denying the truth of what has just been told in an attempt to obliterate the fear and chaos inspired by the life-threatening diagnosis and to restore equilibrium.Usually the individual does not maintain the stance that the incident never happened, and asks a series of questions that help to confirm the new reality. With a life-threatening illness, most will breach their denial to some degree but will often shore it up again with the aid of family members who are terrified at the prospect of loss and hide behind the possibility of doing something—anything at all—to dissipate the helplessness and fear.

Some physicians are models of sensitivity as they speak of that which is difficult to hear and still remain fully present and available. Others protect themselves by disgorging unpalatable facts over the phone or even in hospital corridors. Medical schools give scant attention to teaching students how to digest painful information and reframe it for their patients simply, clearly, and compassionately. We need to give only as many of the facts as the one with ALS needs at the moment, all within a framework of compassion and gentle hopefulness, not the false hope of the blusterer who dangles insubstantial half-truths with the justification that he does not want to take away all hope. He does not understand that real hope and optimism are always appropriate in life-threatening illness; not that the condition will be cured, but that in a loving atmosphere, with truthful communication and connectedness, we will experience the hope and preciousness of each day, and the peace that comes from having settled our technical and emotional affairs.

Bereavement is defined in the Oxford English dictionary as the state of being deprived, robbed, or stripped, usually of immaterial possessions. Thus, if we feel that we own someone or something that is then lost, we will believe that we have been robbed. The feelings that accompany this robbery usually include all manner of rage and outrage.

If we believe that we have a birthright to good health, and that muscular power, control, and integrity which have been painstakingly promoted and learned from our earliest days are "ours," we will experience bereavement with rage, outrage, and bewilderment when it is taken away by ALS. If we believe that a loved one belongs to us, then the death threat and gradual taking away of that person will cause us to go through all the pain of the bereaved. Since we are human and have been brought up to believe in ownership, we will feel bereaved many times in our lives. Those who are able to love without attachment and are not tied to goods, chattels, or the inalienable right to good health are less apt to become engulfed by anger and more ready to accept whatever comes their way.

Rage is a word associated with being mad, going berserk, running amok, and losing control. When we say that we are mad, we do not usually imagine that we mean it literally, that we are really insane or are out our minds. But the fact is that if we maintain rage, we are insane and incapable of responding in a healthy manner to the realities of the moment.

A well-respected physician, who had authored several books and was a wonderful teacher and observer of others, was wheeled into my office by his wife. I had no idea he was physically sick until that moment, but one look at his intense jaundice and emaciated state and it was clear that he was close to death. He said that he had asked to see me because he was afraid that he was going out of his mind and wanted my opinion. His story was that carcinoma of the pancreas had been diagnosed several months earlier, and since then he had been involved in a continual technological nightmare of surgery, chemotherapy, and tests. In his words, he barely had time to catch his breath. It was as if he had been holding his breath and suspending his feelings for the past months, aided and abetted in this denial by his intellect, his family, and a horde of physicians. Now he was beginning to experience feelings of rage, translated by this cultured man into feelings of loss of control and fear of losing his mind or going mad. With a little gentle nudging and a couple of family meetings the following week, he was able to acknowledge his rage and leave it behind. At that point, he was ready to grieve with his family, share stories, and express tender feelings, all of which had been a lifelong difficulty for this logical, controlling man. He died a few hours after the second family gathering, peacefully, with all said and done.

> *Charles was a fear-filled man who raged against the diagnosis and manifestations of ALS. His rage and fear were such that he developed unremitting angina that was uncontrollable with medical treatment. This created a dilemma between the risk of surgery in one whose respiration was already affected by ALS and the prospect of pain for the rest of his life.He elected to undergo surgery, which completely*

relieved the angina, but then he was compelled to face his bereavement and address the rage over the perceived rape of his physical integrity. The rage and madness over his state and the outrage that this happened to him abated as he gave it voice. Years before, his teenaged son had died in a climbing accident, and at that time and subsequently he avoided his grief and dealt with bereavement by banning all thought and talk of his son. With his own life-threatening illness, he initially avoided having to deal with his feelings by almost killing himself with angina, breaking his heart rather than allowing himself to feel broken-hearted. The next year provided him with the time to experience his bereavement and grief over the loss of his son, and this in turn gave him the courage to mourn his own losses and impending death. Six weeks before he died, his younger sister was killed in a motor vehicle accident. He attended her funeral in a wheelchair and appeared to be fully present to his outrage and sadness over her death. It seemed as though her death gave him permission to let go and die, and the last few weeks of his life were relatively comfortable and peaceful.

Outrage at being the subject of life-threatening illness is rage that is more focused and controlled. The one outraged screams "Why me?" or the relative cries out against this happening to a good person like mother when there are so many worse people out there who are perfectly free of illness. Outrage blames an unjust God or sees the illness as a punishment. It storms against a missed diagnosis or fastens blame for what is happening on anyone or anything. It is like paranoia as it projects the insanity of the situation on to an outside source, unwilling or unable to understand or accept the randomness and impersonal nature of terminal illness. It is an attempt to avoid the impotence of medicine and its regular inability to control outcomes. Rage and outrage disconnect us from each other and our world just at the time we most need connectedness and love. Its main purpose is to stave off grief, which is the necessary prelude to connectedness, acceptance, and integration.

Betty was in her early sixties when she came to see me following surgery for what proved to be metastatic colon cancer. She said that she had foregone chances to live independently or get married in order to take care of her chronically ill mother, who eventually died twelve years before the diagnosis of her colon cancer. Her mother never said a word in gratitude and seemed to be in a perpetual state of rage, outrage, or their internalized associate, depression. The thirty years of care giving produced little joy and a constant stewpot of anger, and mother's death offered little emotional relief since they had never shared anything but rage and had not allowed themselves to connect through grief, which in turn leads to integration, permitting the exchange of love. The stewpot continued to simmer for the next decade, during which she looked after her meek and mild father until his death. The long awaited peace and happiness, expected as a birthright, especially with the departure of her parents, never happened. Two years after her father's death, she was diagnosed with colon cancer, and I remember the spirit of her words, if not their actual form, as she raged and bubbled in my office: "It is not fair. After all I did for my parents. Now I expected to enjoy myself and travel, and look what has happened. If there is a just God in heaven, He will take this cancer away, and I am going to sit here until He does!"

That is exactly what she did. She sat on her stewpot of rage with her spiritual arms folded and did little else for the nine months until she died. No softness, no grief, no letting go. No kindness to herself for her service to her parents even though it was reluctantly given. No tears for the little girl within her who never felt loved. She died as she lived; a stony monument to self-righteousness and outrage, fending off the comfort and love that was within her reach.

Bewilderment is the state of losing one's way or being unable to grasp what is happening. It is beyond denial in that there is an understanding that all is not well. But there is a numbness or apathy that does not admit to feelings, especially rage, outrage, or grief.

Distancing results from not wishing to become too emotionally involved. Some family members and friends keep their distance from the one with ALS, and so never accompany the dying person though grief to acceptance and a place of new intimacy born of having gone through the emotional refiner's fire together. If we keep our distance, we protect ourselves from grief but do not experience intimacy. We will not have to say goodbye, which many of us believe too painful, but this ensures that we will be forever nagged by the wish that we had made some expression of love; that we had told our loved one that she was important to us and would be sorely missed. It is paradoxical that such an expression is a necessary prelude to letting go, and it is only after we let go that we are free to be nourished by the everlasting images and stories that are the real essence or soul of the one who has died.

Physicians, nurses, and other caregivers frequently distance themselves from their patients. We have been taught by words or example that it is not good to become too involved. How much is too much has never been clearly defined other than the proscription related to sexual behavior with patients. Are we permitted or do we permit ourselves to love a patient or mourn her loss? If we grieved for each of our patients who died, there is the fear that we would burn out or go mad. Oddly enough, it is our resistance to mourning and our stubborn maintenance of distance that is a frequent cause of chronic anger and burnout among caregivers. If emotionally we will go the whole distance with patients and their families and be prepared—or unprepared—to weep and also to attend the wake or funeral, we will have done everything possible so that we can then let go and move on. Those who distance emotionally and feel that their work is done, as soon as they run out of technical tricks, never experience completion and peacefulness with their patients who die. This, like any form of interrupted intercourse, is, by definition, incomplete and unsatisfying. It is the failure to accompany the family to the end that creates in caregivers a continuous sense of bereavement. Burnout means being consumed by the fire of rage, and this in turn precipitates fight or flight. We will fight by becoming even more angry and distanced, and we will fly by changing specialties, leaving medicine, or committing suicide.

Grief: We will go to any extreme in our attempts to avoid grief. We have been admonished to hold back tears and be brave. Little John Kennedy saluting the coffin of his Dad. The show must go on. Keep the stiff upper lip, and be "strong."

We are uncomfortable with feelings, and being emotional in a male-ordered world is considered little short of sinful, and most certainly weak. In the face of grief, many physicians, especially the pseudo-masculine, macho ones, will provide and encourage tranquilizers and sleeping pills so that its expression is muted. Others will prescribe antidepressants rather than listen to the rage and outrage and assist their patients in the delivery of their grief. There is the fear that being very emotional in grief will lead to breakdown and this inspires the fear of madness and even the fantasy of incarceration in a mental hospital. It is not always accepted that grief is the normal final expression of loss and being out of control.

The story of Dante's *Inferno* is a vivid reminder that the pain of grief cannot be avoided if we wish to emerge from mourning. The Inferno was imagined as a round pit with steep sides, and almost all of the sufferers tried to escape the flames by scrambling toward the periphery and attempting to get out by clawing their way up the steep sides. Just a few realized that the only way out was through an opening in the middle of the pit. The flames of grief will end only if we travel into their midst.

We are uncomfortable with grief because it is both the harbinger of death and the beginning of its acceptance, and in our society death is hopeless, a failure, and the greatest of all possible negatives. We may never say die. So it is common in families for each of the members to experience grief but to do their crying alone. Over and over again I have heard variations on the theme of a daughter who was heartbroken over her mother who had advanced ALS. When I asked if she had shared her fears with mother, she was shocked, saying that she did not want to upset her and that she needed to remain strong for her. What a sad dissipation of soulful feelings. I will always remember a daughter who was the devoted caregiver for her much-loved mother: "When I am down, she holds me while I cry, and when she is sad and tearful, I am able to hold and comfort her. We are each there for the other." If we share grief and be witnesses for one another, we experience the connectedness that we crave, and it becomes the prelude to acceptance and peace. Mourning does not end while grief is in the closet.

We often wonder whether children should witness our grief and we attempt to protect them from feelings, both ours and their own. It is a real gift to share our tears and sadness with children. We are telling them by example that the loss of grandmother to ALS is painfully heartbreaking, and that these feelings are both appropriate and very much worth sharing. Children who are "protected" from feelings are fundamentally deprived, and are being taught that the feelings induced by loss are dangerous and not to be expressed. When feelings of loss are pushed underground, they do not disappear and may be transformed into chronic fear and anxiety to emerge in full force at the next appearance of life-threatening illness.

Integration and acceptance may be at hand when we have ceased fighting and raging against the coming of the night. Tears have been shed for the child within, and she is at peace. We have grieved with our family and have ceased to hide behind endless procedures and other doings. We have let go of family and friends and are now able to be a human being rather than a human doing, simply being with ourselves and our family for whatever time remains.

I remember Melba, a marvelous, energetic, humorous woman I had the privilege of knowing at different stages of ALS. In the early days she raged, but in listening to herself and being listened to, the anger seemed to evaporate in a mist of wit and wisdom. She grieved for her husband and children, and she wept for herself, and there was a wealth of healing and love between them all as they laughed, cried, and told stories. As her breathing became very shallow, talking was almost impossible, but at that point, all had been said and done. There was nothing more to say. She died quietly and peacefully, simply breathing out-expiring.

I had several taped interviews with Joan, a most remarkable woman who had lost the ability to speak and swallow a few months before my last interview. She had been living independently, but profound muscular weakness had made it necessary for her to leave the area and move in with family. She was able to type with one finger on a word processor and her words conjure up images of acceptance and letting go that move me beyond words: ". . . it is not easy to part from each other. That is why we should make the most of our time and be open and trusting. I'm not saying anything new. I want to say that it seems to me since I am no longer verbal, I talk a lot! It is ironic and a little sad. I don't feel sick. I keep thinking it's a big mistake and I'm waiting for someone to correct it. At least God has big shoulders, but I still think or rather I wish he had overlooked me! It is amazing. I am still struggling to hold on to life, and at the same time there are those who throw theirs away. How sad for them who have never known joy of life.

Do not feel sorry for me; I have peace and love. At times I get a sense of life slipping away and it is frightening, but at the same time I know I will be fine.

What is important is never to let ALS be a person instead of seeing your loved one as the person with ALS. I have seen time and time again when family members become isolated from one another. It is a gift of love that we remain connected. It is an obligation for both the person with ALS and the caregiver. It is not ALS that cuts us off. It is our fear and lack of love for one another.

Finally, I want to thank you all for your generosity, friendship, and love. For being there with me, sometimes in silence, sometimes with soft suggestions, but always dealing with me as a person, as an individual. I wish I had the ability to tell you all how much you have given me. I'm not alone, traveling in uncharted waters. You have kept me safe, close to shore, and when I've drifted too far, you have gently guided me back to safety. I thank you, all my friends. You are my heroes.

Caring for Those Who Mourn

Caring for the Patient

The prerequisite for care giving is that the caregivers understand the process of mourning for the one with ALS and are also able to articulate how this process is affecting themselves. If we are frightened of rage, we will discourage its expression in the families to whom we are giving care. If the expression of sadness rocks our need for self control, and we have been raised to worship the stiff upper lip and the belief that any public expression of grief is not positive or is an admission of defeat, then we will be routed by the tears of our patient and so be of little help.

Openness and connectedness among all involved are essential to good care. Family connectedness is enhanced and encouraged by the family meeting, which should be held soon after the diagnosis and repeated at the request of the family or whenever they appear to be stuck in the journey of mourning. It is important to address technical questions and any symptoms that may arise, but it is tempting to remain focused on these practical issues and not give voice to the responses to loss. Anticipation of the losses of ability to talk, swallow, and breathe, and skillful discussion of these issues over time will usually avert a crisis response, born of widespread denial, which may well lead to the patient being impelled into a course of action which, on greater reflection, he would not want. A peaceful death, when all has been said and done, is much more likely when all involved have given their full attention to both body and soul.

Caring for the Family

Isadora Duncan (1), reflecting on her own grief following the death of her two small children:

The next morning I drove out to see Duse, who was living in a rose colored villa behind a vineyard. She came down a vine covered walk to meet me, like a glorious angel. She took me in her arms and her won-

derful eyes beamed upon me such love and tenderness that I felt just as Dante must have felt when, in the "Paradiso," he encounters the Divine Beatrice.

From then on I lived at Viareggio, finding courage from the radiance of Eleanora's eyes. She used to rock me in her arms, consoling my pain, but not only consoling, for she seemed to take my sorrow to her own breast, and I realized that if I had not been able to bear the society of other people, it was because they all played the comedy of trying to cheer me with forgetfulness. Whereas Eleanora said: 'Tell me about Deidre and Patrick,' and made me repeat to her all their little sayings and ways, and show her their photos, which she kissed and cried over. She never said, 'Cease to grieve,' but she grieved with me, and, for the first time since their death, I felt I was not alone.

Isadora might have said: "Don't cheer me with forgetfulness nor keep me in denial nor drug me into apathy and distance. I need to grieve. I need to be held, so that my anger and hurt flows out of me, and I need love to help me cry. Don't tell me to get on with my life and cease to grieve because at that moment we become disconnected and I am plunged deeper into loneliness."

The family will have mourned to a greater or lesser extent while the patient was alive. Few will still be in denial or "in shock" at the time of death. Most will have left their rage and anger behind, but some will experience bereavement after the death of their loved one even though they were the most meticulous and loving of caregivers. Mrs. B told me that the 18 months after the death of her husband from ALS were quite awful. Their marriage was intimate and unusually exciting, but the year of his illness was filled with losses that seemed to follow one another without respite. He coped with each crisis with dignity, humor, and compassion for all right up to the moment of his death, which followed removal from a respirator at his request. But Mrs. B, caught up in her husband's crises especially toward the end, never allowed herself to feel the rage and anger while he was alive, and after he died she was engulfed by overwhelming resentment at the disease and the turmoil it created in her life. She had worked alongside her husband, and that ceased. Recreationally, physically, emotionally, sexually, her life was turned upside down, and after his death some of her rage was vented toward her image of him and toward the "selfish" decision he made to disconnect the respirator. After his death, when the hubbub of family and friends quieted down, she became almost paralyzed by anger and depression. Gradually, through talking about her feelings over and over again with a handful of nonjudgmental friends, she was able to move from rage to grief. She stressed to me how important it was for her to solicit these few friends to come and share their feelings about her husband and invite them to listen to her. Without her encouragement, they would not have come and shared painful feelings, which was the necessary prelude to moving on.

Self-help groups are very good for some of those whose loved ones have died. The death can be a precious opportunity to mourn many other losses that have gone unmourned. If this happens, the individual's life may take on a new zest, freed from a dark pall of unremitting bereavement and grief from the past. I frequently advise and encourage counseling for those who have been involved with a death since many are ripe for change at that moment.

Caring for the Caregiver

We look for and are expected to provide answers even when there are none. There is great uncertainty in medicine, and yet we are not taught how to deal with it, emotionally and interpersonally. ALS offers caregivers the perfect opportunity to confront helplessness and to go beyond it and realize we are only helpless in doing but never in being. Because of our illusions of professionalism we will be bereaved by ALS. We will be angry at the disease, the patient, or the family, or else distance ourselves behind a proclamation that there is nothing to be done. It is not a waste of valuable professional time for a physician to be with someone afflicted with ALS, although it may be one of our most difficult challenges because of our own discomfort, not the patient's. Our grief and sadness will be evoked, and we may wish to flee, especially if there have been significant others in our lives who have died and for whom we never mourned.

I believe that all caregivers who provide care for the dying, including all physicians and nurses as well as many others, need to participate in a workshop that focuses on their mourning, past, present, and future, and the workshop needs repeating at least once or twice during a career. The "soul searching" workshops I have given for several years last two or three days and include time for visualizing or imagining our own death so that we can experience some of our fears and apprehensions about death, and so be more in touch with what our patients are experiencing. Workshop participants also experience a simulated family meeting when they are the ones who are dying and are finishing up their business with those they love by saying what needs to be said. There is also time in the workshop to mourn other losses, and there are many opportunities to experience the art of being an impeccable listener and witness. Being a nonjudgmental, fully present witness is difficult and unfamiliar. We are so practiced in half-listening, interrupting, and dispensing advice. Experiencing the power of witnessing and being witnessed is one of the great surprises for workshop participants. They also learn a few techniques on how to nudge and encourage others to move along the route of mourning. The workshop is extremely personal, and in experiencing and processing the personal we become more empathic caregivers who are less prone to fight and flight.

Since death is still considered as failure and technology is becoming ever more insistent in medicine, it is doubtful that medical and nursing schools will give the lead by having this kind of workshop experience as an essential part of the curriculum. This should not deter smaller groups from introducing such workshops, and the collaboration, interpersonal connectedness, and skills of individuals who are members of care giving groups for ALS and cancer will be much enhanced as a result.

Another suggestion for ALS care giving groups is that there be an hour, every week or two, when caregivers gather together to discuss the process of their own mourning and that of the patients and families with whom they work. This is a time when personal reactions to care giving, families, helplessness, the anger of others, and a box full of other feelings may be aired and witnessed. If we work with the dying for long, we will certainly be reminded of the past or future deaths of our own mothers, fathers, brothers, lovers, and of ourselves. We will have the opportunity to rehearse a little what it might be like when someone close to us dies, and we need a safe place where we can discuss this. Having been part of such a "process group" in St. Peter's Hospice for the past 14 years, I know of its usefulness. But I also know that these meetings can be filled with feelings, and that many care giving groups abandon them because of discomfort with exposing their vulnerability before colleagues with whom they have to work every day. I believe the intention behind any process or support group is the key to failure or success. If the intention is confrontation and analysis, then sooner or later the group will self-destruct. If the intention is to encourage the expression of feelings that will be lovingly witnessed without judgment and without being pulled apart, the group may become a vital force in the care of the caregiver.

Reference

1. Duncan I. *My life*. New York: Liveright, 1927.

31

The Role of the National Voluntary ALS Associations

Mary Lyon

You Are Not Alone

This chapter introduces the national voluntary organizations and what they offer to people with amyotrophic lateral sclerosis (ALS), their family members, and their caregivers. The functions and services provided by the two national organizations are described to send a strong message that people with ALS and their families are not alone. There are hundreds of volunteers and staff from the national organizations standing ready to help them and provide needed services.

The national voluntary organizations exist only to serve people with ALS and their families. The ALS Association (ALSA) and the Muscular Dystrophy Association (MDA) are the two national organizations that provide programs and services to benefit people living with ALS.

The ALS Association and the Muscular Dystrophy Association are important partners in the multidisciplinary team approach to the clinical management of ALS. Having these associations dedicated to fighting ALS and working to improve the lives of people struggling with this disease sends a clear message to patients and families that they are not alone.

411

Where to Go for Help

- The ALS Association
  - National Office
    27001 Agoura Road, Suite 150
    Calabasas Hills, CA 91301-5104
    (800) 782-4747 toll-free information and referral service for patients and families
    (818) 880-9007 business number
    (818) 880-9006 fax
    www.alsa.org (web site). alsinfo@alsa-national.org (e-mail).
    Information and Referral Service for patients and families.
  - 34 Chapters
  - 38 Freestanding support groups
  - 14 certified ALSA centers
- The Muscular Dystrophy Association
  - National Office
    3300 East Sunrise Drive
    Tucson, AZ 85718-3208
    (520) 529-2000
    www.mdausa.org (web site).
  - MDA ALS Research and Clinical Centers

About the MDA

The Muscular Dystrophy Association is a voluntary national health agency—a dedicated partnership between scientists and concerned citizens aimed at conquering the 40 neuromuscular diseases in the Association's programs. ALS is one of the 40 diseases the MDA covers in its services. Patients are referred to their local MDA office for medical services and clinical care. The MDA provides research grants into the cause and treatment for the 40 diseases it represents, and it offers professional and public health education.

About the ALS Association

The ALS Association is the only not-for-profit voluntary health agency in the United States dedicated solely to ALS. Having a single focus assures that all of ALSA's resources are directed exclusively to ALS. The vast majority of ALSA's funds go for research (42 percent in 1998) and patient services (25 percent in 1998), while only 6 percent of expenses were allocated for administrative costs in 1998.

The people who provide leadership for ALSA by serving as members of the national and chapter boards of trustees are volunteers whose personal lives have been touched in some way by ALS. Working diligently to make scientific discoveries and improve the lives of people living with ALS, ALSA is committed to engaging patients and families in the process of setting and achieving organizational goals. Along with the volunteers, ALSA has paid staff at the national office, and many of the chapters have full-time executive directors and patient services coordinators.

The ALS Association is fortunate to have physicians, nurses, and other clinicians who graciously serve as voluntary members of ALSA's Medical Advisory Committee. The purpose of the Medical Advisory Committee is to provide ALSA with information and advice on clinical and research issues of importance.

Purpose

The ALS Association seeks to discover the cause and cure for ALS (Lou Gehrig's disease) through dedicated research while improving the lives of people with ALS by providing patient support, information/education for health care professionals and the general public, and advocacy for ALS research and health care concerns.

What Does ALSA Do?

I. Research—working to find the cause, cure, and treatment for ALS

II. Patient Services—providing information, care, support, and services to patients and families

III. Advocacy—making change at the local, state, and federal levels to benefit people with ALS

IV. Awareness—increasing public knowledge about ALS to foster more research and services

I. Research.

- The ALS Association has an organized program of scientific research that includes encouraging, identifying, funding, and monitoring relevant and cutting-edge research into the cause, means of prevention, and possible cure for ALS. Through an application and review process that is patterned after the National Institutes of Health's rigorous process, abstracts and proposals are peer-reviewed and ranked by ALSA's Scientific Review Committee consisting of renowned neuroscientists. Each year nearly 200 abstracts for scientific study are submitted for consideration.

- ALSA holds scientific workshops that bring together ALS researchers and non-ALS investigators renowned in their respective specialties to explore specific ALS-relevant topics such as "free radicals and programmed cell death," "the biology of motor neurons," and "glutamate toxicity and its role in ALS."

- Clinical Management Research Grant Program—In 1998 the ALS Association began a program to stimulate and support research that will help patients deal with the symptoms of ALS and improve the quality of their lives. Examples of funded projects include an evaluation of the effects of exercise in people with ALS and a study to determine if beginning noninvasive ventilation earlier in the disease will prolong life.

What Kind of Help Is Available?

II. Patient Services

Feelings of hope, a positive mental attitude, and knowledge are powerful weapons in the battle against ALS. ALSA's materials and services are designed to offer hope, give needed information about living with ALS, and encourage people to live their lives to the fullest.

The generosity of ALSA's donors ensures that all patient and family services and materials are provided without charge.

A. Information—What to expect and how to live with ALS

- Toll-free Information and Referral Service—By dialing 800-782-4747, patients and family members are connected to informed, caring people who answer questions, mail literature about ALS and offer hope and support.

- E-mail—The Information and Referral Service is also available by e-mail, fax, or letter.

- Web site—ALSA's web site (www.alsa.org) includes information about the disease, resources for clinical care and second opinions, and how to get more information.

- Manuals—The most popular source of information for patients and families is ALSA's Living with ALS manuals—a set of six paperback books designed to take the patient through each of the stages of ALS offering ways to cope and therapies to treat the many of the symptoms of ALS. Manuals are provided without charge to patients and families and can be ordered by calling the toll-free number or writing to ALSA.

  - *What's It All About*

  - *Coping with Change*

  - *Managing Your Symptoms and Treatment*

  - *Functioning When Your Mobility Is Affected*

  - *Adjusting To Swallowing and Speaking Difficulties*

  - *Adapting To Breathing Changes*

- FYI Information Index—A series of brief flyers on 38 specific topics including swallowing tips, minimizing fatigue, and speech devices.

- Research news—Twice a year, new research grants awarded by ALSA are described in Scientific Update. Chapter and support group newsletters keep patients aware of breaking news from the research front.

- Clinical drug trials and *Drug Development Update*—Information on the drug trials and where they are being conducted as well as what is new in the development of drugs for ALS are included in the *Drug Development Update*. It is available in print and on ALSA's web site.

- Recommended reading, videos—A suggested reading list can be sent to patients on request and ALSA's library includes a variety of videos that are loaned to patients.

B. ALSA Center Certification Program—Along with medical experts, the ALS Association developed standards for ALS clinics to encourage quality care that is interdisciplinary and includes clinicians who are knowledgeable and experienced in making the diagnosis and taking care of people with ALS. Clinics that pass the rigorous application and site visit reviews are certified as ALSA Centers. It is ALSA's intent that the every-two-year recertification requirement helps to improve the quality of the ALSA Centers. Another benefit of the ALSA Center Program is the facilitation and fostering of information exchange among the medical directors and staff of the ALSA Centers. There are 14 ALSA Centers at the present time.

Standards and Requirements:

- Active support for the ALS clinic from the local ALSA Chapter or Freestanding Support Group

- An existing multidisciplinary and interdisciplinary ALS clinic

- A clinic director with well-recognized expertise in ALS

- A full availability of neurologic diagnostic and other necessary medical services

- A number of established ALS patients seen and a pattern of new ALS patients added to those being seen, sufficient to justify ALSA Center status

C. Someone to talk to—Sometimes people with ALS, their families and caregivers just need someone to talk to—someone who will listen and who understands the day-to-day challenges they are facing. ALSA provides telephone contact with concerned, knowledgeable people from both the national office (800-782-4747) and each ALSA chapter.

D. Patient and family education programs—Many ALSA chapters sponsor patient–family education programs covering general information about ALS as well as specific tips and hints that make living with this disease easier.

E. Support groups—Talking with other people who are living the same experience can help decrease the common feelings of depression and isolation. ALSA's chapters and freestanding support groups conduct hundreds of support group meetings across the country every month. Support groups range from an informal sharing of successful ideas of how to solve problems of daily living to formal medical presentations. There are support groups for newly diagnosed patients, caregivers, and, in some areas, groups for children of people with ALS. In all cases the emphasis is on helping people maximize their physical function and maintain quality in their lives.

F. Equipment loan programs—ALSA chapters provide equipment on loan to patients for activities of daily living—wheelchairs, walkers, bedside commodes, and so forth. Many chapters also have a variety of augmentative communication devices that are made available to patients.

G. Respite programs—Family caregivers have demanding and often overwhelming jobs. A break from caregiving to go shopping, see a movie, or spend a day with friends can provide a needed change and rest. Many ALSA chapters offer respite care to families to help them cope with the demands and burdens of ALS.

H. Transportation programs—Patients requiring sophisticated wheelchairs and modified vans may need more help in getting from home to an ALSA Center or to support group meetings than family and friends can provide. Some chapters are able to offer transportation services to patients.

I. Caregiver support—The ALS Association recognizes the needs caregivers have for information and support. Through the Information and Referral Services provided by the national office and chapters, literature, support groups and respite programs, ALSA is reaching out to help and support caregivers.

J. Patient Bill of Rights for People with ALS—When people are knowledgeable about their rights regarding health care they are more likely to get the services and patient care they need. ALSA's Patient Bill of Rights for People with ALS is an information and advocacy tool for patients and families as they negotiate the health care system.

III. ALSA as ALS Advocate

The ALS Association advocates on behalf of ALS patients through its year-round, network-wide advocacy program centered in its capital office in Washington, D.C. The overall goal is to advocate for public policy in support of ALS research and ALS-related health issues, including accelerated treatment development and access to proper care and treatment. Current legislation before Congress will waive the two-year waiting period for Social Security disability for Medicare coverage, and it will allow Medicare coverage for all FDA-approved drugs prescribed for use in the treatment or alleviation of symptoms relating to ALS.

IV. Raising Awareness

Raising general awareness about ALS will lead to an increase in research funding and support for clinical and support services. Everyone has a part to play in increasing ALS awareness—from talking with community friends and neighbors to writing a letter to the editor of a local newspaper. A public awareness campaign including articles, features and public service ads in major newspapers and magazines and on radio and television is led by ALSA's national office. Although the awareness campaign is year-long, special emphasis is given to awareness events in May—National ALS Awareness Month. LINK is ALSA's national publication. Distributed quarterly to nearly 90,000 people, LINK reports on research findings, clinical trials, and services and programs for patients. To be added to the LINK mailing list, call 800-782-4747 or write to ALSA.

ALSA strives to involve and engage patients and families in the process of raising awareness and advocating for legislative changes. A broad base of committed people in communities across the country can create a powerful voice for increasing research funding and improving care and treatment.

Other ALSA Activities

- Over the past three years, ALSA has met twice a year with representatives of the pharmaceutical industry who have developed or are developing ALS drugs. Ten companies have participated in the Drug Company Working Group first established to encourage combination medication therapy. Recent accomplishments include development of the Bill of Rights for people with ALS, the Educating Payers Project to provide managed care companies with information about ALS and the health care benefits people with this disease need.

- Representatives of ALSA regularly attend scientific and neurologic professional meetings to keep abreast of the most current research and treatment news and to raise awareness about ALS by sponsoring exhibit booths.

- Every other year ALSA sponsors an ALS Clinical Conference for nurses, social workers, and therapists who work with ALS patients.

- ALSA provides financial and human resources to support many ALS professional activities such as the International Symposium of ALS/MND and the ALS Clinical, Assessment, Research and Education (ALSCARE) program—a North American database intended to improve care for people with ALS.

- The ALS Association maintains communication and working relationships with federal and private agencies. Examples include the Food and Drug Administration (FDA), National Institutes of Health (NIH), Health Care Financing Administration (HCFA—Medicare), National Health Council (NHC), and the Paralyzed Veteran's of America (PVA). Efforts with these groups are directed to creating changes and making improvements that benefit people with ALS.

The Amyotrophic Lateral Sclerosis Association's Patient Bill of Rights for People Living With ALS

As a person living with ALS, you have the right to:

1. Receive comprehensive information about ALS, including treatment options and resources for your health care needs. This includes the right to communicate with your government representatives regarding policies and practices of the Food and Drug Administration (FDA), National Institutes of Health (NIH), Department of Health and Human Services (DHHS) and other agencies that affect ALS.

2. Participate in decisions about your health care including the right to accept, discontinue or refuse treatments and therapy.

3. Receive ALS specialty care in a timely manner.

4. Receive health care that is coordinated and individualized for you across the spectrum of home, hospice, hospital, nursing home, outpatient, and work-place and throughout all the phases of your illness.

5. Access health care benefit coverage and life insurance coverage without discrimination based on your ALS diagnosis or disability.

6. Obtain clear, timely information regarding your health plan including benefits, exclusions and appeal procedures.

7. Review your medical records and have the information in your records explained to you.

8. Prepare an advance directive to state your wishes regarding emergency and end-of-life treatment choices.

9. Receive care that is considerate and respects your dignity, your cultural, psychosocial and spiritual values, and your privacy. You

have this right no matter what choices you make about treatments and therapy, what your disabilities related to ALS might be, or what your financial circumstances are.

10. Know that information about you and your medical condition are held in confidence.

11. Receive support to maintain or enhance the quality of your life and have your family involved in all aspects of your health care.

32

Resources for Patients and Support Services

Mary Wooley, LSW, and John Sharp, MSSA

This chapter will help you, your family, and your friends become knowledgeable about ALS support services that are available worldwide. Supportive services are very important for several reasons. Services can lessen some of the emotional strain you and your loved ones are enduring by giving your mental feelings a boost from knowing you are not alone and that there are ways to help you based on the experiences of ALS patients. This information can give you a feeling of control that you can contribute to your own well-being, which in turn increases your quality of life.

MDA/ALS Research and Clinical Centers

This list was current at the time this book went to press; updated information may be obtained from http://www. mdausa.org/clinics/alsserv.html

CALIFORNIA
Robert G. Miller, MD
Forbes Norris MDA/ALS Research

Center
California Pacific Medical Center
2324 Sacramento Street, Suite 150
San Francisco, CA 94115
(415) 923-3604
(415) 923-6567 (fax)
E-mail: rmiller@cooper.cpme.org

W. King Engel, MD
Jerry Lewis MDA/ALS Clinical and
Research Center
University of Southern California

School of Medicine
637 South Lucas Avenue
Los Angeles, CA 90017
(213) 743-1611
(213) 743-1617 (fax)
E-mail: not available

Michael C. Graves, MD
MDA/ALS Center at UCLA
UCLA Neurological Services, Suite
B200
300 UCLA Medical Plaza
Los Angeles, CA 90024-6975
(310) 825-7266
(310) 825-3995 (fax)
E-mail: mcgraves@ucla.edu

COLORADO
Hans E. Neville, MD
Steven P. Ringel, MD
The University of Colorado
MDA/ALS Center
Health Sciences Center
4200 East Ninth Avenue, Box B-185
Denver, CO 80262
(303) 315-7221
(303) 315-6797 (fax)
E-mail: hans.neville@uchse.edu;
steven.ringel@uchsc.edu

CONNECTICUT
Jonathan M. Goldstein, MD
Yale University MDA/ALS Center
Dept. of Neurology
PO Box 208018
New Haven, CT 06520-8018
(203) 785-4867
(203) 785-5694 (fax)
E-mail: jonathan.goldstein@yale.edu

FLORIDA
Walter G. Bradley, DM, FRCP
Kessenich Family MDA/ALS Center
The University of Miami

1150 NW 14th Street, 7th Floor,
Suite 700
Miami, FL 33136
(800) 690-ALS1
(305) 243-7400
(305) 243-1249 (fax)
E-mail: wbradley@med.miami.ed

GEORGIA
Jonathan Glass, MD
MDA/ALS Center
Emory University School of Medicine
Woodruff Memorial Bldg.,
Suite 6000, Drawer V
Atlanta, GA 30322
(404) 727-3818
(404) 727-3157 (fax)
E-mail: not available

ILLINOIS
Raymond Roos, MD
MDA/ALS Center
University of Chicago Hospitals
Department of Neurology/ MC2030
5841 South Maryland Avenue
Chicago, IL 60637
(773) 702-6390
(773) 702-9076 (fax)
E-mail:
rroos@drugs.bsd.uchicago.edu

KANSAS
Arthur Dick, MD
MDA/ALS Center
The University of Kansas Medical
Center
39th and Rainbow Blvd.
Kansas City, KS 66103
(913) 588-6997
(913) 588-6595 (fax)
E-mail: kpeters@kumc.edu

MARYLAND
Daniel B. Drachman, MD

Jeffrey D. Rothstein, MD, PhD
MDA/ALS Center
The Johns Hopkins University School
of Medicine
600 N. Wolfe Street Meyer 5-119
Baltimore, MD 21287-7519
(410) 955-6435
(410) 955-1961 (fax)
E-mail:
ddrachm@welchlink.welch.jhu.edu

MASSACHUSETTS
Robert H. Brown, MD
MDA/ALS Center
Massachusetts General Hospital
15 Parkman Street
Boston, MA 02114
(617) 726-5750
(617) 726-8543 (fax)
E-mail:
brown@helix.mgh.harvard.edu

MISSOURI
Alan Pestronk, MD
MDA/ALS Center
Washington University School
of Medicine
660 S. Euclid, Box 8111
St. Louis, MO 63110
(314) 362-6981
(314) 362-2826 (fax)
E-mail: pestronk@kids.wustl.edu

NEW YORK
Hiroshi Mitsumoto, MD
The Eleanor and Lou Gehrig
MDA/ALS Center
Columbia Presbyterian Medical Center
Department of Neurology
710 West 168th Street
New York, NY 10032
(212) 305-1319
(212) 305-8398 (fax)
E-mail: alscenter@columbia.edu

C. Warren Olanow, MD, FRCP
Dale J. Lange, MD
MDA/ALS Center
Mt. Sinai Hospital & Medical Center
One Gustave Levy Place, Annenburg
14-94
New York, NY 10029
(212) 241-8674; (212) 241-8435
(212) 987-7635; (212) 987-3301 (fax)
E-mail: warren.olanow@mssm.edu

Jeremy M. Shefner, MD, PhD
MDA/ALS Center
SUNY Health Sciences Center
750 East Adams Street
Syracuse, NY 13210
(315) 464-4627
(315) 464-5006 (fax)
E-mail: shefnerj@vax.cs.hscyr.edu

NORTH CAROLINA
Jeffrey Rosenfeld, MD
MDA/ALS Center
Carolinas Medical Center
PO Box 32861
1437 Scott Avenue
Charlotte, NC 28232-2861
(704) 446-6257
(704) 446-6255 (fax)
E-mail: jrosenfeld@carolinas.org

Richard S. Bedlack, Jr., MD
MDA/ALS Center
Duke University Medical Center
PO Box 3403
Durham, NC27710
(919) 684-5422
(919) 660-3853 (fax)
E-mail: bedla001@dellnet.com

TEXAS
Richard J. Barohn, MD
MDA/ALS Center / University of
Texas

Southwest Medical Center at Dallas
5323 Harry Hines Boulevard
Dallas, TX 75235-8897
(214) 648-6419
(214) 648-9311 (fax)
E-mail:rbaroh@mednet.swmed.edu

Stanley H. Appel, MD
The Ronny & Linda Finger
MDA/ALS Center
Baylor College of Medicine/
Neurosensory Center
6501 Fannin Street, NB302
Houston, TX 77030
(713) 798-4072
(713) 798-3854 (fax)
E-mail: sappel@bcm.tme.edu

UTAH
Mark B. Bromberg, MD, PhD
MDA/ALS Center
The University of Utah/
Dept. of Neurology
50 North Medical Drive
Salt Lake City, UT 84132
(801) 581-6873
(801) 585-2054
E-mail: mbromberg@hsc.utah.edu

WISCONSIN
Benjamin Rix Brooks, MD
MDA/ALS Clinical Research Center
University of Wisconsin–Madison
600 Highland Avenue , CSC H6-563
Madison, WI 53792-5132
(608) 263-9057
(608) 263-0412 (fax)
E-mail: brooks@neurology.wisc.edu

SUGGESTED READING RESOURCES

Amyotrophic Lateral Sclerosis
A Comprehensive Guide to Management

Edited by:
Hiroshi Mitsumoto, M.D.
Forbes H. Norris, Jr., M.D.

Demos Publications
386 Park Avenue S., Suite 201
New York, NY 100 16
$39.95 per copy
$4.00 shipping & handling
(NY State residents add sales tax)

Realities in Coping with Progressive
Neuromuscular Disease

Edited by:
Claire F. Leach
Leon I. Charash
Robert E. Lovelace
Stewart G. Wolf
Austin H. Kutscher
David Price Roye

The Charles Press
P.O. Box 15715
Philadelphia, PA 19103
(215) 545-8933
$34.95 per copy
$5.50–UPS, 1st copy
$2.00–UPS, add'l copies

Communication and Swallowing Solutions
for the ALS/MND Community

By: Marta S. Kazandjian

CINI
250 Mercer Street, Ste. B1608
New York, NY 100 12
(516) 874-8354
$7.95 paperback
$1.50 shipping & handling
ISBN 1565938089

We Are Not Alone—
Learning to Live with Chronic Illness

By: Sefra Korbin Pitzele

Workman Publishing
708 Broadway
New York, NY 100 13
(212) 254-5900
$10.95 per copy
$3.00 shipping & handling
ISBN 0894801392

Family Caregiver's Guide

By: Joan Ellen Foyder

The Futuro Company
5801 Mariemont Avenue
Cincinnati, OH 45227
(513) 271-3782
$14.95 per copy
$2.50 shipping & handling

Home Health Care

By: JoAnn Friedman

W. W. Norton & Company, Ltd.
550 Fifth Avenue
New York, NY 10010
$22.50 per copy, plus postage
(in local book stores)

Handbook of Living Wills
(free Living Will available)

Choice in Dying, Inc.
200 Varick Street
New York, NY 10014
(800) 989-9155

Caring and Coping When A Loved One
Is Seriously Ill

By: E Grollman

Beacon Press Order Dept.
25 Street
Boston, MA 02108
(800) 706-2220
$10.00 paperback
plus shipping & handling

Share the Care

By: Cappy Capossela and
Sheila Warnock

Simon & Schuster
Fireside
1230 Avenue of the Americas
New York, NY 10020
$13.00 paperback
(in local bookstores)
ISBN 0-684-811367

Avoiding the Medicaid Trap
How Every American Can Beat the
Catastrophic Costs of Nursing Home Care

By: Armond D. Budish

Avon Books
1350 Avenue of the Americas
New York, NY 10019
(800) 238-0658
$15.00 trade paperback
plus shipping & handling
ISBN 0-380-72771-4

Beyond Rage—
Mastering Unavoidable Health Charges

By: JoAnn LeMaistre, Ph.D.

Alpine Guild
P.O. Box 4846
Dillon, CO 80435
(800) 869-9559
$24.95 per copy

$2.50 shipping & handling
ISBN 0-931712-11-4

How Will They Know If I'm Dead?

By: Robert C. Horn, III

GR/St. Lucie Press
100 East Lincoln Blvd., Ste. 403B
Delray Beach, FL 33483
(561) 274-9906
$12.95 paperback
$4.95 shipping & handling
ISBN 1-5744-071-3

It Helps To Talk About It
Living, Not Dying, with Lou Gehrig's
Disease
By: Bob MacLean

The ALS Association
21021 Ventura Blvd., Ste. 321
Woodland Hills, CA 91364
(800) 782-4747
$18.00 oversize paper

Living Well with Chronic Illness

By: Gayle Heiss

Gayle Heiss
P.O. Box 210
Mendocino, CA 95460
$2.00 each
$.60 shipping & handling

Help Yourself: Problem Solving for the
Disabled

By: Douglas R. Bucy

Macmillan Publishing USA
1633 Broadway
New York, NY 10019-6785
(212) 654-8500
$14.95 paperback
plus shipping & handling
(in local bookstores)
ISBN 0028610598

Meeting the Challenge
Living with Chronic Illness

By: Audrey Kron, M.A., CGP

Audrey Kron
7466 Pebble Lane
West Bloomfield, MI 48322
$16.00 each
$3.00 shipping & handling
(will donate $2 of each book sale to
ALSA)

In Sunshine and In Shadow

Edited by: Judy Oliver

(out of print—available for loan only)
$3.00 shipping & handling
The ALS Association
21021 Ventura Blvd., Ste. 321
Woodland Hills, CA 91364
(818) 340-7500
(800) 782-4747

Non-Chew Cookbook

By: J. Randy Wilson

Wilson Publishing, Inc.
P.O. Box 2190
Glenwood Springs, CO 81602-2190
(800) 843-2409
$23.95, 1–9 books

(free shipping & handling)
$16.77, 10 or more books
(30% discount, postage paid)

Pot Holders and Love Handles
(cookbook)
By: Lynda Cabela

Cabelas Furniture Store
602 Second Street
Cappell, NE 69129
$5.00 per copy
$1.25 shipping & handling

Meals For Easy Swallowing

By: Vickie Appel, Sandy Calvin,
Gena Smith, Donna Wolhr

MDA
3300 East Sunrise Drive
Tucson, AZ 85718
Attn: Patient Services
(520) 520-2000, (520) 520-5300—Fax
$6.00 per copy

VIDEOTAPES

What Is ALS?

An educational video presenting
information about ALS

Purchase: $15.00
including shipping & handling
Loan: $5.00 shipping and handling
charge—2-week loan
The ALS Association
21021 Ventura Boulevard, #321
Woodland Hills, CA 91364
(818) 340-7500
(800) 782-4747

Reason for Hope

An educational video about ALS and
The ALS Association for someone new
to ALS

Purchase: $19.95 including shipping &
handling
Loan: $5.00 shipping & handling
Two-week loan period
The ALS Association
21021 Ventura Blvd., Ste. 321
Woodland Hills, CA 91364
(818) 340-7500
(800) 782-4747

It's Your Choice
An education video presenting
information to people who need to make
an informed decision whether to use a
ventilator.

Valona Productions
5105 E. Los Angeles Avenue, #E-178
Simi Valley, CA 93063
(805) 527-8557 (message)
(805) 527-9366 (home)
Also loan
$19.95 per copy, including shipping &
handling

*Ventilation: The Decision Making
Process*

Loan: $5.00 shipping & handling
Two-week loan period
By: The Les Turner ALS Foundation

The ALS Association
121021 Ventura Blvd., Ste. 321
Woodland Hills, CA 91364
(818) 340-7500, (800) 782-4747

Caring for the Caregiver

An educational video and workbook that
explores ways caregivers can take better
care of themselves, reduce stress, make
life easier and more enjoyable, and find
help when it's needed.
By: Ismail & Cheryl Tsieprati

Program Development Associates
5620 Business Ave., #B
Cicero, NY 13039
(800) 543-2119

$69.00 per copy plus shipping &
handling

The Cutting Edge Medical Report

Discovery Channel—June 1996
Educational video about ALS including
a visit to an ALSA Center geared to
health care professionals

Loan: $5.00 shipping & handling
The ALS Association
21021 Ventura Blvd., #321
Woodland Hills, CA 91364
(818) 340-7500
(800) 782-4747

*When Bad Things Happen to Good
People*

By: H. Kushner

Avon Books
1350 Avenue of the Americas, 2nd Floor
New York, NY 100 19
(800) 223-0690
Fax: (212) 261-6895

*How to Help Children Through a
Parent's Serious Illness*

By: Kathleen McCue, M.A., C.C.L.S.
with Ron Bonn

St. Martin's Press
175 Fifth Avenue
New York, NY 100 10
ISBN 0312113501

Tuesdays with Morrie

By: Mitch Albom

Doubleday Books
P.O. Box 5071
Des Plaines, IL 60017
(800) 223-6834
Fax: (212) 492-9770

Letting Go

By: Morrie Schwartz

Doubleday Books
1540 Broadway
New York, NY 10036
(800) 323-9872
Fax: (212) 492-9700

MANUAL

Living with ALS
A series of 6 manuals, each of which can
be ordered separately:
1) What's It All About

Request order form from:
The ALS Association
21021 Ventura Blvd., Ste. 321
Woodland Hills, CA 91364

2) Coping with Change
3) Managing Your Symptoms & Treatment
4) Functioning When Your Mobility is Affected
5) Adjusting to Swallowing and Speaking Difficulties
6) Adapting to Breathing Changes

(818) 340-7500
(818) 340-2060
Persons with ALS and their families need only pay shipping & handling costs.
Patient Difficulties and physician names need to appear on order form

CATALOGS FOR DAILY LIVING

Enrichments
Catalog of everyday aids for daily living

Bissell Healthcare Co.
P.O. Box 579
Hinsdale, IL
(800) 323-5547

Fred Sammons Catalogue for Healthcare Professionals
Catalog of equipment, orthotics, ADLs, etc.

Box 32
Brookfield, EL 60513
(800) 323-5547

Accent
Catalog of books, products, magazines

Box 700
Bloomington, IL 61702
(800) 787-8444

TRAVEL

SATH
SATH is a volunteer unfunded non-profit organization that maintains lists of tour operators and travel firms that cater to the disabled. It also has info on accessible facilities worldwide. Quarterly newsletter

Society for Advancement of Travel for the Handicapped
347 Fifth Avenue, Ste, 610
New York, NY 10016
(212) 447-SATH

Amtrak
Amtrak has special cars adapted for wheelchair travelers. Reservations should be made well in advance.

(800) USA-RAIL

Flying Wheels Travel, Inc.
Arranges travel plans for people with disabilities. Knows accessible hotels, motels, resorts, cruise ships, etc.

P.O. Box 382
Owatonna, MN 55060
(800) 533-6790

Travel-Ability, A Guide for Physically Disabled Travelers in the U.S.

By: Lois Reamy

Macmillan Publishing Company
Front & Brown Streets
Riverside, NJ 08370
(609) 786-9778

Travelin' Talk
An information network providing assistance

P.O. Box 3534
Clarksville, TN 37043-3543

to the disabled traveler worldwide. Connects
people with others in area they are traveling
to.

(615) 552-6670

Central Reservation Service
Hotel reservations service, provides info
on accessible hotels and books accessible
rooms.

7000 S.W. 97th Avenue, Ste. 205
Miami, FL FL
(800) 950-0232

Easy Access to National Parks: Sierra Club
Guide for Disabled

Sierra Club Books
(800) 935-1056
$16.00 per copy
$4.00 shipping & handling
(in local bookstores)
ISBN 0-871566206

Directory of Travel Agencies for the
Disabled
Lists travel agents specializing in
arrangements for people with disabilities.

Twin Peaks Press
P.O. Box 129
Vancouver, WA 98666
(360) 694-2462
$19.95 paperback
$3.50 shipping & handling
ISBN 0933261048

Golden Eagle Passport
Free lifetime pass to federally-operated parks,
historic sites, recreation areas, wild-life
refuges for persons who are permanently
disabled/blind.

P.O. Box 37127
Washington, D.C. 20013

COMMUNICATION, ADAPTIVE AIDS, USEFUL ITEMS

AT&T National Special Needs Center
Special communication products for people
with hearing, vision, motion, and speech
impairment

2001 Route 46
Parsippany, NJ 07054-1315
(800) 233-1222
(800) 833-3232 (TDD)

The National Library Service for Blind
Physically Handicapped
or your local Braille Institute

Library of Congress
Washington, D.C. 20542
(202) 707-9275
Free books, periodicals loaned on tape,
with machine provided free

Radio Shack Stores

Sears Home Care Catalog

(800) 948-8800

There are resources too numerous to list—feel free to talk with our Patient Services Coordinator to get lists of companies nationwide for all sorts of assistive aids.

Internet Resources for ALS

The Internet provides a unique resource for those with ALS and their families. Because ALS is a relatively uncommon diagnosis, most hospitals and physician offices lack lay information on diagnosis, the disease process, and treatment. Meeting other patients and families dealing with ALS is difficult for those at a distance from clinical centers specializing in ALS. Family caregivers may have difficultly leaving the patient to attend a support or information group. With the increasing amount of information and support available on the Internet, ALS treatment centers, clinical trials and mutual support are only a click away.

The two most common Internet tools, the World Wide Web (web) and e-mail, provide access to a wealth of information. With a simple search on the letters ALS, a variety of web sites appear which include treatment information, clinical trials, research and treatment centers, national ALS foundations, recommended books, resources for patients and families. Using e-mail, one can subscribe to a discussion group (or e-mail list) and participate in a daily discussion of ALS from a layman's perspective with people from around the world. Those with ALS and their families who have personal computers and Internet access from home can gain a sense of empowerment while reducing the feelings of isolation which often accompanies the disease. For those without home computers, most public libraries now have Internet access with librarians willing to provide some guidance and training.

Some caution needs to be mentioned with relation to obtaining medical information and support from the Internet. First, one must look for reliable sources of information. Major ALS clinical centers and foundations review the information they post carefully. On the other hand, individual postings, web sites or groups which claim to be authorities but have no connection to these primary information sources should be approached with a health skepticism. E-mail discussion groups can also be a helpful source of support and suggestions on living with ALS, however, what works for one person may not apply to everyone with ALS. Finally, regarding alternative treatments which are promoted on the Internet, one should use caution and follow the advise, "if it is too good to be true, it probably isn't."

Following is a list of some of the Internet resources for ALS available at the time of publication. It should be noted that the Internet is a dynamic information tool which changes frequently with new web sites and other resources being added on a daily basis and other sites being removed without notice. For the most up-to-date information, the use of a reliable search engine should bring up the most current web sites available.

Major ALS Organizations

World Federation of Neurology/Amyotrophic Lateral Sclerosis
www.wfhals.org
Includes listing of ALS centers by country

ALS Association National Office
www.ALSA.org
Includes listing of ALS physicians by country

The Muscular Dystrophy Association
www.mdausa.org

The ALS Patient Care Database: The ALS C.A.R.E. Project is a voluntary,
physician-directed program to improve outcomes for patients diagnosed with
amyotrophic lateral sclerosis.
www. outcomes. org

Additional Web Resources

ALS Network: resources and support for people with ALS and caregivers
ALSnetwork.en.com

ALS Survival Guide
www.lougehrigsdisease.net

Drug Infonet on ALS
www.druginfonet.com/lougehrig.htm

Family Caregiver Alliance
www.caregiver.org

Caregiver Magazine
www.caregiver.com

Search Engines

Yahoo: Diseases and Conditions
dir. yahoo. com/Health/Diseases_and_Conditions/Amyotrophic_Lateral
_Sclerosis_Lou_Gehrig_s,_Disease_/

OnHealth/WebMD on ALS
http://onhealth.webmd.com/conditions/resource/conditions/index.asp

Altavista
www.altavista.com/

Index

Note: boldface numbers indicate illustrations; italic *(t)* indicates a table.

A.C.C.E.S.S Program, 358
AARP Pharmacy Service, 338, 339*(t)*
Abiotrophy, 5
AbleData Database, 358
Access methods of communication, 135
Acetaminophen, 57
Acid reflux, treatments for, 55
Action Mail Order, 338, 339*(t)*
Activities of daily living (ADLs),
    76, 86–87, 100, 105, 279
Acupuncture, 206–207
Adaptive devices (See also Assistive
    devices), 100–101, 105, 110
Addiction, 314
Advance directives, 307, 309, 312
Advocacy groups, 74
Aerobic exercises, 85–86
Age of onset of ALS, psychological,
    social, spiritual factors of, 286–287
AIDS, 212
Allopurinol, 204
Alpha lipoic acid in, 232
Alpha-motoneurons and, 21
Alphabet boards, 135, 136, 136
ALS Association, 145 ALS Association
    (ALSA), 74, 143, 278, 336, 344*(t)*, 345,
    350, 358, 411–419, 421–432
Alternative and complementary treatments,
    202
    clinical therapeutic trials and, 218
ALS Functional Rating Scale (ALSFRS),
    76, 234
ALS-like diseases (See Differential
    diagnoses for ALS)
ALSA Center Program in, 74, 75*(t)*

ALSCARE databases (See CARE
    Database)
Alternate funding sources, 338, 339*(t)*
Alternative and complementary treatments,
    9, 49, 201–209, 311
    acupuncture as, 206–207
    addiction and, 314
    allopurinol in, 204
    alpha lipoic acid in, 232
    antioxidants in, 49, 203–205, 223
    bee pollen in, 204
    beta-carotene in, 203–204, 223
    brain-derived neurotrophic factor
        (BDNF), 223, 228, 230–231
    calcium supplements in, 204
    ciliary neurotrophic factor (CNTF) in,
        202, 227–228
    coenzyme Q-10 in, 204, 223, 232
    creatine in, 205–206, 232
    diet in, 227
    energy supplements in, 205–206
    flaxseed oil in, 204
    free radicals and, 203–204, 223
    ganglioside in, 227
    ginkgo biloba, 338
    glial cell-derived neurotrophic factor
        (GDNF) in, 228–229
    glutamate, 222–223, 229, 231, 232
    grape seed extract, 204
    herbal remedies, 207–208
    insulin growth factor (myotrophin) in,
        202
    insulin-like growth factor 1 (IGF-1) in,
        228
    insurance coverage of, 337–338
    L-threonine in, 227
    lecithin in, 204
    magnesium supplements in, 204

433